clean

clean

a history of
personal hygiene
and purity

virginia smith

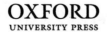

OXFORD
UNIVERSITY PRESS

OXFORD

UNIVERSITY PRESS

Great Clarendon Street, Oxford OX2 6DP

Oxford University Press is a department of the University of Oxford.
It furthers the University's objective of excellence in research, scholarship,
and education by publishing worldwide in

Oxford New York

Auckland Cape Town Dar es Salaam Hong Kong Karachi
Kuala Lumpur Madrid Melbourne Mexico City Nairobi
New Delhi Shanghai Taipei Toronto

With offices in

Argentina Austria Brazil Chile Czech Republic France Greece
Guatemala Hungary Italy Japan Poland Portugal Singapore
South Korea Switzerland Thailand Turkey Ukraine Vietnam

Oxford is a registered trade mark of Oxford University Press
in the UK and in certain other countries

Published in the United States
by Oxford University Press Inc., New York

© Virginia Smith 2007

The moral rights of the author have been asserted
Database right Oxford University Press (maker)

First published 2007

British Library Cataloguing in Publication Data

Data available

Library of Congress Cataloging in Publication Data

Data available

Typeset by SPI Publisher Services, Pondicherry, India
Printed in Great Britain
on acid-free paper by
Clays Ltd, St. Ives Plc.

ISBN 978–0–19–929779–5

1 3 5 7 9 10 8 6 4 2

This book is dedicated to

Roy Porter
(1946–2002)

acknowledgements

I would here like to acknowledge and sincerely thank all those people who have listened, given advice, answered endless strange questions, responded to letters and telephone calls, lent books, read chapters and papers, put up with harangues or monologues and shown kind interest generally, with patience and curiosity, over the years. They know who they are. They certainly include all my supportive friends, and my family. In particular, I would like to thank my supervisors Brian Abel-Smith (in memoriam) and Charlotte Erikson, both at the London School of Economics, where the project began; and above all, to Roy Porter (in memoriam) at the Wellcome Institute for the History of Medicine, who gave such support and encouragement throughout my Ph.D. and well beyond, and was so close to actually seeing it all in print. Especially grateful thanks go to Peter Burke, Roger Cooter, Logie Barrow, Margaret Pelling, Peregrine Horden, Andrew Darnell, Susan James, Hannah Charlton, Jane Hutchings, Will Sulkin and Jörg Hensgen for commenting on manuscript drafts; and to Barry Lewis for the photograph. Very great thanks go to Virginia Berridge and all at the Centre for History in Public Health, London School of Hygiene and Tropical Medicine, for their support and comradeship; also to the Wellcome Trust for giving me early financial assistance to browse and work my way through their library's extensive popular health collection, and later towards costs for completing the project. Finally, I cannot thank Luciana O'Flaherty and Matthew Cotton at Oxford University Press enough, for helping to turn it all into a book. The award for sheer patience, however, goes to my dear husband, John Cumming, who has very rarely complained; and to our darling daughter Kate, who has had to suffer two obsessed parents under one roof.

contents

list of illustrations

introduction

In our hall hangs a nineteenth-century framed handbill, hand-blocked in red and blue, printed by the 'Inmates at the Prevention and Reformatory Institute, 237 Euston Rd, London'. It used to hang in the parlour of a farmhouse near Louth in Lincolnshire, close by the chair in which, according to family legend, John Wesley sat when he came to tea one memorable afternoon. It says:

RULES
To Be Observed By This Family.

Waste Not, Want not

Gather up the fragments that remain that nothing

be lost—John vi.12.

Do everything at its Proper Time

To everything there is a Season, and a time to

every purpose—Eccls.iii

Put everything in its Proper Place.

Use everything for its Proper Purpose.

Rise early. Be industrious.

Let all things be done decently and in Order—Cor. xiv.40

BE PUNCTUAL. BE REGULAR. BE CLEAN.

The chair still has a place of honour; but the Rules have been relegated by the next generation to a lowly space next to the coat rack. We no longer need to be told 'Be Clean'—being clean is hardly worthy of comment. Even so, there are still some visitors who look at the Rules and say simply: 'I agree with that.' That handbill speaks with distant voices that can still be heard, but are growing fainter.

There is a certain timelessness about cleansing and cleanliness that seems to intrigue all of us—and even horrify us, when ancient purification mentalities crop up in modern politics—but there is no real mystery about cleansing and cleanliness. Historically speaking, all of it comes from somewhere, and has a reason for being. This book starts from the premiss that everything about cleanliness is datable, and traceable, and tackles its well-hidden history head-on, across all fronts. Cleansing was such a universal subject, and so obviously consisted of any number of different histories, all of them probably interrelated in various ways which we knew very little about, that it would have been unwise to leave out any scrap of evidence.

Seek and ye shall find: under every rock that was turned over were fresh sources, new angles, new events, and new people waiting to be disinterred. Hygiene was almost virgin soil, a historian's dream. The work originally started in the nineteenth century, and many years later ended up in the Neolithic; I then slowly worked my way back again towards the twenty-first century. The trawl gradually started to turn into a coherent story. Inevitably, many of the details have had to be cut; and individual histories and close historical interpretation very much reduced, painfully, sometimes to a mere half-sentence. But half a loaf is better than none.

A few preliminary comments will be helpful. I have gradually come to think of the words 'clean', 'purity', and 'hygiene' as representing three—possibly even four—historical dimensions piled on top of one another, overlapping through time (for reasons I will touch on later). Simple 'cleanliness' I think lies at the bottom of everything, and seems to me to represent our animal and human side—not only the demands of our extremely ancient biology, but also our very 'Neolithic' love of grooming, orderliness, and beauty. Purity was man-made, but also lies in deep levels of time as a psychology that produced certain refined religious, or supernatural, ideologies of divine perfection and pollution that were socially imposed on animal nature and the material world. 'Hygiene' derives from the classical Greek word for wholesomeness and human healthiness, which then became a shorthand term for the Greek natural science of preserving and extending life. The first half of the book sketches out these main themes in some detail; while the second half deals with the subsequent literary and social history of European personal hygiene in its original, and much broader, ancient Greek sense, popularly known as 'the regimen of health'—what we did (and do) for ourselves in order to preserve our bodies, with or without trained doctors, or publicly provided facilities. You could call it a social and cultural history of preventive medicine.

There was a lot of solid material evidence involved in all of this; but it was always obvious that there was an 'immaterial' world that was just as real, if not more so, to many of the actors concerned—cleanliness is, after all, next to godliness. To the religious mind the two worlds were fused as one, and could not be separated: it is called holism. This is why there had to be a history of personal hygiene *and* purity. The religious mind also revealed a further secret: patriarchal ascetic Puritanism had effectively wiped the history of grooming and cosmetic care from the European records, certainly from the history of hygiene. They genuinely despised its very close and happy associations with beauty, women and sex. Yet grooming and cosmetic care are two of the most intensive and regular forms of bodily cleansing that we do to ourselves, and fully deserved to be rescued.

Readers will be familiar with some parts of the story, but probably not the whole—it is not the normal view of personal hygiene. This is scarcely your fault. In fact there hasn't been a book on the general history of hygiene for over fifty years. One historian complained in 1974 that 'there has been no serious scholarly study of personal hygiene. The subject has been treated as a source of amusement and has been presented in the context of social history as entertainment.' Heaven forbid. He was of course referring to the large genre of jocular coffee-table books on the history of the bath and toilet, each one a labour of love and wit, from the immortally named *Flushed with Pride: The Story of Thomas Crapper* (1969) by Wallace Reyburn, to the international best-seller Lawrence Wright's *Clean and Decent: The History of the Bath and Loo* (1971).[1] The serious nineteenth- and twentieth-century work on hygiene had gone into Victorian sanitary public health; and into numerous inconclusive attempts to measure the rate of hygienic Progress through economic statistics. The real death-blow in the 1970s was the switch to demography, which concentrated on the causes of birth, death, and population increase, and emphasized the importance of food supplies and marriage rates, but which provocatively reduced all types of hygiene (public or private) to a late, and minor, demographic factor. It did not look good. Now at the beginning of the twenty-first century, the whole landscape has changed. Hygienic behaviouralism has crept back onto the agenda. The range of potential sources had grown significantly, largely owing to the sociological historian Norbert Elias, who built a psychological theory of decreased dirt tolerance (and increasing bodily refinement) into his influential study *The Civilising Process*; and to the anthropologist Mary Douglas, who revealed the politics of pollution in *Purity and Danger*. We can now study hygiene without necessarily asking whether it was 'successful' or not; and can put the hardline models of demographers and economists (temporarily) to one side.

But if you get rid of the myth of Progress, what are you left with? Why do hygienic standards so frequently and confusingly overlap? Why (as Lawrence Wright put it) has 'a living Englishman complained of his Oxford college that it denied him the everyday sanitary conveniences of Minoan Crete'; why has the design of baths scarcely changed in 3,000 years; why do we still have rats, lice, and fleas despite all our advances in antibiotics?[2] The problem really lies in our old-fashioned philosophy of time. The March of Hygiene was traditionally thought of as an undifferentiated, linear flow of Time—also known as 'true' time or, as Marx called it, 'Absolute' time. Time as a regular succession of physical events, flowing steadily like a river. Or time measured mechanically—clock time. Traditional Western thought was strong on linear time, easily described by drawing a line on a piece of paper. If you were an ancient Greek you would have drawn a circle. If you were Hegelian you would have drawn a spiral. If you were a Victorian 'positivist' you would have drawn a gently rising line, a single path stretching ahead to a utopian infinity: the social philosopher William Morris gave a full account of this wonderful hygienic world to come (somewhere around the year 2003) in his famous utopian novel *News from Nowhere* (1890).[3] Reading this work now brings a strange sense of temporal dislocation, and wry amusement. Real life is so much grubbier and unpredictable than it is in the imagination, and far more heavily weighed down with burdens from history.

But there is a more modern philosophy of time, derived from Einstein and developed by early twentieth-century European historians, which solved these temporal problems at a stroke. Norbert Elias thought of time as a river flowing at three different speeds and levels: deep, slow biological time; quickening human socio-historical time; and right at the surface, the flickering ephemera of individual memory. This became the basic structure and principle of the book.[4] The *Annales* historian Fernand Braudel also described multidimensional time as an 'orchestra' of different histories, each with its own score, acting in concert. These succinct descriptions ended up providing the basic theory and chronology of the book, because, empirically speaking, comparing all the evidence from all the sources, multidimensional time-theory was the only philosophical principle that actually appeared to work. Multidimensionality accounts for all the historical continuities as well as all the historical changes. It allows the processes of Nature and Nurture to be complementary and coexistent, rather than mutually opposed; and it makes all ideas of hygienic 'progress', 'modernization', or even 'evolution', suddenly look like one-dimensional tunnel vision.

It would certainly take an orchestra of histories to deal with such a multifaceted phenomenon as cleansing, over such long periods. There are just two further points to be made here. I am unashamedly looking for universal trends, but do not claim to be anything other than a local European (in fact a British) historian. Potentially every part of the world—or any social group—has its own unique profile and history of cleansing, purification, or hygienic practices, and its own cultural mix. Like chess, human hygiene is played out with a set of basic options, giving rise to a very wide variety of situations. Secondly, I am not looking at dirt, but at standards of cleanliness and the reformers of cleanliness; which may make it appear as if I am taking an 'optimistic' historical standpoint, which is not the case. The science of hygiene is far too complex for that. Food, water supply, clothing, housing, climate, seasons, geographical location, height above sea level, size of settlement, drainage, building styles, earth floors, occupations, work patterns, immunity levels, age, sex, status, professional medical help, standards of midwifery, maternal child care, and now genes, have all been cited as 'variables' which could shorten—or lengthen—the lives of individuals. You could also add handkerchiefs, toothpaste, or soap. Multidimensional, multi-causal, multi-variable—how do you judge a moving bio-system?[5]

I recently came across the seventeenth-century scientist Robert Boyle's classic definition of 'The Requisites of a Good Hypothesis': 'That it be consistent with itself... [and] at least be consistent with the rest of the Phaenomena it particularly relates to, and does not contradict any other known Phaenomena of Nature, or any manifest Physical Truth'. That was all right; but on the next page was a rather more alarming list of 'The Qualities and Conditions of an Excellent Hypothesis': firstly, 'That it be not Precarious, but have sufficient Grounds in the nature of the thing itself or at least be well recommended by some Auxiliary Proofs'; and secondly, 'That it be the Simplest of all the good ones we are able to frame, at least containing nothing that is superfluous or impertinent'.[6] Acutely aware of the many gaps in evidence and constant reliance on the expertise of so many others, I can only hope that the hypothesis and results coming from these first few exploratory trenches are neither too precarious nor impertinent.

chapter 1
bio-physicality

Dirt is only matter out of place, and is neither 'good' nor 'bad'. Nature does not care what we think, or how we respond, to matter in all its forms. But as a species we do care, very deeply, about our own survival. A dense mass of human history clusters around the belief that dirt is 'bad', and that dirt removal (cleansing) is always 'good'. The old Anglo-Saxon word 'clean' was used in a wide variety of situations: it was often blatantly human-centred or self-serving in a way we might call 'moral'; but it was also used more objectively as a technical term, to measure or judge material things relative to other things. It was thoroughly comprehensive, and unquestioned.

Preceding all human cultural history, however—certainly before any human history of personal hygiene—were billions of years of wholly amoral species development. The exact date one enters this endless time-line is almost irrelevant; what we are really looking for are the time-spans or periods when things speed up, which in the case of *Homo sapiens sapiens* was somewhere between *c.*100,000 and 25,000 BCE, followed by another burst of development after *c.*5000 BCE. Throughout this long period of animal species development, all of our persistent, overriding, and highly demanding bio-physical needs were evolving and adapting, and providing the basic infrastructure for the later, very human-centred, psychology, technology, and sociology of cleanliness.

It is difficult not to use ancient language when describing the egotistical processes of human physiology—routinely described as the 'fight' for life—and in particular, our endless battle against poisonous dirt. Much of this battle is carried out below the level of consciousness. Most of the time our old animal bodies are in a constant state of defence and renewal, but we feel or know nothing about it; and the processes are virtually unstoppable. We can no more stop evacuating than we can stop eating or breathing—stale breath, of course, is also an expulsion of waste matter. Ancient scientists were strongly focused on the detailed technology of these supposedly poisonous bodily 'evacuations'; and modern science also uses similarly careful technical terminology when describing bodily 'variation', 'elimination', 'toxicity', or 'waste products'. In either language, old or new, inner (and outer) bodily 'cleansing' is ultimately connected to the more profound principle of 'wholesomeness' within the general system of homeostasis that balances and sustains all bodily functions.

Inner Cleansing

There can be no disputing the link between cleansing and survival. Survival is the main aim of the organism. External attacks or accidents apart, the most common and constant threats to its survival are internal poisoning, and premature decay. The body defends itself from these vigorously: firstly, through the complex filters and waste-disposal system which make up most of the innards; secondly, by the judicious use of the internal–external sense organs; and thirdly, by manipulating the outer limbs to attend to the external body surfaces. Without this massive tripartite, self-defensive, self-cleansing, physiological system we would quickly die.

'Biological cleansing' is a biotechnology of perpetual motion, common to all species. Bio-perpetual motion runs on its own time. As in all other plants and animals our bodies respond obediently to the macrobiological rhythms of our solar and lunar 'body clocks', that prompt us through the years, months, days, and hours, ordaining the time to eat, sleep, give birth, grow, or die.[1] Human body-cleansing also has its own physical calendars and clocks. Powerful daily circadian cycles regulate our total energy flow and all the major bodily processes, particularly the arrival and passing of the menses, the fetus, and the faeces. Micro-second cellular activity is constant—but it is when we are asleep, or resting, that microbiological 'cleansing' can take place relatively uninterrupted. It is no accident that we cleanse ourselves in the morning from the evacuated remnants of our night's sleep; just as we cleanse ourselves in the evenings from the remnants of the day's work.

Poison or dirt removal—cleansing—starts in the cell. Modern immunology records the great cellular battles that are fought by the organic 'Self' against mutation, malfunction, and the physical invasion of lethal pathogens—cells which bring about the death of whole cells, or whole organisms, before the genetically determined time.[2] Not all 'foreign bodies' destroy their host cells, but some of them do it rapidly and spectacularly, and the most lethal of these travel the globe, creating epidemics of infectious diseases. Normal healthy cells, on the other hand, reproduce exactly to order, in order, with all parts functioning correctly, time after time. Any disorderliness is a clear threat to their survival, and a rigid cellular discipline prevails—a sort of constant cellular 'housekeeping' is carried on in which wholeness or 'wholesomeness' of the cell is the great aim, and anything that is 'foreign' (or 'alterior') to the cell is rejected. The pool of circulating water that bathes the working cells is kept pristine at all times, within a chemical variation of only 1 per cent: any more variation and the cells would start to die.[3]

You are what you eat—and your body takes the best, and leaves the rest. This job is done by the larger organs in the hydraulic system now called 'elimination' (formerly known as 'the evacuations'). Everything we eat or drink goes into the stomach and slowly passes through the small intestines, by which time most of the nourishment or 'goodness' has been absorbed. The liver rearranges the products of digestion that are distributed to the other tissues by the blood supply; the kidneys filter the blood and keep the cellular water pool clean, excreting waste products as urine. By the time the food reaches the colon whatever remains is surplus to requirements, and ready to be ejected through the bowels via the anus. Human excreta or dung consists mostly of water, dead bacteria, and cells, indigestible matter, and various gases and chemicals, such as bilirubin, which is made when the body takes old blood cells apart— bilirubin is a brown colour. Watery fluids also seep out of other orifices such as the mouth, nose, and eyes, but also with great consistency through the pores of the skin, which act like one-way valves, keeping us cool—and moist, and scented—with oily waste matter (hold your arm against a sunlit wall and you can see the vapours of perspiration steadily evaporating from it). Dead dry matter is also continually falling away from our outer bodies. We shed skin, hair, and toenail clippings, and generally dispose of quantities of waste matter minute by minute, day by day, year in year out—normally between 3 and 6 ounces a day, or 4 tons in the average lifetime. Between 75 and 80 per cent of vacuum cleaner dirt consists of human skin cells.

The Senses

The next layer in the body's homeostatic self-defensive response system are the delicately built sense organs, hard-wired into our psyche: the eyes, ears, nose, mouth, and skin—sight, smell, hearing, taste, and touch. This is where the psychology of cleansing comes in. The sense organs are the brain's external antennae, connecting the body to the outside world, and it is they that detect all foreign or alterior bodies approaching or entering the organism, and ruthlessly guide our responses. The brain supports one particularly formidable physiological safety net: the nervous reflex of disgust and repulsion. Disgust is certainly a primary reaction. Most mammals show their nervous reactions of distaste or disgust by turning away, averting the eyes, shaking the paws, or wrinkling the nose—though with less of the more extreme reactions of disgust such as a spitting or vomiting. In humans actual loathing is nervous and immediate, triggered by any or all of the senses. Odours, for example, send their message directly to the 5 million receptor cells in the nasal mucus and down into the olfactory regions that 'are yellow, richly moist, and full of fatty substances...the deeper the shade, the keener and more acute the sense of smell...The effect is immediate and undiluted by language, thought, or translation.' (Or as one fourteenth-century scientific encyclopedia put it: 'And the air with the likeness and quality of fumiosity comes suddenly unto the sinew of smelling and presenteth thereto the likeness of the vapour of the fumiosity that is printed in that air.')[4] In one famous experiment, a group of volunteers were given a full-face blast of animal excrement (*skatole*) and paid good money to withstand it as long as they could. None lasted more than five minutes. The nostrils flared, the face turned away and went pale, the heart rate went down, blood pressure up, sweat poured onto the skin, and finally the stomach started to convulse. It was the pure disgust response in action, located deep in the insula, the area of the brain that malfunctions in patients with obsessive-compulsive disorder, which causes them to wash and clean things endlessly, or vacuum endlessly, most of the day. It is the total opposite of the gross self-neglect that is often a sign of clinical depression.[5]

Biologically speaking, the neurology and chemistry of 'delight' plays a crucial part in animal grooming and nurture. The opposite of sensuous disgust is sensuous 'delight'—all those things 'that pleaseth and comforteth the brain wonderfully'. Delight is a psychology—we crave our delights. True delight, according to the poets and philosophers, consists of things that pleasure all the senses: good food, fine music, sweet smells, soft caresses, sheer beauty. The effects of cleansing and cleanliness can genuinely be counted as one of life's great pleasures—gladdening the eye, sweetening the taste, inviting the touch, and delighting the nose. Delight has not yet been as much studied as disgust; but the 'attractive' sense chemistry and sense neurology is apparently just as necessary to the body as the more negative feelings of repulsion or fear.

We display the release of the body's pleasure-giving chemical opiates, the endorphins, through broad smiles, a lowered heart rate, relaxed muscles, widened eyes, increased eloquence, or speechless laughter. The welcoming smile is as universal as the repulsing frown, and babies have the smile very quickly after birth. Most of the early delights we feel as babies are directly related to the sense of touch, and are all to do with being fed, nuzzled, handled, and enveloped in adult arms in that close tactility we call 'love'—and much of that is parental grooming; later on, we also take delight in touching and grooming our sexual partners. Zoologists have artificially stimulated grooming bouts by using hormones and peptides; but a soft caressing touch is all that is needed to stimulate the production of the opiate endorphins and damp down the pathways in the nervous system: the heart rate goes down significantly. In other words, being groomed produces mildly narcotic effects; and the longer it carries on, the more swooning or relaxing effects it achieves.[6] These periods of relaxed 'de-arousal' are carefully timed. Generally speaking, animal grooming occurs in gaps between energetic primary activities: i.e. before or after social contact, sexual activity, or eating, after exploratory or defensive behaviour or gaps in work, and before or after sleeping. During these resting periods peace is restored, and ruffled fur or feathers can be rearranged, repaired, and brought to their normal state of readiness. Grooming thus helps animals relieve stress: it is a useful way of going off duty, of taking a break. Grooming therefore does double duty as work and play (and a surprising amount is play).

The sense of smell is, again, right at the forefront of attraction. Good or 'fresh' smells, in particular sweet floral smells, have always been a crucial indicator of wholesome, welcoming cleanliness; to be 'as fresh as a daisy' or 'as sweet as a rose' is high praise. Attractive smells, lavishly applied, can become an important part of one's own self-identity: people often choose perfumes, or perfumed toilet soaps, for life. Our body involuntarily produces its own strong and attractive natural odours. Pheromones, discovered with delight in the 1970s, are human sexual scent-markers belonging to the odoriferous glandular system that serves as a mammalian communicator (stink glands, recognition glands, rutting glands, marking glands), which are contained within the apocrine glands under the armpits in particular, coating the long underarm hairs with their oils. Odourless in themselves, their scent is triggered through bacterial decomposition, which produces the sweet or musky smell. The pheromonal sweat of other animals has long been a constituent of musk-based perfume, bringing a feeling of delight that is clearly deeply ingrained in the mammalian psyche. Animal researchers trying to encourage endangered wild cats to breed 'stumbled on the secret powers of [Calvin Klein's perfume Obsession] during experiments with ocelots ... In captivity the cats are hard to mate, but a little dab of "Obsession" sent the cats into a sexual frenzy.'[7]

Training and Adaptation

A relatively recent physiological discovery strongly suggests a vital link between human nature and nurture, built into the anatomy of the senses. The human sense organs are pre-wired into our brain—but they are also preconditions 'waiting to be learnt'. In other words, they take on the 'primary imprint' of the local environment at birth, and are subsequently fine-tuned by personal cultural experience.[8] Only primary imprinting can explain the wide range of sense cosmologies throughout the world. There is not even any universal agreement on the physical existence of the five senses: some population groups have always thought there are more, or fewer; the Tzotzil of Mexico judge things by heat quality; other peoples prioritize the sense of smell, or hearing, or touch; the famous five-sense European classification was laid down by the ancient Greeks.[9] Cultural anthropologists and psychologists now detect different degrees of sensual tolerance in all sorts of different social situations. It has become obvious, for example, that the tolerance of strong smells and tastes has declined among the world's wealthier populations, for whatever reason; in much the same way, possibly, as visual and aural sensitivities (and particularly the sense of inviolable personal private space—when to touch or not to touch) can evidently become more refined or acutely sensitized (or desensitized) under certain conditions, or with certain individuals.

All we know for sure is that there is obviously a deep psychology of slime, dirt, and stickiness that all hominids apparently share, in different degrees. Close physical contact with other people's bodily wastes is generally and universally thought to be rather repulsive, and it is for precisely these reasons that extended contact with human waste matter (laundering, rubbish clearance) is commonly assigned to the lowest human rank, class, caste, or gender.[10] Jean-Paul Sartre noted that different individuals, as well as different age groups, can have

different 'thresholds of tolerance' to dirt. To a certain extent
this can be seen in the developmental psychology of children
and food-taking. Babies are not born with a full sense of disgust
to 'dirty' foods, but only a vague sense of danger, distaste, or
simple aversion, rather like animals. By the age of 4 they are
more suspicious but still fairly casual, but by the age of 8 they
react just like adults.[11] By adulthood our dislike of dirt, or any
other signs of deadly decay, is so strong that we tend to avoid
touching, tasting, smelling, looking at, or even speaking or
writing about, dirt and dirty things. No doubt there is also a
genetic component connected to each individual's dirt threshold—we all know people who seem to have been born clean and
tidy, those who acquire cleanness and tidiness, and those who
definitely have to have it thrust upon them. The anthropologist
Mary Douglas freely acknowledged that 'my other source of
inspiration has been my husband. In matters of cleanness his
threshold of tolerance is so much lower than my own that he
more than anyone else has forced me into taking a stand on
the relativity of dirt.'[12]

By adulthood we are more or less trained to reject dirt in any
form, and to practise some basic cleansing habits—in the
twenty-first century, teeth-cleaning, hair-combing, going to
the toilet, face- and hand-washing (young humans also have
to learn how to get dressed). The role of human parenting in
passing down information, and establishing routine patterns of
personal hygiene behaviour, should not be underestimated
either in prehistory or later. Trained habits inculcated by
human parents during the early years are essential social skills:
children can physically survive without them, but without
human rules and etiquette they behave more like sensuous
animals. The sociologist and historian Norbert Elias for one
was convinced that toilet-training was the initial stage of
human civilization, and seemed to him genuinely to explain
a gradual bio-psychological refinement of human manners

and habits over time—of thousands of generations of parents repeating or improving on what their parents had shown and told them.[13]

Care of the Body Surfaces

Toilet-training—or in adults, the act of performing your 'toilet'—is in fact part of a whole repertoire of grooming behaviour, common to all species. 'Grooming' is the old generic word that was commonly used to describe everything that we would now call personal hygiene. Grooming is our final physiological defence system, taking place 'outside', on the exposed surfaces of the body, in direct response to the environment. It is a behaviour trait that employs all the senses and looks after all the body parts. External surface grooming is so central to the history of human cleanliness (and medicine) that it is strange we know so little about it. Even social anthropology has studiously ignored human grooming; and although we so often see animal grooming live, close up, on screen, sadly no one has yet filmed similar behaviour with human subjects. It is grooming that saves the body from falling into disrepair, the same grooming that induces respect, or perhaps finds us a mate. As medicine it is both foreseeing (preventive) and healing (therapeutic). As a social system it is mind-boggling.

Animal grooming habits are the only possible model for human grooming behaviour, and help fill the inevitable gaps left in the historical record. The detailed observation of animal grooming systems in zoology originated some forty years ago from small specialist studies of COBS (care of the body surfaces). COBS grooming patterns are now routinely mapped out, and the animal ethology of grooming has become one of the main methods of establishing species group dynamics—physical hygiene is regarded as almost a minor function.[14] Significantly, our primate cousins have the biggest 'grooming budgets' of all

mammals, grooming between 10 and 20 per cent of their time—
'an enormous commitment' given the amount of time they
need to find food, and far more than they need simply to
control infestation.[15] Like other animals they not only 'auto-
groom' (grooming one's self); they also practise long hours of
'allo-grooming' (grooming by or for someone else). They may
even be practising 'vocal grooming'.

The basic routine for land animals is the 'dry grooming' of the
outer hide, or *pelage*. In most animals each body part is invariably
treated in a certain order (generally head to toe) and becomes a
separate grooming zone. Each zone has specific requirements
and allotted time. Typically, grooming bouts in mammals vary
in length between thirty seconds and ten minutes, with the
longest bouts in the morning and special attention given more
randomly to different parts, at odd moments.[16] When the time is
right for grooming, the hands and sense organs automatically
take over, looking or feeling for encrustations, living parasites,
minor lesions, or breaks in the structure—bumps, bruises, scrapes,
small wounds, pustules. Primate hands are exceptionally flexible
and have a wide range of *techniques du corps*: scratching, scouring,
picking, pricking, probing, pressing, stroking, rubbing, wiping,
combing, shaking, tugging, stretching.[17] Mammals without hands
or forepaws more commonly use their mouth orifices to groom:
the main primate mouth-grooming actions are licking, spitting,
sucking, nibbling, eating, nipping, and biting. Primates, humans,
and certain other mammals also have the curious 'toothcomb'—
the pair of long, pointed, semi-lateral canine teeth which seem
to be part of the 'nibbling' and 'scratching' grooming apparatus,
being more sensitive and less rigidly anchored than the other
teeth.

Animal grooming has many observable links with later
human history. Semi-automatic primate grooming actions are
still used today in what we call 'first aid'—the quick instinctive
attention given to oneself by oneself, or to others by parents

or intimates. It is difficult to ignore the grooming 'alert' that scratches an itch. 'Relic gestures' in modern populations include shaking, flicking, or smoothing hair; stretching and rubbing the limbs; feeling and absent-mindedly scratching the skin; brushing, or straightening or adjusting the clothes that form our artificial *pelage*.[18] We still use our tongue and toothcomb publicly to nibble and clean our nails, and pick off skin, or lick small wounds with our anti-bacterial saliva. The well-known practice of removing and then eating 'snot' from the nose is always denied or laughed off (by adults); but it is strange to note that while the evacuatory sneeze is instinctive, blowing your nose is a skill that will have to be acquired (sucking obstructive snot from the noses of cold-ridden young babies is a well-known folk remedy, discreetly practised).[19]

We also still pick out nits. This ancient human occupation, only occasionally documented, has become increasingly shameful and only performed in private. Getting rid of poisonous or unwelcome parasites is, across virtually all species, a primary function of grooming: they can damage the hide and multiply fast unless checked, and only constant vigilance keeps the parasite-load down. Parasites are remarkably host-specific and highly adaptive, even down to their colouring—small white lice try to become invisible in well-groomed fur, while large dark lice wallow luxuriously in poorly groomed fur—and they cannily concentrate themselves in the hard-to-reach areas, where the animal cannot see.[20] Human flea and bedbug populations have only very recently been reduced. The human head louse is a remarkably persistent and successful species, hanging on despite combing or brushing, and only losing grip when lathered with conditioner or dying under an onslaught of chemicals. But the chatty social occasions when we all sit around allo-grooming and picking nits out of each other no longer exist. A rare twentieth-century description from an isolated Russian

village billeting Second World War refugees revealed a symbi-
otic relationship between the village lice and the village people:

> The village was full of lice. Hannah poured petrol on their clothes
> and burned them. They put paraffin on their hair to get rid of the
> lice. But for the villagers, lice were part of their daily life. Every
> Friday after they bathed, they would put their heads in someone's
> lap, look for lice, and squash them between a knife and a fingernail.
> 'That was their pastime' says Rosa.[21]

The phenomenon of animal (and human) 'group allo-grooming'
gives weight to the distinct possibility that the grooming may
have helped to develop human speech skills. With primates
especially, it has been found that the larger the group, the
more time is spent grooming—mainly because they are literally
having to 'stay in touch' with more individuals. But for any
bigger population groups (say over 120–30 bodies) touch and
eye contact alone would become unfeasible, and may have been
supplemented by a type of grunting, cooing, or muttering
speech form that has been described as 'vocal grooming'.[22] It
is tempting to see vocal grooming as the precursor of human
'gossip'—the sort of mindless nattering, chattering, or free-
association vocal sessions that assert status and relay the most
intimate news and views. Young hominid females have it in
abundance. Certainly in later periods of history, gossip was
inextricably linked with key grooming areas: bathhouses,
barber's shops, roof terraces, courtyards, and bedrooms.

Equally fascinating are the group dynamics of animal grooming—the social politics of grooming. Allo-grooming may have
been vastly more important in the past than it seems to be now
(though it still reappears before festive occasions) and human
history is replete with grooming hierarchies, life-cycle grooming, allo-grooming, and medical mutual aid. In the animal
world, an individual's chances of a safe passage through life
increase hugely through being assisted and generally cared for

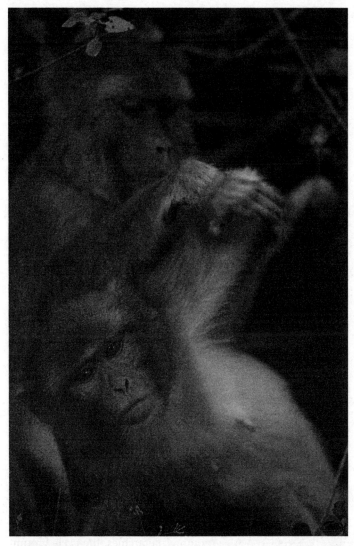

1 Primates grooming—an intense and loving experience. Careful observation and nit-picking is essential grooming care for all animals, including primates.

by others, and solitary animals are at a grave disadvantage in this respect. Allo-grooming is the basic technique behind all nursing care: the fact that another pair of eyes can often detect small problems before they become large ones, keep watch on your back—or help you through a major medical crisis.[23] Nothing more strongly suggests social cohesion in prehistory than the discovery that many skeletons and well-preserved ancient bodies had obviously been groomed, nursed, and given medical aid. The prime example of medical mutual aid would have been childbirth: there is a 20,000-year-old cave picture of a pregnant woman in labour, surrounded by a circle of figures, in northern Brazil. A surprising number of Neolithic skeletons had been 'trepanned' (a hole made in the skull) while still alive; yet others have survived broken limbs that have been set, and limbs that have been amputated. The business of rearing infants and nursing adults would have been (as in tribal communities today) very much the work of the entire family, extended kin included; and all life-and-death decisions would have been tackled on the spot (as they still are in isolated areas). There were no specialized 'doctors' then, but a great many carers and allo-groomers with time on their hands. At one Neolithic cave site it was estimated that food-gathering took up as little as twenty hours per week per person, or roughly three hours a day.[24] The famous traveller who froze to death on a Tyrolean pass in c.3300 BCE was aged 25–40, had worn teeth and arthritis but excellent internal organs (with lungs blackened by fire smoke), had survived severe illnesses, was healing several broken bones, and had small tattoos set in groups on either side of his spine, possibly for back pain. He was also shaved and beardless, and had recently had his hair cut.

All regular animal grooming bouts are finely tuned to the politics of social status. It appears that grooming is such a valuable skill—perhaps the only resource the giver has to trade with—that it is often politic and self-seeking. Primates in particular use grooming as a way up the social ladder, and as part of a social reward system: the more powerful you are, the more attention you will get. Through grooming friendships are sealed, and intimate groups are formed: 'a light touch, a gentle caress, can convey all the meanings in the world... Knowing which meaning to infer is the very basis of social being...'.[25] The choice of grooming partners is highly deliberate. The most important social divisions in the primate world are between young and old, kin and non-kin, and male and female. Rank and power go to the strongest member of the family (and to whichever natal gender group is in charge). There is some flexibility, but on the whole a top-down grooming hierarchy prevails. The powerful 'A' ranks—alpha males and alpha females—are groomed more than others, by others, and allo-groom less than others. 'B'-ranking groups, male and female, are usually the busiest overall, grooming both up and down the chain. 'C'-ranking males and females—often outsiders or unmatched males or females—get least attention of all. But even such powerful social divisions seem to be as much for guidance as a rigid rule; it ultimately all depends on circumstances, and self-interest.

Grooming 'peaks' occur over the life cycle, and the very young get preference over all ranks. After the birth, primate mothers allo-groom incessantly, up to 20 per cent of their time (approximately twice that spent on their own grooming needs) but maternal concern quickly eases off. The second most important grooming peak in a young primate—and young human's—life is the time of sexual maturity, courtship, and sexual display. For sexual success, health and beauty are a winning combination—females especially like to get good value from their mate. Good grooming enhances the sexual signals, and both sexes will attempt to display themselves as well groomed and well kept, and often select their partners by giving or soliciting grooming. In the last phase of the life cycle, old age and death, both auto and allo-grooming drop to a new low. Among elderly humans, a poor sense of smell (and reduced vision) is often the prelude to a decline in personal grooming. Powerlessness and helplessness are a lethal combination. High-ranking males and females are displaced, and themselves become supplicants, at the mercy of the new rank-holders. Again, survival depends largely on individual circumstances and ability. In one chimpanzee group one old male was groomed by the alpha male, but never returned the grooming—he was still a key player in the group's politics.[26] At the end, though, primate death is a private affair, a last retreat into the bushes. It would be inconceivable for other primates to 'lay out' or publicly groom the body after death, as hominid primates do.

Place, Space, and Order

In the very earliest periods of human society, grooming was governed only by biology; but the next sedimentary layer in the history of personal hygiene was the arrival of human artificial technology. By slow degrees the biological body of early *Homo sapiens* became refined, retuned, towards a range of new sensory experiences—smells, sounds, textures, colours, tastes— most of which are now wholly taken for granted, but at the time must have seemed miraculous. They were certainly deeply embedded in the Late Neolithic spiritual world. Medical materialism, on its own, is never going to be a sufficient explanation of human attitudes towards cleansing. Cleansing is a mechanical physical process, but in the human psyche it developed imaginatively and gained an invisible moral dimension that we have lived with ever since—cleanliness as a moral virtue. Moral cleanliness was and is inevitably a subjective or qualitative assessment; but the judgement between the 'right' way and the 'wrong' way of proceeding through life is the point where natural technology and human morality (or psychology) overlap. Technology has its own inviolable rules and cleansing disciplines; so does religion. Human cleansing behaviour has long been ruled by strict personal discipline, orderliness, and regimen, and some history of human routines, spatial rules, and the psychology of 'order' has to be invoked if we want to track down these long historical changes.

The great achievements of Neolithic peoples were the artificial or 'applied' technologies (or *techne*) created by their hands and brains, which they used to safeguard and enrich their domestic lives. There was a definite surge of technical (and religious) innovation in personal hygiene and cleansing following the Cro-Magnon migration from Africa into Eurasia and beyond, from around 40,000 to *c*.3000 BCE—a dynamic period normally known as the Neolithic, or Late Stone Age.[27] During this period *Homo sapiens sapiens* developed a strong physical dependence on specific places and artificial objects, shared with other animals, that zoologists call 'environmental physiology'. Many if not most of our domestic artificial cleansing skills were developed during the Late Stone Age, alongside the vernacular architecture that emerged in innumerable varieties, on all continents. Protective artificial nesting-places snugly surrounded the throbbing human body organism, filled up with 'belongings', and became the body's known habitus—which, like anything else in close contact with the body, had to be cleansed and kept whole.[28] Manual surface-grooming, food preparation, and domestic cleaning took turns in ministering to the body and its needs; many of the actions, indeed, were the same.

The social division of space, and the separation of domestic functions, are at the root of all house- and body-cleaning operations. Inasmuch as the brain has an innate spatial and visual 'ordering' ability—otherwise we could not physically perform at all—it is usually concerned with snap-second judgements; but these instincts clearly also extend to the wider environment. In Anglo-Saxon the verb 'to order' (Middle English *ordren*) has two distinct meanings—prioritization and soundness: 'to give order or arrangement to; to put in order; to set or keep in proper condition; to dispose according to rule; to regulate, govern, manage; to settle'. (As a noun, it is rank order or full classification: i.e. the order of all things.) The philosopher Plato once described cleansing (*katharmos*), logically, as the science of division—'of the kind of division that retains what is better but expels the worst'—and commented that 'every division of that kind is universally known as purification'. This is an almost exact philosophical description of housework, which deals with the orderly inflow and outflow of matter, and the purification of 'matter out of place', on a daily basis.[29]

Having a sense of space and place is obviously psychologically important for humans, who will still mark out and divide even the tiniest of corners, under the most difficult of conditions (as, for example, during imprisonment). Neolithic nesting arrangements would have been rather similar to those still used in the small spaces of a modern tent, boat, or caravan: small rooms, severely functional, holding just a few well-used basic objects, but with each object in its exact place.[30] At the famous Neolithic settlement on the island of Skara Brae in the Orkneys between 3100 and 2500 BCE, six small interlinked stone-built houses were built to a remarkable standard of Stone Age convenience and comfort. Each contained a large amount of stone-built furniture: stone 'dressers' with several shelves, stone water tanks, bed-shelves and built-in hearths, and a drop-latrine built into an outside wall (they also had complete command of a beer-brewing technology).[31] Our knowledge of the history of Neolithic domestic surface technology, and domestic cleaning tools, is negligible; all we know for sure is that housework has to be connected to the worldwide history of building materials. The Sumerians, for instance, invented glazed mud bricks (ceramics); the ancient Egyptians (and the Chinese) coated their interior house walls with anti-verminal plaster. Stone or wooden habitats were perhaps easier to keep clean, but earthen floors and woven vegetation (with or without a smooth cladding) were probably the norm. In addition, there is the insufficiently analysed effect of the so-called string revolution—a 'joining' technology that neatly complemented the more-famous 'cutting' stone technology. First came the single twisted thread of some vegetable fibre, then the double or triple twisted string, then the weaving of the plait, the rope, and the net—all with multiple uses for storage, hunting, adornment, and, of course, the eventual development of brushes, cloths, and clothing.[32]

Storage—on shelves or in nets, pots, bags, or boxes—is an efficient and inherently 'ordered' system, and one that the people of the Late Stone Age apparently invented out of sheer necessity. Cleanness, neatness, and tidiness in 'stowing' or storing and maintaining objects would always have been necessary not only for their own survival, but for their owner's survival, if they were essential objects. Cleaning up is a sign of finishing the job. Modern machine manufacture is also dependent on a cleansing work discipline—and even a modern building specification can yield a rich mix of historic terminology: 'Cleaning: chip, scrape, disc sand and grind surfaces to remove all fins, burrs, sharp edges, weld spatter, loose rust and loose scale. Clean out all crevices. Thoroughly degrease . . .'.[33]

In Old English, 'clean' itself appears to have been a rather overworked generic word that was used, initially, to describe dainty physical forms. The root word *clene* is derived from the Old High German *clacne* or *clani*, in turn derived from the verb stem *kli-klai*, meaning 'to stick'; the Old High German root firmly gives the meaning as 'clear' with an additional meaning of 'littleness'—neat, delicate, fine, tiny, small, and puny (see also sweet, cute)—with similar echoes in Icelandic. The moral definitions evidently arrived later. 'Clean-liness' is definitely a later, suffixed word that seems to embody a new level of cultural generalization; as do the well-known later 'compound' pairings such as 'clean 'n' decent', 'clean 'n' tidy', or 'sweet 'n' clean'. (For the record, 'pure' is a Middle English French–Latin import, while 'hygiene' is a seventeenth-century Greek–Latin import.)[34]

Human rubbish radiates out from the source, and putting human faeces 'outside'—anywhere immediately past the *domus* threshold—is universal behaviour. Neolithic middens were typically located directly outside the habitation, with further rubbish dumps on the outer boundaries of the settlement. The near-universal and ancient 'dry' sewage sanitary system, still found in isolated rural areas, consisted of indoor sand, ash, or earth buckets that were dumped on outdoor middens, and subsequently scavenged for fertilizer or fuel. Toilet habits apparently divide universally into 'washers' or 'wipers'—and most ancient peoples were wipers: 'These words refer to how people clean themselves after they have excreted. Washers use water, wipers use some solid material like grass, leaves, paper, sticks, corncobs, mudballs, or stones.' The drop-latrine at Skara Brae was yet another example of advanced Neolithic hydraulic technology. Drop-latrines were vertical hollow shafts built on an outside (stone) wall down which the solids dropped and the water flowed, with a receptacle or pit to collect the final waste.[35]

On Skara Brae the middens grew so large that the famous stone-lined and covered corridors were actually built in order to drive a clean and sheltered passageway between the huts, which later themselves became completely enclosed by their middens.

To appreciate the level of comfort and containment eventually reached we can look at the traditional ground plan and furniture of the tented Mongolian *ger* (or *yurt*). Inside the *ger*, the circular space was divided not only into halves but into quarters, according to categories of gender and purity. Men and women sat and slept on opposite sides of the tent; the dirty cooking and cleaning area was on the women's side in the quarter nearest the exit flap, and the sacred space was on the men's side in the quarter at the back. The domestic artefacts in the *ger* were packed into boxes, chests, nets, and bags; and as a further flourish it was decorated with glittering and crafted objects, including decorative traditional clothing produced on important occasions.[36] This was a survival kit—a life that could be packed within hours and hauled across plains, rivers, and mountains, all based on Neolithic technology. In the end, domestic cleanliness is always entirely relative, and psychological. Although you could not ignore the muddy, weather-beaten, and extreme conditions of life in the wilderness, you could if you were lucky mitigate them—soften the harsh surfaces, add touches of refinement, and keep things separate, dry, and unsoiled. In theory, even in the Neolithic the most makeshift accommodation could have been to its owner (in the words of a twenty-first-century migrant refugee living in a hut made of flattened oil-cans, hung with embroidered cloths) 'my beautiful house'.[37]

Pollution

Distancing yourself from poisons, dust, and dirt is one thing; but distancing yourself from invisibly 'unclean' people and objects is quite an achievement of the imagination. Animals maintain certain social boundaries and distances, but they have no conception of a dirt demon. The metaphysical or sacred dimensions of the *ger* were clearly just as important to its inhabitants as its physical dimensions, which were so carefully arranged to reflect their cosmological beliefs in the workings of the universe. Religious purity has a distinct role in the history of personal hygiene. It was not functional, not rational, and more often than not completely illusory; but it was a key cultural component that determined the lives and cleansing behaviour of very large numbers of people.

Religious purity rules and prohibitions are a social phenomenon that developed over many millennia, and still exist worldwide. For a long time they were looked on as a sideline to theology— irrational or magical superstitions that somehow arose from the instinctive or 'hygienic' sense of disgust. In her classic work *Purity and Danger* (1966), Mary Douglas reanalysed their social significance, and showed decisively how and why it was that 'pollution fear' came to be universally developed as a method of social control. There was nothing irrational about purity rules: they were a form of social legislation. Pollution psychology, Douglas suggested, is still very much alive today, even in our modern, technological, and highly 'differentiated' societies.

Purity and pollution rules vary worldwide in their complexity and intensity, and have always been subject to different geographical, economic, political, and historical processes. There are some societies that place almost no emphasis on metaphysical pollution, like the remote twentieth-century Pygmies; or societies where pollution rules are hierarchically ordered, highly differentiated, and closely regulated, as in the Indian and South-East Asian caste systems. Even within a given geographical region, tribal religious rules could frequently change completely within the space of a few miles; it was the later written religions that imposed common practices over large regions. The dirt-avoidance religious practices that evolved in early societies performed two particular functions. Firstly, they were a type of metaphysical insurance policy, a defence against the physical cracks in the universe. Secondly, they held the body politic together in an orderly set of social relationships.

Purification was an attempt to control the universe through forethought and active intervention. By patrolling and constantly defining the spiritual boundaries and keeping the supernatural defences secure, everything was done to ensure the safety of the group, ward off death, and lengthen the chances of survival. Cosmic harmony was ensured by a series of sacred purificatory rituals directly linked to universal biorhythms (often dedicated to a particular god, goddess, or spirit). Virtually all early cosmologies were rooted in philosophical dualism: the observation of moral 'polarities' or opposites in nature—day–night, sun–moon, right–left, man–woman, hot–cold, above–below, inside–outside, life–death.[38] In extremely hierarchical systems, dirt slopped and hovered around the bottom rungs of the ladder of creation and was given supernatural physical form: no religious system has such lively dirt demons as the coprophiliac, shit-eating, 'hungry ghosts' of Indian, Chinese, and Japanese Buddhism—the thirty-six *gaki zoshi* ghosts, and the seven *po* spirits that live in the body, who delight in filth, turn their back on life, and are fixated on death: 'the ones with bodies like cauldrons, those with needle-thin throats, vomit eaters, excrement eaters, nothing-eaters, eaters of vapours in the air, eaters of the Buddhist *dharma*, water-drinkers, hopeful and ambitious ones, saliva eaters, wig-eaters, blood-drinkers, meat-eaters, consumers of incense smoke, disease-dabblers, defecation-watchers'.[39]

Naming and isolating the various dirt dangers through regulation and classification reduced them and made them manageable; and elaborate purifications were devised using every element—hot, cold, wet, or dry—with other materials judged by their porosity (from 'hard and pure' to 'soft and impure') or potency.[40] Each local sacred technology was unique, and might remain so under isolated conditions: there is only one tribe of cattle-keeping Todas, 'the whole basis of whose social organisation is directed towards securing the ceremonial purity of the sacred herds, the sacred dairy, the vessels, the milk [and] the priest-dairyman'.[41]

People used their eyes, hands, and noses when they took part in these rituals, but by definition, the supernatural was not of this world. As Douglas discovered, lists of ritual dirt 'abominations' such as those in the Hebrew text of Leviticus, or those of the tribes of the Lele, Dinka, or Ndembu, held a contradictory message: 'suddenly we find that one of the most abominable or impossible is singled out and put into a very special kind of ritual frame that marks it off from other experience ... Within the ritual frame, the abomination is then handled as a source of tremendous power.'[42] So in Judaism *hatat* blood purged the sanctuary; being scattered with funeral dust cleansed Nyakyusa mourners; in Hinduism all the waste products of the cow were considered holy, and were therefore pure, and purificatory. Many 'dirty' but potent ingredients were and still are used in indigenous systems of polypharmacy, including the widespread use of many different dead animal parts as charms (such as the wearing of a rabbit's foot, or the dung hung in a bag round the neck in ancient Mesopotamia). Hence the imaginative phenomenon that rationality finds so strange—that ritual purity and impurity laws do not refer to observable cleanliness or dirtiness, but to a classified purity status: 'If you touch a reptile, you may not be dirty, but you are unclean. If you undergo a ritual immersion, you may not be free of dirt, but you are clean.'[43]

Death was always a major defilement. Physical contagion ('catching' a poison through air, liquid, or by touch) may have been a recognized phenomenon; but ancient *Homo sapiens* clearly thought there was far more to death than that. Stringent isolation and purification rites were imposed on the polluted corpse, its home, and its relatives, after death. Widows and widowers, or anyone who had to touch the corpse, were especially unclean. In some societies, the death of a chief could cause defilement so great that it sometimes entailed the abandonment of the settlement; while death defilement could even affect family members who were nowhere near at the time; or was even inherited through several generations. There was another gamble with death contained in the ritual of scapegoating—the 'transference' of badness or bad luck to another body, thereby purging and renewing your own; and, with a similar motive, in certain types of ritual wounding or ritual murder (such as the killing of kings).[44]

The opposite of death and decay was life and goodness; wholeness and purity were supernaturally linked to regeneration and fertility. Agricultural rebirth or regeneration was marked in many New Year equinox ceremonies. All early gods, goddesses, and spirits were elemental, and usually fecund; but fertility goddesses were particularly associated with the earth, spring, and water, especially running water. Spring-time bathing festivals have everywhere been used to signify new-year renewal; anyone who has watched the (televised) mass purifications of the Kumbh Mela festival that take place by the Ganges in India each January can easily appreciate the potential scale of these ancient water rituals.[45] 'Hypogenic' or sacred water architecture from 16,000 BCE has been found in Sardinia, where the Nuraghi peoples worshipped their enormous Great Goddess in round stone temples built over sacred wells; as the distribution of the famous so-called 'Venus' figurines show, the very early Neolithic worship of fertile female 'fat goddesses' covered most of western Europe from Scandinavia to the Mediterranean.

In the emerging world of 'Homo hierarchicus', to be born a polluting low-caste 'untouchable', or a chosen excluded one (the living human equivalent of a dirt demon), was a fairly nasty fate.[46] Transitional states—which represented formlessness, dirt, and disintegration—messed up the tidy divisions of holiness. Thus unusual anomalies in nature, or marginal people who crossed social, physical, or metaphysical boundaries— 'outsiders'—were especially likely to be polluted, or polluting. Primate *Homo sapiens sapiens* was also well aware of the times and occasions when extra care was required in the human life cycle, particularly those parts of the cycle where the body was in some form of major transitional (and dirt-ridden) relationship with the external world—as at birth, puberty, pregnancy, or death.

Every substance that issued or fell away from the body was transitional and therefore suspect (saliva, blood, urine, sperm, sweat, vomit, faeces, hair, and nail clippings). Food intake was closely monitored.

According to these rules of transition women were the main polluters. Menstruation was contained and controlled by purity rules and seclusion, while menstruating women were often believed to be contaminators of food; pregnant or post-partum women were frequently separated off from the entire community as well as their own household, sometimes for months. Sex pollution or chastity rules (such as purdah) required ritual seclusion inside the home, both before and after marriage, even though these politic rules that so carefully protected fertile women on behalf of the male line could easily be self-defeating if not enough females were allowed to procreate, or indeed do useful work.[47] For both males and females, however, the puberty initiation ceremonies that marked the arrival of new sexual emissions were often severe tests of bodily endurance, cathartic privation, and ritual purification. After the rites the young adult was, like chrysalis to butterfly, transformed into his or her new adult 'skin', fully displayed in the ceremonial dancing and sexual peacocking which followed—among the South African Xhosa, the red ochre painted on your newly purified body was supposed to be rubbed off in the arms of your future wife.[48] Betrothal and marriage ceremonies were more festive occasions: the worldwide rituals of preparatory purification, grooming, bathing, and dressing up of the bride and groom were yet another time of extensive group bonding, when every effort was made to bring about good luck, and expel evil influences.

There can be no such thing as 'total holiness', and the religious imagination frequently collided with hard reality.[49] Whatever happened to you depended to a large extent on your immediate circumstances—religion, age, gender, or purity status. But everyone was involved in the duty of self-patrol. On a day-to-day level, ritual purifications stopped anything 'bad' from entering the body, and protected the body from what it touched: from casual contact, formal contact, contact between old and new, contact with strangers, contact with strange things. If you were not vigilant (or were deceitful) most likely someone would be vigilant for you. It was part of politics, a way of living within, and not outside, your own society. Although there have always been certain societies, places, and occasions, where religious writ did not run and human life continued along older paths, so that more people lived outside elite circles of spiritual purity than lived within them, nevertheless it seems that once the sense of a metaphysical or psychological purity danger was alerted or imprinted on a group, it could become a source of communal tension that was difficult to eradicate or deny, and created a new source of power that could be exploited for political ends. To read purity rules fully, Mary Douglas once said, 'you must always ask who is being excluded'; adding 'the only thing that is universalistic about purity is the temptation to use it as a weapon'.[50]

Tools, Adornments, and Body-Art

We come back to earth with the human toilette, which was very much a celebration of the living human form and a constant reminder of the endless human labour that was going on behind the scenes. We have already investigated the biology of personal hygiene; and purity rules have shown how the skin could become a significant cultural boundary between the self and the world. But for many people today there is one sole and sufficient reason for practising personal hygiene that eclipses all others: self-representation. It was at some time during the Neolithic that the body became an artwork. The human capacity for aesthetics must surely have been one of those ontological pre-wired conditions waiting to be learnt, ready to be sharpened and inspired by all the sensuous colours, smells, and forms displayed in nature. Neolithic technology gave us most of the cosmetic body-art we have today, including the specific decoration of the different body parts, and the clothing styles and adornments that became, in effect, an artificial 'second skin'. Washing and bathing the human body also required artificial technologies all of their own, and are only partly natural.[51]

Although it was technological expertise that perfected high-art Neolithic body culture, there were a number of animal grooming techniques around that could have been observed, copied, and refined. Animals regularly use water, mud, or dust baths. Apes and chimpanzees are especially fond of tools (and toys) and frequently use stones for massage, twigs for cleaning teeth, or bundles of leaves like towels or napkins. Animals also scent and oil themselves; a whole new world of zoopharmacognancy—the discovery and use of natural drugs by animals—opens up when we consider the small white-nosed coati who go to a particular aspen tree to wallow or rub themselves with camphor resin once a day; or the spider monkeys who use a citrus tree in much the same way.[52]

But the unique methods of human skin decoration only worked on a clean or naked canvas. The gradual loss—or adaptation of—human body hair (fur) over millions of years gave the final shape to human grooming habits. In the tropical and semitropical zones where bipedal hominids originated, hairlessness is supposed to have been a heat advantage; though in colder regions, artificial clothing became another adaptive heat advantage as a replacement furred hide—which of course is what such costumes were made of, in the days before artificial cloth. Growing population numbers may have been another cause of change. Lacking other natural markings on their *pelage*, the body-painting, hairstyling, and other adornments that distinguished human beings from other beasts presumably made

them more readily and easily identifiable to each other, especially from a distance.

All Neolithic body-art was and still is an 'art for the parts', in
that each different body part or grooming zone goes to make up
the decorative whole, and any or all of the grooming zones can
be emphasized for special artistic attention. Thus the eyes, nose,
ears, mouth, hair, neck, arms, hands, fingernails, breasts, waist,
navel, legs, feet, ankles, and toes have all been given decorative
forms everywhere. Particularly elaborate hand and nail art, for
example, still survives in South-East Asia; and hair art in Africa;
but nothing quite matches the cosmetic dental art of tooth-
filing and coloured tooth-inlays—tooth art—practised among
the ancient Aztecs.[53] The condition of the skin was always
considered especially important. It was either well oiled and
glossy or (as in Namibia and many other places worldwide)
carefully rubbed over with the ochre-coloured earth; both treatments also help against infestation and sunburn. The African
Nuba tribe have words to describe each different style of body
movement, every visible muscle on the body (and even the
indentations between them), and five different types of skin
abrasions: 'if a man has ... a minor abrasion, he will not paint
or call attention to his body in any way; dry, flaky skin is not
merely considered unattractive, it signifies that a person has
removed himself from normal social intercourse'.[54]

The earliest human body idols from southern Europe, Africa,
and the Middle East are ubiquitously painted with red ochre,
over-painted by stripes of other colours, particularly chalk
white, and the blue, yellow, and black vegetable dyes (woads).
One 42,000 BCE cave settlement on a beach at the tip of southern Africa has revealed evidence of red ochre paints and a paint-
grinding stone set just within the cave entrance.[55] Other forms
of radical body manipulation—tattooing, circumcision, body-
branding, the stretching of earlobes, necks, mouths, and
noses, ring-piercing, the binding and moulding of arm and leg

bones, waists, feet, and skulls—depended entirely on the specialized skills of whatever community you were born into.
Skin-tattooing had appeared on all continents by the Late Neolithic, but found a particular home in the southern Pacific; in
New Guinea today the Roro people will describe the untattooed
person as 'raw', comparing him unfavourably with uncooked
meat. Contemporary Melanesian body-art involves tattoos,
scarification, teeth-blackening, penis gourds, noseplugs, ear-
plugs, and much casual ornamentation of leaves, flowers, fur,
or feathers.[56]

From around 30,000 to 40,000 BCE the ornamental layer
seems to have developed fast, as the string revolution started
to kick in. The world's earliest rock art and sculptures show
figures with head ornaments, fringed armbands, beaded girdles,
and braided hairstyling; while a large industrial bead-making
site from c.30,000 BCE at Dolní Věstonice, in the Czech Republic,
has been described as the 'New York of the Palaeolithic': finds
there included exotic beaded costumes, braids, hats, ropes, nets,
and a very extensive ceramics industry.[57] One of the most
spectacular early Eurasian burial sites is at Sunghir' in Russia,
dated around 24,000 BCE, where the bodies of two high-status
children were found wearing full-length costumes sewn with
3,500 mammoth ivory beads; other graves contained ivory
bracelets, pendants, necklaces, and rings. Such graves prove
beyond doubt that, 'weather permitting', as one archaeologist
rather quaintly put it, 'Ice Age people may have been dressed
and decorated with more elegance than generally imagined.'[58]
In fact the children must have been dazzling in life as well as in
death. Cloth and clothing technology developed even faster
during the 'secondary products revolution' of the Eurasian
Bronze Age from c.4000 BCE, when ivory, stone, pottery, and
wood products were rivalled by metal.[59] Fine cosmetic tools
became prestigious grave goods—especially the burnished
bronze mirrors that enabled people to study their own face

and hair closely and conveniently for the first time, alongside well-made combs, knives, paint palettes, and small metal water buckets. One of the best-preserved bodies we have from the ancient past is the ice mummy, or 'Ice Maiden', from the Iron Age Pazyrick tribe in Siberia, a high-class female buried around 400 BCE. Her whole body was tattooed with stylized trees and flowers all over the neck, back, and chest, with two deer, whose antlers flowed wavelike up both arms. Her next ornamental layer was a white silk embroidered blouse, a red dress, a long red sash, thigh-length red leather boots, necklaces, and a 3-foot-high headdress—which took up a third of the coffin—carved and coated with golf leaf. Also buried with her were her horses, her drinking cup—and her face mirror.[60] By that time the new metal technology was simply an extra bonus.

Water, Springs, and Stoves

And what of water, that supreme ingredient of modern personal hygiene? And how do we account for the rise and ubiquity of hot water? Clean drinking water was of course the first human necessity: anything else was a luxury well beyond the norm. The long story of washing and bathing water began in the Neolithic at some indeterminate date, but probably (since it required extra resources and labour) during the later periods of relative prosperity and economic surplus. Later Neolithic technology seems to have risen to the challenge of water, with ingenious solutions to the problems of both fresh water and drainage. The large, square, stone water containers of the Late Neolithic (like those at Skara Brae) were the first form of domestic water supply, and were also quite capable of boiling a large amount of water when heated with hot stones from the fire. Water could be brought from the source in leather, pottery, wood, or shell containers; but the more convenient light and portable metal basins and buckets only start to appear in the records during the

Bronze Age. Bath-tanks, using even larger quantities of water for full-body bathing (not to mention clothes-laundering), seem to have accompanied the civic hydraulic sanitary engineering that was certainly one of the wonders of Late Neolithic technology—in Mohenjo-Daro, Knossos, Carthage, or Rome.

There was also a natural template for the human use of luxurious heated baths. Neolithic tribal groups undoubtedly discovered most of the world's extra-ordinary natural waters during their nomadic wanderings. Cold-water springs, rivers, and lakes might be innately sacred and healing; but the world's naturally heated waters must have been even more fascinating and awe-inspiring. There are hot springs worldwide in Africa, North and South America, Australia and New Zealand, Siberia, Iceland, Japan, and elsewhere. The planet's volcanic geothermal systems produce water in many different temperatures and forms, ranging (in Europe) from the 'sweating grottoes' in the rocks near the Greek *thermae* of Aedepsos, to the calcium hot pools circling the extinct volcano of Monte Amiata in central Italy, and the hot mud wallows at Dalyan in Turkey. It is likely that nomadic routes developed around the hot-spring systems on all continents (like the aboriginal 'walkabout' water-hole routes known to have existed in Australia), and the hot springs seem to have played a significant part in human settlement patterns. For instance, many if not most of the highly decorated Upper Palaeolithic sacred cave systems in the French Pyrenees and the Cantabrian Mountains of northern Spain are within walking distance of important hot-spring sites, also later exploited by the Romans.[61]

Japan, of course, is the outstanding example of an ancient hot-spring folk culture, and has some of the world's most lengthy and fastidious bathing rituals. In Japan hot springs even come up under the sea, as on the westernmost island of Kyushu, where the ocean reaches temperatures of 32° C (104° F) and where (in later times and as in thermal Iceland) almost

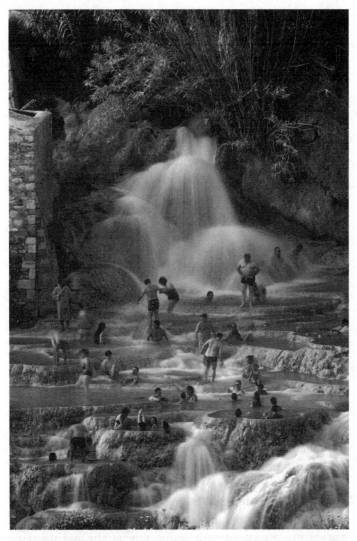

2 The Terme di Saturnia in Tuscany, one of many springs surrounding the extinct volcano Monte Amiata that local people have used for thousands of years, creating the bathing-basins. The chalky water is pale blue–green, and hot.

every house had a thermal bath. Remnants of Japan's past could still be witnessed in the early twentieth century, when the Kamchadales tribe still took long annual treks to the hot springs, putting up their tents and staying for several weeks.[62] Similar ancient tribal gatherings and parties around hot springs were witnessed in nineteenth-century central Africa (and North America) where 'the inhabitants came in large groups, and the business of bathing, washing, and idling was interspersed with joyful scenes, instrumental music, and barbaric songs'. The same things happened in any Roman *thermae*—or Finnish sauna.

Artificial 'stoving', or sweat-bathing, may have been another of the skills that the Cro-Magnons took with them from place to place. Sweat huts were common throughout Africa and the Americas, and were particularly favoured in the cold northern zones of western Asia (especially Finland, Russia, Poland, Denmark, Sweden, Norway, and the Germanic and old Celtic regions; a few ancient Irish sweat huts still existed in the nineteenth century). At its simplest, the person was wrapped up next to a fire; or covered with hot earth; or put into a sealed hut or tent, and steamed with hot stones and water. The intensive heat therapy relaxed the body and opened the pores of the skin so that the sweat poured out. A bunch of twigs could be used (as in the Finnish and Russian saunas) to further 'raise the blood', and stones, shells, or other abrasives used to scour loosened scurf off the skin. Cold air—or a sluice of cold water—restored the body's median temperature.[63]

Communal stoving or 'allo-stoving' not only made you well, it provided relaxation and 'good times'. Later on, stoving was particularly associated with spring celebration and marriage parties, or even with burial rites. The remarkable Scythian stoving ritual reported by the Roman author Herodotus was a riotous wake that also served as a purification ceremony:

> After a burial the Scythians go through a process of cleaning them-
> selves; they wash their heads with soap, and their bodies in a
> vapour-bath, the nature of which I shall describe. On a framework
> of three sticks, meeting at the top, they stretch pieces of woollen
> cloth, taking care to get the joints as perfect as they can, and inside
> this little tent they put a dish with red-hot stones in it. Now hemp
> grows in Scythia, a plant resembling flax but much coarser and
> taller... They take some hemp seed, creep into the tent, and
> throw the seed on the hot stones. At once it begins to smoke, giving
> off a vapour unsurpassed by any vapour bath one could find in
> Greece. The Scythians enjoy it so much that they howl with pleas-
> ure. This is their substitute for an ordinary bath in water, which
> they never use.[64]

People obviously dealt with their temperature problems in
idiosyncratic ways, and some of them actually embraced the
cold. There was a particular practice, or ceremony, of deliberately 'hardening' or training the body that seems to have been
common among some northern European tribes. The Romans
famously noted the Teuton or Germanic habit of cold-dipping
their children and babies into streams; and something of a
similar sort occurred among the people of the isolated Lofoten
peninsula off northern Norway, in a ceremony observed by the
Italian mariner Pietro Querini, in 1432. The round wooden
houses of 'these beautiful and immaculate people', as he called
them, 'have only one opening to the light, up in the middle
of the arch of the roof... They take their new-born when they
are four days old and place them naked under the peephole,
remove the fish skin and let the snow fall on them to get the
children used to the cold.'[65]

Modern cultural sociologists rightly describe the human body
as an 'unfinished body'—a body created by nature but finished
by humans—and, by following this line, have rediscovered all
sorts of different 'social' bodies (gendered, emotional, regulated, dominant, reproductive, economic, civilized, consuming,

narcissistic) with human culture imprinted firmly all over them. This would be an excellent description of the Late Neolithic body—except that it is usually applied to 'modern' bodies only. But human evolution may not be the one-dimensional, one-way process we usually take for granted. Humans are highly adaptive, and we often see comfortably bred urban populations reverting to 'prehistoric' practices and levels of awareness whenever there is a technical breakdown (just as other populations can rapidly learn to wear clothing, handle cars, or surf the Internet).[66] The idea of the 'unfinished body' should perhaps also be seen as a very old and self-regarding, or self-conscious, species theory. Back in the Neolithic the word 'naked' was presumably given to people without any bodily adornments, in order to distinguish them from those who had, and certainly by *c.*3000 BCE personal cleanliness had become an established feature of human society. As Bronze Age societies saw it, the extra 'polish' or 'finish' given by their grooming and adornments separated them from all other animals, and, as we shall see, they wore them with pride.

chapter 2
the cosmetic toilette

This is really the story of *'ellu'*, an ancient Mesopotamian word meaning a type of glittering, strikingly luminescent, or beautiful cleanliness—a powerful, non-ascetic, pre-Christian image of beauty that was entirely guilt-free. The cosmetic routine now called 'pampering'—baths, aromas, facials, manicures, pedicures, hairstyling, and costuming, conducted in sensuous surroundings with or without groups of friends—emerged at both ends of Eurasia during the Bronze Age from *c.*4000 BCE, along with most of the necessary tools and raw materials. Cosmetics is the underbelly of personal hygiene, usually ignored, often much reviled, but even now forming an essential part of personal health care and self-identity. The sensuous beauty of *ellu* turns out to be an integral part of the long history of royal court culture, which ran more or less unbroken from this period through five millennia to the present day. Thanks to the Neolithic revolution in technology and trade, Eurasia's fertile sub-tropical river valleys, coasts, islands, and hinterlands had produced some tribal societies that had grown very rich indeed.

Stratification and Outcome

The Eurasian Bronze Age is famous for an entirely new cast of characters: the super-rich. High kings and queens, high priests and priestesses, pharaohs and emperors—chiefs of the local tribal chiefs, traders, empire-builders, all huge hoarders and displayers of luxury goods. Their urban-based civilizations are the founding myths of Eurasian history; a story told quite simply with a roll-call of their famous cities scattered throughout the fertile subtropical zones, all of which provided the context (and the cash) for their expensive lifestyles. In western Eurasia the Fertile Crescent in Mesopotamia supported the Sumerian and Assyrian dynastic cities of Ur (*c.*5000–2000 BCE), Babylon (*c.*1792–800 BCE), and Nineveh (*c.*883–612 BCE); Egypt had created the Nile river port cities of Memphis (*c.*3000 BCE), Thebes (*c.*2060 BCE), and Alexandria (*c.*323 BCE); in central and eastern Eurasia the Harrapans built the stone cities of Harrapa and Mohenjo-Daro (*c.*2550–1550 BCE) along the Indus valley; the early Bronze Age Shang dynasty founded the Yellow River valley cities of Zhengzhou and An-yang (*c.*1554–1045 BCE), and the Chou dynasty on the Wei River founded a grid-planned city at Chou-tsung (*c.*1027 BCE). The large continental 'inland seas', with their ports and volcanic-island archipelagos, produced the Mediterranean cities of Knossos (2000–1200 BCE), Sidon (*c.*1000 BCE), Carthage (814 BCE), and Rome (753 BCE); and the various early volcanic-island civilizations of ancient Japan, Indonesia, and the peninsula of Burma, Thailand, Cambodia, and Vietnam. Bronze tools and weapons had accelerated one imperial phase in Eurasia; iron tools set off the next round of warring states. Isolated thousands of miles away across the Pacific Ocean, in *c.*2000 BCE the Mayans and other Meso-Americans were just getting to grips with their Stone Age, to be followed by a prosperous 'Gold Age'.[1]

Surplus wealth and increasing populations irrevocably brought about increased social stratification and widening social divisions between city, town, village, and countryside. A pyramid of social ranks rose from a broad agricultural base to a small urban–palace elite (thought to be roughly 10 per cent or less of their populations).[2] A similar social stratification can be seen in religious politics. It was around this time that the Indus valley or Vedic caste system (*jati*), which was heritable down the bloodline, developed as a purification theology which divided the whole of society from top to bottom, into four separate orders or clans (*varna*) according to a hierarchical order of purity—holy priests (Brahmans), noble warriors (Kshatriyas), wealthy merchants (Vaisyas), and obedient servants (Sudras). (The aboriginal Dalits, or Untouchables, were excluded from this classification by their Aryan conquerors, becoming socially invisible.)[3] But whether you were rich or poor, there were three important reasons to groom in the ancient world: bodily protection, social status, and divine protection—the proverbial state of 'health, wealth, and happiness' (or peace of mind).

The main regional hubs of the ancient Asian beauty trades scattered along the Eurasian subtropical latitudes served the city civilizations. Within these stratified, centralized societies, grooming had become a 'high' art form associated with the modern urban era, clearly distinguishing their populations from earlier or peripheral tribal groups—those without towns, houses, clothing, cookery, kings, or religion. The importance of grooming to the social elites is proved by the quantities of high-class cosmetic evidence they left behind them, leaving the personal grooming (toilet, or toilette) of the remaining 90 per cent of their populations something of a blank. Body-art was not confined to the wealthy; but as you moved up the social scale, you got every extra bit of grooming that time or money could provide (the same strict principle of unequal access that also applied to purification rituals). The old Neolithic nursing and grooming routines, however, were probably insufficient to protect fully those in the bottom ranks, living on bare subsistence, from significant environmental change; particularly those living in increasingly dense urban sites, who were the likely victims of proliferating parasites, (worms, flies, lice, fungi, bacteria), and new species of epidemic disease (malaria, dysentery, bilharzia, tuberculosis) already on the move.[4] Each individual may have had similar needs, but there was a wide variety of outcomes.

The Cosmetic Trades

All these imperial-sized chunks of land carved out by local dynasties were centres of cosmetic excellence, with fragile trading links. A strong dynasty was a definite commercial asset. Dotted about the landscape in strategic positions, massive palaces and temples towered over the rest of the population, and drove the luxury economy. Beauty was a powerful display of rank order; and it was just as true in *c.*3000 BCE as it was to the Roman author Herodotus later 'that the countries which lie on the circumference of the inhabited world produce the things which we believe to be most rare and beautiful'.[5] If a thing was rare and beautiful, the kings, queens, and chieftains wanted it (which created a trade); and then so did everybody else (which created an industry). Palaces and temples not only created demand, but also refashioned raw materials in their own farms or workshops, turning themselves into middlemen and 'adding value' to local resources or cheap imports. At Pylos (*c.*1550–1200 BCE) in Mycenaean Greece, the palace administrators ran an extensive perfume industry by importing crude oil, recruiting local labour to add imported spices and local herbs, then selling the product either in locally made bulk jars or in small expensive phials, in exchange for all the gold, silver, Egyptian faience, copper, ivory, and wool that the local community and the palace required.[6] For the local palace, its suburban 'service city', and the local hinterland farmers and gatherers, cosmetics and beauty goods were, literally, a golden trading opportunity: small, portable, and profitable—if you had the technical know-how.

Thanks in part to this sustained demand for beautiful and rare things, almost every useful rock, tree, shrub, plant, fruit, root, flower (or animal part) in Eurasia was gradually discovered and exploited during the Bronze Age between *c*.3000 and *c*.1500 BCE. Beautiful and desirable 'goods' (i.e. good things) were created from local wood, stone, metal, and animal products, or from the heaps of leaves, seeds, and flora that the gatherers brought in; while already domesticated plants like olives, grapes, corn, flax, and wool were grown, harvested, and manufactured in bulk on an ever-increasing scale. Natural materials exploited for a specific cosmetic purpose around this time included the soft volcanic rock called pumice stone, used for filing or scraping the skin; and the natural sponges found in warm seas, used for sluicing the body. The ornamental cut-flower trade was one of many specialized luxury trades that underwent a long transition. From at least *c*.3000 BCE the Egyptians gathered two types of native lotus flower, the white and the blue; by *c*.AD 200 the Indian pink lotus had been introduced, and bulk quantities of roses, narcissus, and lilies were artificially cultivated and shipped off to flower and garland traders in Rome (who were also importing artificial silk garlands from India). It was said that 2,000 lilies were needed for 3 pounds of flower oil: 'The more times you repeat with fresh lilies, the stronger the ointment will be.'[7]

Over the course of several millennia Egypt emerged as the main hub of the western Eurasian cosmetic trades. The Egyptian upper classes alone consumed the products of thousands of villages, thousands of miles away. To meet demand and serve their perfumed unguent industry, the Egyptians invaded and developed the 'Land of Magun' (ancient Oman) as a spice region. In *c*.3000 BCE the coastal village of Ras al-Junayz in Oman was apparently connected not only with Old Kingdom Egypt, but with Mesopotamia and the Indus valley:

the inhabitants of the village traded their own products—large mollusc shells, as well as shell rings—with crews of incoming vessels...a manganese oxide of local origin, pyrolusite, was

ground to make a black powder used as an unguent (kohl) and kept
in shells of small molluscs of the genus 'Anodara'—and Anodara
shells containing a black powder have also been found in the Royal
Tombs of Ur... [and there were] other exports, for example the
operculi of molluscs, which when ground up, were an essential
ingredient in perfumes for incense.[8]

That all these trading and manufacturing skills should have been
contained in one small village in 3000 BCE is a sobering thought.

Cosmetic equipment was now routinely included in the trip
to the land of the dead, and grave goods are a main source of
evidence outside the imperial courts—even beyond the subtropical zones. That the north-west Eurasian Celts were always well
barbered and groomed is underlined by the grave of one Celtic
chief, buried honourably with a small bag laid on his chest
containing his most essential personal belongings: three iron
fish-hooks, five amber beads, a wooden comb, and an iron razor.
The Russian Pazyricks were buried with their bronze mirrors.
In China the preference was for ivory hairpins. Well before 3000
BCE Egyptian pre-dynastic graves contained long-toothed
combs, hairpins, and an especially revered tool among the
Egyptians, the eye palette, a thin stone oval or rectangular
slate used for grinding up eye paint that became increasingly
elaborately decorated and ceremonial in character, and is consistently found in tombs up to the Nineteenth Dynasty and
beyond. The most expensive consumer item of all was probably
the cosmetic travelling-case; an unusually well-preserved Egyptian Eighteenth Dynasty case gives us just a glimpse of this new
batterie de toilette. A well-packed traveller's kit, this resinous
cedar box has four compartments containing one terracotta
and two alabaster vases for oils and unguents; a piece of pumice
stone; two (joined) 'stibium' tubes for eye and face paint, a
wood and an ivory stick; an ivory comb; a bronze shell for
mixing ingredients; a pair of pink gazelle-skin sandals; and
three red cushions.[9]

For valuable cosmetic products especially, the container was now part of the product. Container designs multiplied, and were lavishly decorated with the new range of pigments: Egyptian blue-glass, for example, and Egyptian blue-glass ceramics (faience) were made into small and elegant jars, jugs, and bottles of all sizes, all with handles, stands, lids, and spouts. They were high-class *bijoux* gifts which were widely traded (and copied) for centuries. Kohl eye paste was normally packed into reeds; but the luxurious kohl tubes of the princess Meritaten, found in her bedroom suite at the royal palace of El Amarna, were made of red, white, and apple-green painted pottery with her name inlaid in white and blue; other kohl tubes found there were 'made of glass in the shape of a small hand-sized column with a spreading palm-leaf capital, with the column then decorated by bands of different coloured glass, dragged into loops around the stem'. Cosmetic tools and containers now often came in sets; complete sets of tubs and basins were a traditional marriage gift in China.[10] For water and other liquids there were bronze or wooden shells, saucers, finger-bowls, hand-basins, foot-basins, small buckets, large buckets, and bathtubs; for drying the skin, bath towels, hand towels, and face cloths; for scraping the body, gold, bronze, and ivory combs, toothpicks, brushes, knives, files, and scissors. Some of these ancient toilette items have survived better than others: wooden, leather, or cloth items were all highly perishable, and the crystal, marble, gold, silver, and bronze baths of which the poets speak were either highly breakable or highly recyclable, or mythical. Only some sturdier stone or pottery baths have survived.[11]

Cosmetic Receipts

The serious point that the ancients understood about cosmetic or beauty care was that it kept you well and healthy: 'such, indeed, are human means of embellishment, and therewith they keep off death from themselves', as one Vedic author put it.[12] A more comprehensive view of the connection between cosmetics and health care can be obtained from some of the very earliest medical texts. Many of these simply recorded a folkloric pharmacology of herbal, animal, and mineral 'receipts' (ingredients) for the treatment of various conditions, that continued to be recycled for centuries to come; ancient Indian cosmetic receipts in particular were preserved uninterruptedly from 600 BCE to AD 1600 and onwards to the present day. All these early receipt texts show an overwhelming medical interest in the care of the body surfaces. Egyptian cosmetic receipts appear in medical papyri next to skin salves, eye salves, and tooth remedies; similarly in the early Anglo-Saxon leech books. In the Indian herbals, cosmetic receipts for hair dyes, hair promoters, hair oils, depilatories, and hair-disentangling cream jostle with recipes for the treatment of grey hair, dandruff, lice, and nits. Face paint, lip dyes, and perfumed unguents were set side by side with face salves for moles, blemishes, pimples, and peeling. There were teeth-cleaners, mouth deodorants and washes, nose deodorants (fumes through the nose), and armpit deodorants. There were any number of aromatic oils, unguents, pastes, bath waters, and bath powders for the body—things that 'will make the bodies of the males and females gold-like, beautiful, fragrant and lovely'.[13]

The basic common senses—especially vision and touch—that were used to check the general state of the body were natural methods that took no notice whatsoever of any formal division between preventive and curative medicine. It is perhaps easiest to think of this external COBS medicine as operating along a continuum of self-care, ranging from the ephemeral to the urgent—from painting to cleansing; from cleansing to emollients; from emollients to remedies. The Romans clearly regarded cosmetics as a legitimate branch of medicine; for example, Crito, personal physician to the emperor Trajan (AD 98–117)

wrote an exhaustive four-volume work on cosmetics, all lost
except for its table of contents:

> *For care of the skin*: cleansers, emollients, bleaches, paints, remedies
> (dryness, wrinkles, freckles, white spots, sunburn, warts, scars,
> double chin, superfluous hair, deodorants). *For the care of the hair*:
> hair-dressings, bleaches, dyes, scalp lotions, remedies (scaliness,
> falling hair, baldness, lice). *For the care of the parts*: manicure,
> pedicure, mouth care, teeth care, throat, remedies (washes, tooth
> powder, pastilles), bust developers, perfumes (powders, liquids,
> ointments). *Cosmetic tools*: mirrors, brushes, combs, fancy pins,
> hair-bands, razors, tweezers, false hair, curling irons, tongue
> scrapers, breast binders and false teeth.[14]

Graded Holiness

The divine 'means of embellishment' took cleansing into a
different dimension. In order to understand anything about
the full political significance of the toilette and its relationship
to society, one needs to understand the workings of ancient
courts and palaces—and of temples. In Mesopotamia the earliest kings were simply successful political candidates, *primus inter
pares* (first among equals), but by the end of the Early Dynastic
this had been superseded by the doctrine of divine kingship.
Throughout Eurasia successful clan dynasties bolstered their
credentials not only by appealing and sacrificing to the gods
in the traditional manner, but by annexing sacred authority as
the gods' representative on earth, 'God's Steward' for the welfare of the people, and therefore the sole arbiter of rule. Under
divine kingship, the king officially had 'two bodies': one corporeal, the other spiritual. The purity rules of the courts were a
pale echo of those in the temples.[15]

As formal temple cultures developed throughout Asia, religious purification reached new standards of magnificence and
thoroughness. Religious historians have described temple

purity rules as a form of 'graded holiness', or a 'Holiness
Spectrum'. The central source of ineffable 'holiness' was the
spiritual presence of the god in the inner sanctuary, radiating
divinity outwards far into the wide world up to heaven, pro-
tecting the temple and ceaselessly guarding it from the touch,
sight, sound, or smell of impure things.[16] In third-millennium
Sumeria the royal temple ziggurat of the alpha god Nanna at Ur
was particularly richly endowed. But before even a brick had
been laid at Nanna, a complex series of rituals, omens, visions,
meditations, and sacrifices had already been performed in order
to determine the site and to protect it with holiness, and many
more rituals were to follow. Archaeology confirms what literary
evidence suggests, that temple sites were physically purified first
by burning over the site and digging the foundations down
'eighteen cubits' to clean soil; then filling these pits with clean
sand, to receive the first brick, which had already been prepared,
purified, and poured by the king into a pure and anointed
mould, and exposed to the pure burning sun. On the right day
for good omen the local town was cleansed and purified 'with
fire', and the local townspeople cleansed and purified themselves in order to witness the ritual of the foundation brick. At
exactly the right time of day it was struck out, and the freshly
purified and abluted king placed the sacred brick-hod over his
head and shoulders, and reverently carried the holy brick to its
holy resting place: 'he took for E-ninnu the pure head-pad,
and the true brick-mould [of] the decision of fate. Gudea performed completely the proper rites . . . [And] took on his head the
head-pad for the house, as though it had been a holy crown'.[17]

Elsewhere the sacred statue of the temple, adorned with gold
and jewels, was being prepared for the god to enter into it
through the ceremony of 'opening the mouth', which was followed by the night-long riverside purification ceremony of
'washing the mouth'. The next morning the eyes of the statue
were ritually 'opened' and the now living god was led by the

hand to his temple and placed in his sanctuary, his resting-place on earth. Thus the ceremonies that worshipped the now living Nanna were reverently, even enthusiastically, tended to by many generations of royal personages, and faithfully preserved by each new generation of priests (as they were all over Eurasia, in very similar rituals). Each morning in Nanna's sanctuary the god–statues were offered food and were brushed, rubbed, oiled or painted, garlanded, and robed as necessary, each 'presentation' of body services and unctions given as a separate grooming ritual. Sweet tamarisk scent perfumed the air, and the holy objects were set out, decorated or made from gold: the sacred bowl, the holy table, the holy kettledrum and *balag* musical instruments, and the holy water pail. Outside the ziggurat holy trees had been planted in the holy gardens, and the gods had the use of a holy wagon and a holy barge.[18]

Deep religious reverence was attributed to beauty. It had a strong metaphysical role. In ancient Greece the word *kosmos* originally meant 'to order, to arrange, or to adorn'; *kosmetikos* meant 'having the power to beautify'; and the high priestess–goddess Kommo was the beautifier and arranger of the temple. The Mesopotamian definition of *ellu* was 'free from physical impurities'; anything could be beautifully *ellu*—a jewel, clean linen, a person, or a sacred place. The sacred books of the Veda laid down *kama* (the appreciation of beauty) as a religious commandment for the right conduct of life; described in Vatsyayana's classical version of the *Kama Sutra* as 'the enjoyment of appropriate objects by the five senses of hearing, feeling, seeing, tasting, and smelling, assisted by the mind together with the soul'.[19] In temples everywhere, the sacred *ellu, kosmeticos, kama,* or divine cleanliness came from the daily labours and skills of temple servants charged with keeping good order within the precinct. High priests and priestesses supervised lower orders of 'keepers', 'washers', and 'anointers', and chose the most beautiful (or talented) temple servants for ceremonies adorned with musicians, singers, and dancers.

Precise degrees and definitions of what was holy to the touch, taste, sight, sound or smell—the most or least sacred materials, food, colours, objects, animals, and people—were all graded according to the laws handed down. White robes were sacred to the Babylonians and Egyptians; Judaism favoured sky blue; yellow was sacred in eastern Eurasia. Gold was everywhere considered the purest and most beautiful metal. Later Greek authors reported that the temple of Marduk in Babylon used over 20 tons of gold; also that the rituals required over 2 tons of imported frankincense each year.[20] In Egypt the exact method of making the sacred holy incense and unguents was a closely guarded secret, written in stone on the walls of the priestly inner sanctum. There was even a holy soap—a carbonate of soda called *natron*—which was used to purify everything in the temple. Mostly *natron* was dissolved in water to clean the body, clothes, and furniture; sometimes it was ignited with incense; and to achieve fullest purity, the priests chewed it and drank it internally. It was particularly associated with the purity of the mouth.

The Holy Toilette

The flesh rubbers, kohl pots, rouge pots, lipsticks, razors, and mirrors found in the great water tank and temple courtyard at Mohenjo-Daro (2500 BCE) are evidence of the very early religious grooming traditions in the Indus valley, a thousand years before the incoming Indo-Aryans re-established a Vedic theocracy which abhorred body dirt.[21] In Vedic theology any touch or sight of the prohibited bodily secretions—such as sweat, saliva, hair and nail clippings, vomit, urine, blood, sperm, faeces, and afterbirth—was closely monitored, and the Vedic toilette rules were laid down for all classes as a religious duty; their thoroughness (or lack of it) served as an indicator of religious status. Washermen and barbers were especially impure, but played a vital role as the polluted intermediary in all purification ceremonies, including the personal toilette. Public outdoor barber's shop services that provided shaving, hair-cutting, manicures, pedicures, nose- and ear-cleaning, existed in ancient India at the same time as public *tonsors* flourished in ancient Rome. They are still observable on the pavements of Indian cities, or near the religious bathing places (*ghats*) along the holy River Ganges, where barbers provide traditional grooming to accompany the client's lustral dip: shampooing (massage) sitting on special shampooing stools; 'frictions' (scraping) using the stone columns and walls; hot baths, shaving (designs on the stomach hair a speciality), flower garlands, and every type of face paint and body powder.[22]

The Egyptian population's strict adherence to purity rules, and the strength of their religious belief, were considered especially remarkable by that indefatigable traveller and folklore collector Herodotus. It was not just, he said, that they abided by the normal purity rules that any Greek might follow—such as purification at birth, after sexual intercourse, during the menses and sickness, and after childbirth (in a birth-house, or 'House of Purification'), with minor attentions on minor occasions of possible impurity (before meals, after evacuation, after journeys)—but that he felt they were 'religious to excess, beyond any nation in the world, and here are some of the customs which illustrate the fact: they drink from brazen cups which they scour every day—everyone, without exception. They wear linen clothes that they make a particular point of continually washing. They circumcise themselves for cleanliness's sake, preferring to be clean rather than comely...'.

The highest degree of personal cleanliness was reserved for direct contact with the deity. In addition Egyptian priests were required to 'shave their bodies all over every other day to guard against the presence of lice, or anything equally unpleasant, while they are about their religious duties...They bathe in cold water twice a day and twice every night—and observe innumerable other ceremonies besides.'[23] They shaved their heads, oiled their bodies, kept their feet, hands, and nails clean (with nails kept short), rinsed their mouths, and fumigated all their orifices. The Egyptian priest–pharaohs were excused the more onerous priestly requirements, and enjoyed considerably higher standards of decorative cosmetic care, but had other unique obligations: they were purified at birth, at coronation, before any temple rite, and even, while still alive, and as a precaution, given a purification ritual for the afterlife. After death, it was imagined, the Pharaoh would be bathed, fumigated, shaved, and oiled by the goddesses— after which, not merely cleansed but revived, 'he received "his bones of metal" [and] stretched out his indestructible limbs . . . his body came together again [and] was entirely refashioned'.[24]

Goddesses were themselves the divine high priestesses of the arts of beauty and seduction. The Mesopotamian alpha female fertility goddess Inanna-Ishtar was eulogized as 'the divine harlot' and credited with taking 120 men without tiring; at the New Year festival of the Sacred Marriage, the current high king and high priestess acted out the parts of the fertility god Dumuzi-Tammuz and his wife, Inanna, on the sacred bed in the temple—a ceremony that naturally aroused the imagination of poets and gave rise to a special genre of love songs (and toilette descriptions) of Inanna: 'When I have washed myself...When I shall have adorned my body...have put amber on my face, [and] mascara on my eyes . . . When the lord who sleeps with the pure Inanna . . . shall have made love to me on the bed, Then I in turn shall show my love for the lord; I shall fix for him a good destiny...'.[25] The Greek poet Homer was obviously on his mettle when it came to his own 'white-armed' goddesses, with a

similar but especially luscious description of the toilette of the
wife–goddess Hera, before her seduction of Zeus:

> She began by removing every stain from her comely body with
> ambrosia, and anointing herself with the delicious and imperish-
> able olive-oil she uses. It was perfumed and had only to be stirred in
> the Palace of the Bronze Floor for its scent to spread through
> heaven and earth. With this she rubbed her lovely skin; then she
> combed her hair, and with her own hands plaited her shining locks
> and let them fall in their divine beauty from her immortal head.
> Next she put on her fragrant robe of delicate material that Athene
> with her skilful hands had made for her and lavishly embroidered.
> She fastened it over her breast with golden clasps and, at the waist,
> with a girdle from which a hundred tassels hung. In the pierced
> lobes of her ears she fixed two earrings, each a thing of lambent
> beauty with its cluster of three drops. She covered her head with a
> beautiful new headdress, which was bright as the sun; and last of
> all, the Lady goddess bound a fine pair of sandals on her shimmer-
> ing feet.[26]

In Homer beauty was a sacred gift to favoured individuals, and
was absolutely not a power or a favour to be taken lightly. When
Athene made Odysseus divinely handsome she added vibrant
sex appeal: she 'gave him ampler stature and ampler presence,
and over his head made his hair curl and cluster like a hyacinth.
It was as when a man adds gold to a silver vessel . . . Then he
walked to the water's edge and sat down apart, radiant with
handsomeness and grace.'[27]

How many story-loving Greeks had read or knew by heart
Homer's description of the toilette of Hera? Or Babylonians
the toilette of Inanna? There are similar descriptions in almost
every language and stories about divine beauty in every mythology, and they must have been at least partly aspirational.
Religious eroticism in general cut across all classes, ranks, and
gender, and was an occasion for serious sexual display—and a
very careful toilette. Purposeful erotic diversions, orgies, and

sexual rituals often involved entire cities and populations in licensed communal mating exercises on behalf of the gods, ranging from fertility bull cults to phallus worship and love goddesses.[28] The Indian god Shiva was the god of youth, sensuous delights, and erotic activity and Lord of the Dance of Life; in Greece, Aphrodite was the goddess of love, beauty, and fertility, honoured by women, and was also the patron goddess of the public concubines—the *heterae*. During the annual regenerational bath, or 'Aphrodisia', at her supposed birthplace in Paphos, Aphrodite's statue would be attended by hundreds of girls and women purifying themselves for her rites; it is reported that the renowned *hetera* Phyrne of Paphos, though usually very closely gowned in public, would at this festival time walk into the sea fully naked with her hair loose and flowing, as a living image of the goddess (also that the famous sculptor Apelles made her the model of his Aphrodite Anadyomene, a genre which later produced the famous sea-bathing Venus by Botticelli).[29]

Palace Purity

Back at the palace, divinity mingled with more earthy considerations. For the tribal leader and his household the palace complex was a fortress, a regional entrepôt, a cultic headquarters, and a home. Its main function was to defend and protect the body, family, and kin of the tribal chief or tribal alpha male (or female) from every possible catastrophe, in all possible senses—not just military ones. The royal presence created a sacred space; so it was deemed absolutely essential that the king or queen's 'two bodies'—their private selves and their public godlike selves—should be ceaselessly protected not only with layer after layer of palace stonework, but with an invisible web of palace purity rules, working like a comprehensive security system, with various different checkpoints and access levels.

The internal architectural layout of the palace of Knossos illus-
trates the basic spatial arrangements in many Eurasian palaces
then and thereafter, carefully designed to express architecturally, step by step, the spiritual, social, and dynastic intentions of
the reigning king. Here the monarch was heavily guarded by a
long Corridor of Procession, a Central Court, a Great Hall, and
various lustral basins and pools that also decontaminated anyone entering the adjoining antechambers and shrines of the
Temple of Rhea. The royal suite was the sanctuary at the heart
of the complex: a pillared tower block, four storeys high, containing the private domestic quarters of the royal household,
guarded by a purificatory royal shrine and a lustral bath at the
threshold. This tower block was divided by gender as between
husband and wife but also shared, as in a nuclear family. A large
staircase (one of five in the private wing) led up to the royal
megara, or living suites, of the king and queen, one on either
side of a large corridor paved with white gypsum and green
schist, ablaze with frescoes. The king's apartments were larger,
but the queen's suite had a bathroom; both had private stair-
ways to a shared rooftop loggia. The public and private 'two
bodies' were represented symbolically: the king's doorway was
open and imposing, while the small door to the queen's apartments, her *megara*, was guarded and concealed by a private,
narrow, crooked corridor. The superior privacy, intimacy, and
safety of the queen's suite was further underlined by the presence of the king's personal treasure room housed in an annexe
off it.

The Babylonian palace at Eshnunna in 2300 BCE had five
bathrooms and six lavatories, with seats of glazed brick; apparently all Babylonian palaces had elaborate drainage systems,
and used hydraulic engineering to bring in clean water, and to
recycle grey or dirty water (onto gardens or middens). In 2000–
1200 BCE Knossos was also supplied with a white-/grey-/black-
water drainage system that was connected to the queen's

famous bathroom and its plumbed annexe, usually described as a flush toilet (though it may have been a shower room); the king's suite had plumbed, wall-mounted washbasins.[30] The queen's whole suite (which had been expensively redecorated many times) was what the Egyptians called a 'Cabinet of the Morning'—a bedroom, bathroom, and reception room acting as a grooming area, later called the boudoir. The boudoir, or the Cabinet of the Morning, is central to any history of cosmetics— and to most court political histories.

The royal nuclear family was small, but it built a large extended family around itself, and leant on a close trusted circle of lesser kin, 'unique friends' or companions, and body servants, for its physical needs. The bulk of the people who actually inhabited palaces on a daily basis were the servants who kept the building and all its numerous contents clean and sound, and managed the inflow and outflow of its supplies. Thanks to scrupulous tomb and temple records, we know how royal households, especially, ran to a strict calendar and daily timetable of events as demanded by custom or ritual. The more intimate daily body services of the royal boudoir, however, were determined by the strict rules of palace behaviour and status that came to be called etiquette. The age-old question of precedence—who shall be closest to the royal body—was determined in the temple by the chief priests, and in the palace by the chief courtiers, according to the royal will. Body servants came in both genders; but male 'grooms', or young pages, were far outnumbered by the proverbial 'handmaidens', or ladies of the bedchamber, or ladies-in-waiting.

In the worldwide system of 'guest honour'—ways of greeting and welcoming guests—there were many courteous invitations to wash, groom, or otherwise be made clean, at the threshold of the home. On one level greeting cleansing was a mark of politeness and care; on another level, it meant that no dirty, polluted, or unkempt person was actually allowed to disturb the purity, order, and honour of the dwelling-place. In smaller palaces—or even in lowlier houses—the purity precautions might only physically consist of an anteroom or two, a place to remove outdoor garments (especially shoes); or simply a washbasin by the threshold. In the royal Persian courts, guests were given slippers even before their feet touched the threshold, so that they did not tread upon the king's 'holy ground'.[31] Courtiers were not allowed to touch or even breathe upon the king. In the ancient world guest honour was rarely violated, since it was also designed to give 'face' or respect to both parties, and provide 'good report', as Homer's queen Penelope stated:

> For how can you ever know, my guest, whether or not I stand high
> among womankind in thoughtfulness and regard for others if you
> sit down to a meal in this hall with skin unsoothed and garments
> wretched?...But if a man is gracious in thought and deed, his
> guests carry good report of him far and wide over the world, and
> he finds many to call him noble.[32]

In Homer's Bronze Age world, to wash or bathe someone was a particular sign of respect, or of status, or of occasion. In the *Odyssey* the male guests are always washed on arrival (eight times bodily, three for hands or feet only) and occasionally on leaving (twice); often they had 'handsome tunics and woollen cloaks put round them'. Old women washed old men; young women washed young men; the young washed the hands of the elders before eating, and all washed before the feast. Palace servants endlessly cleansed and served in the hall.

The Courtly Toilette

Most people probably started the day with a dawn prayer, a rough comb, and possibly a rough wash, before setting off to work. The rich arose and pottered about their bedroom suites. For the elite classes, life was somewhat different from the norm, even slightly unreal—which of course was the desired effect. Pleasure and play were a serious business in early societies, and pleasuring themselves was what the Bronze Age aristocracy did best, most of their time.[33] For Egyptian aristocrats, the first rising was followed by 'the hour of *i'w*', the hour of the bath, the (unspecified) breakfast–grooming hour which forever afterwards was the mark of the well-to-do; after which they would emerge perfectly fresh, trim, and ready to meet, greet—and administer—the world. Courtly afternoons were usually reserved for outings, games, and sports; but as the sun went down, preparations in the private suite would begin for the full evening toilette, *le grand tenue*, which would outshine everything else.

By *c*.1500 BCE, court and city fashion demanded a highly cleansed and polished naked skin, framed by immaculate cloth; with a carefully modified repertoire of the old adornments of nakedness especially concentrated on the frontal erogenous zones.[34] Personal hygiene consisted of very careful attention to the skin, and equally careful attention to the body's artificially costumed 'second skin'. Hot-water bathing and perfumery went together. Subtly perfumed unguents and oils were used lavishly on all the warm parts of the body, wet or dry—in the bath or out. Oiling the skin was just as important as washing, if not more so. Perfumery reached new technical heights—literally, in Egypt, in the famous head-cone of perfumed wax that was allowed to drip through high-class hair down the neck and shoulders on festive occasions. (When washed afterwards, both the hair and linen would be supple and shining.)[35] The top-of-the-range rubbing oil around the Mediterranean was the famous Egyptian 'Mendesian unguent', originally consisting of rare oil of ben and resinous myrrh, but which by the later Tutankhamun period was made up to a more exotic recipe of oil of bitter almonds, olive oil, cardamoms, sweet rushes, honey, wine, myrrh, seed of balsam, galbanum, and turpentine.

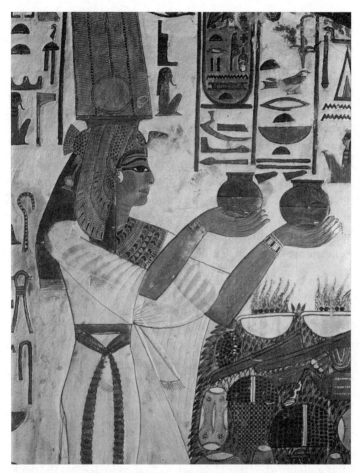

3 The renowned Egyptian beauty Queen Nefertari, pictured on
her tomb in the Valley of the Queens in Egypt, at a feast, wearing her royal
headdress, a figure-hugging sheath tunic and gauze overgarment, face
paint, immaculate nails and hair, with shoulder, wrist, and ear ornaments.

(Cheaper local vegetable oils—castor oil, olive oil—served the poor, and even animal fats would do the job.)[36]

In India both male and female head-hair was treated with a perfumed paste that held it in hundreds of different styles, ready to be garlanded and adorned. The Tamil woman 'bathed her fragrant black hair soft as the flowers till it shone, in the per-fumed oil prepared by mixing up ten different kinds of astrin-gent, five spices and thirty-two herbs soaked in water; she dried it in fuming incense, and perfumed the different plaits with the thick paste [called] musk deer'. Because of all the different perfumes and odoriferous applications, the ordinary morning toilette of an 'affluent citizen' in India, 'desirous of keeping good health', might consist of a dozen or more different operations:

> A man as soon as he got up cleaned his teeth with the toothbrush, washed his mouth and eyes...applied *collyrium* [kohl] to his eyes and chewed a few betel leaves. At the time of his bath he anointed his hair with oil...and his body, thoroughly massaged and rubbed it, took physical exercises and finally took his bath, after which he combed his hair...shaving and paring his nails. [He anointed] the body with scented paste and then he put on gems, flowers, and clean clothes after which he put scent on his face.[37]

Among the treasures rescued from the grave of Queen Hete-pheres were her golden razors. Shaving and depilation was a social insignia in the ancient world. Some societies shaved more than others, or in different ways; according to one Roman author the Celts 'wash their hair constantly in lime-water, and they scrape it back from the forehead to the crown of the head...The nobles keep their cheeks smooth but let their moustaches grow.'[38] From anciently being fully bearded and braided (like the Mesopotamians) the Egyptian male became clean-shaven, kept his hair short or shaven, shaved, plucked, or used depilatory unguents on his entire body, as did Egyptian women. Egyptian and Indian tastes and habits in this respect were very similar. The ten-day cleansing and deodorizing regime for Vatsyayana's 'affluent citizen' (undoubtedly a Brahman) included the full depilatory ordeal:

> He should bathe daily, anoint his body with oil every other day, apply a lathering substance to his body every three days, get his head (including face) shaved every four days, and the other parts of his body every five or ten days [ten days are allowed when the hair is taken out with a pair of pincers]. All of these things should be done without fail, and the sweat of the armpits should also be removed.[39]

Civilized body-art neglected none of the body parts. Tooth care was evidently a problem; tooth decay from excess honey or sugar is one of the so-called 'diseases of civilization' that probably even then affected the wealthy, but many ancient Egyptians (for example) had teeth worn to the quick by poorly milled flour. Aromatic pastes, aromatic gums, leaves and washes, and scented wood (or gold or ivory) toothpicks were used throughout Eurasia. In both Egypt and India the eye paints used on the eyes were considered essential in the same way as we regard modern toothpaste, and used as widely. At some point very early in their history, the Egyptians made a green–blue pigment derived from green malachite, a copper ore which they called *vaz* and used exclusively as an eye paint. All the eye paints of the early dynasties are green; sometime later the fashion changed to a dark grey powder from an ore of lead which they called *mestem* and was later known as kohl. In India it was known as *collyrium*; the Indian author Susruta said that *collyrium* 'alleviated the burning and itching sensation, removed local pain, increased the range of vision... furthered the growth of beautiful eyelashes, cleansed the eyes by removing unhealthy secretions, made the eyes more wide and graceful and also [when a touch of poisonous antimony was added] imparted a brilliant lustre to the pupils'.[40]

High-class bodies were now more often gowned than not; nakedness was reserved for intimate household occasions, or for work, or for the poor. Elite Egyptian women of the Old Kingdom wore clinging, heavily pleated, white linen dresses that revealed every curve of their body; but later high-quality, semi-transparent linen gauzes were worn, and the pictures of Nefertiti and her daughters in the Eighteenth Dynasty (*c*.1575– 1308 BCE) show their beautiful naked skin tantalizingly revealed by gowns that are mostly completely open down the front.[41] Similar, but entirely differently designed, swathes of semi-concealing, semi-revealing, pleated cloth lengths were being created from the new animal and plant fibres discovered in various ecological niches throughout Eurasia, notably the new lightweight linen from flax (and nettles etc.), cotton in India, and silk in China. But when, as so often, we see ancient Egyptian, Greek, or Roman images wearing pure 'white' bleached or undyed robes, we should spare a thought for the expensively coloured cloths of the ancient world, still wonderfully and intensely displayed in ancient costumes on all continents. The Egyptians in particular extended their pigment colour range to include deep blue, green, vermilion, and purple (echoing the colours of the new cut-and-polished precious and semi-precious gems—lapis lazuli, turquoise, emerald, ruby, quartz, and topaz); and were very fond of mixing the pastel colours pale gold, pale blue, and especially pale pink. In the matter of colour the Minoan Cretan islanders were particularly resourceful. They were famous for their dyes: a crimson red dye collected from the 'kermes' insect; yellow dyes from the saffron lily; and a famous deep purple dye, collected from local sea snails. They became the cloth experts of the Mediterranean, developing new dyes, patterned dye stamps, coloured embroidery, and hand-cut tailoring, with a large trade into Egypt.[42]

The perfection, purity, colours, and strong perfume of natural flowers gave the final sensual touch to the Eurasian toilette. You

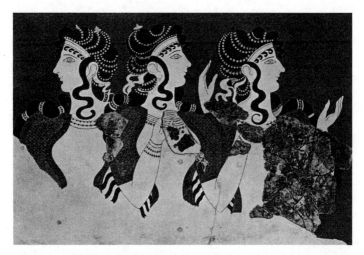

4 *The Ladies in Blue.* These famously decorative Minoan frescoes were also advertisements for high-quality fashion products using local resources and labour.

might set out wearing flowers for a social engagement, but you also would very likely be given flowers or a floral garland when you arrived, as a sign of peaceful hospitality. Flowers were strongly attached to Eurasian religious observances, particularly funeral rites. The lotus was the sacred flower of Egypt, Mesopotamia, and northern India; in southern India, the marigold and jasmine; in Bali and Java the traditional annual religious calendar has a different scent for every season of the year—'a calendar of scents'—and a great deal of money was and still is spent on flowers. All classes in ancient India wore flower garlands, particularly in north-west India, where there were flower chaplets for the waist, flower chaplets for the ears, and 'strings of flowers falling from the back of the hair were known as *prabhrastaka* and those falling from the front as *lalamaka*. *Pralamba* and *rajulamba* were the chaplets falling on the forehead, and the garland worn across the chest under the right arm and over the left shoulder was known as *vaikaksika*.'[43]

Public Women

We have reconstructed a bare outline of the ancient world's large cosmetics industry, some of its social ideologies, and most of its accoutrements—all widely dispersed, and so close to the daily lives of so many people. But there is one other story which has been running subliminally throughout: the position of women at the centre of all this activity.

Originally a biologically determined body-surface treatment, the routines of the cosmetic toilette brought physical aid and comfort to mind and body by clearing up skin diseases, repairing damage, covering up imperfections, and in general enhancing personal beauty and vitality. Whoever did it, allo-grooming was obviously a very valuable skill or service; what-ever went on before, it was clearly already strongly gendered and socially organized in Eurasia by c.3000 BCE; i.e. it was mainly performed by women, for men (and to a lesser extent for them-selves and children). Secondly, it had acquired a new economic status—in fact it had almost become a profession. The Eurasian concubine, courtesan, *geisha*, *bes*, *hetera*, *ganika*, and other 'pub-lic women' were the supreme exponents of the ancient toilette.

From their very first historical appearance in the royal graves at Ur and stretching forward into later court history, we see these massed troupes of courtly women, acting much like 'B'- and 'C'-ranking allo-grooming primate females. At the bottom of it all was the control and exploitation of sexuality—and nothing in the ancient court was more important than royal seduction and procreation. Women, especially beautiful or skilful women, were regarded in law as valuable chattels, and all ancient Indian rulers kept troupes of women for their sexual and social entertainment, taking them along on courtesy calls, or ordering 'all lovely maid-ens' to the gates of the city as a greeting honour for important diplomatic visitors. The Arabic word *harem* originally signified the 'sanctuary or a sacred precinct' of the king's quarters; but the word gradually became synonymous with the female quarters.[44] Unofficially, it was the old custom of polygamy for the chief male; officially, these extra women were servants of the chief female, her sewing maidens, whose youth, *joie de vivre*, and sportiveness gave them the stamina to perform constantly at feasts, picnics, and celebrations—like one Persian monarch whose 'maner is, that watching in the night, and then banketting with his women, being an hundred and forty in number, he sleepeth most of the day'.[45]

Water-play was always erotic, especially banqueting or picnicking by canals, streams, or rivers: 'See', said an Egyptian love poem from 1300 BCE, 'how sweet is the canal in it which you dug with your own hand for us to be refreshed by the breeze, a lovely place to wander.' Or more explicitly: 'I love to go and bathe before you. I allow you to see my beauty in a dress of finest linen, drenched with fragrant unguent. I go down to the water to be with you and come up to you again with a red fish looking splendid on my fingers.'[46] The *Kama Sutra* by Vatsyayana (c.AD 400) was originally written 'at the request of the public women of Pataliputra'—a guild of courtesans. If a public woman mastered the seductive and sexual arts of the Sutra and Shastra, said Vatsyayana, she would become 'a *ganika*, or public woman of high quality', expert in the arts of dress, witty disputation, poetry, game-playing, music, and dance, and a woman universally honoured and praised. Vatsyayana set the seduction scene

> in the pleasure room, decorated with flowers, and fragrant with perfumes, attended by his friends and servants, [he] will receive the woman, who will come bathed and dressed, and will invite her to take refreshment. He should then seat her on his left side, and holding her hair, and touching also the end of the knot of her garment, he should gently embrace her with his right hand. They should then carry on an amusing conversation on various subjects, and talk suggestively . . . sing . . . and persuade each other to drink . . . At last when the woman is overcome with love and desire

[he] should dismiss the people that may be with him, giving them
flowers, ointments, and betel leaves, and then when the two are left
alone, they should proceed as has already been described in
the previous chapters.[47]

These were the chapters that covered the famous sixty-four
erotic sexual positions (derived from already ancient sacred
texts) known as the *Kama Shastra*, which the practically minded
Vatsyayana reduced to eight essential bodily embraces: four to
do with touching, piercing, rubbing, and pressing, and four
which were gymnastic (twining, climbing, lying, lap-sitting);
eight types of kiss, and eight kinds of lovebite with attractive
names such as 'the coral and the jewel', or 'the broken cloud'.
He gave many helpful cosmetic receipts for beautification, and
reported among other things on the adornment of the penis—
'the people of the southern countries think that true sexual
pleasure cannot be obtained without perforating the *lingam*,
and they therefore cause it to be pierced like the lobes of the
ears of an infant pierced with earrings'.[48]

It is not surprising that the beauty of some of these public
women became legendary, or that they apparently enjoyed a
high degree of public support and affection; their fame also
rested on their public performances of religious dancing and
music-making (much like performing stars today), and these
public appearances helped to set popular standards of beauty
and grooming. The skills and accomplishments of the professional courtesan help to illuminate the lives of some of the
famous queens of ancient history; from this perspective Queen
Cleopatra, for instance, can be seen as a royal-born *ganika* playing for high stakes.[49] But for every expensive Queen Cleopatra
(or King Nebuchadnezzar) there were a thousand other prin-
cesses and princes, all with their toilettes to prepare, and marriages to make. Each individual faced a shifting kaleidoscope of
physical and social advantage or disadvantage throughout their

lives which directly affected their grooming habits—and even the poorest had some grooming habits. If they were lucky they had a protective home, family, and kin who performed loving, intimate acts of grooming and gave medical attention 'for free', in their 'free' rest times. Baths, expensive paints, scents, and oils were not essential; simple ingredients, simple tools, and home preparations would do. But even these scanty advantages would be wrecked if the work dried up, or local politics changed for the worse.

Up to around 1700 BCE, Eurasian trade and industry had provided an uninterrupted flood of new capital, high technology, and disposable income. Economically speaking, the beauty trades were an early capitalist success story, a luxury that became a necessity. In eastern Eurasia many ancient cosmetic customs and trades were preserved up to present times; in western Eurasia, however, physical circumstances dictated a different path. Few ancient empires could withstand such natural ecological shocks as the massive eruption at Thera (Santorini) in 1628 BCE, from which the Minoans never recovered; or the deforestation, silting, and salination that destroyed crop yields and created desert in the Fertile Crescent: Nineveh was eventually sacked in 612 BCE and Nebuchadnezzar's fabulous golden city of Babylon was overrun in 539 BCE.[50] But as it turned out, however, the ancient Mediterranean trading system and its luxury trades had not even reached their peak. Around the Aegean archipelago the Greeks were well dug in by 539 BCE. The Greeks are normally where the history of hygiene begins.

chapter 3
greek hygiene

Greek personal hygiene was a philosophy of life that went well beyond good grooming. In the name of their young goddess, princess, or high priestess of health Hygieia, the Greeks ultimately brought another permanent layer of meaning to the idea of cleanliness. We are all hygienic now. Leaving eastern Eurasia and Middle Eastern history behind us, we move west into the Mediterranean and end up on its northern shores: Greece in the Bronze Age, c.1500–600 BCE, followed by an exciting period of transition between oral culture and literacy, and the Greek intellectual and literary renaissance of c.600–400 BCE.

The standard history of hygiene starts in the later classical period, not the earlier Bronze Age; but even with this further addition, one thousand years of cultural change is a relatively short time-span compared with some we have been looking at. It suggests a high-energy society—partly due to the communications revolution of the written word; but also in part because the Greeks were relative latecomers to the high culture of the subtropical zones. After a long gestation, by c.400 BCE Greek 'hygiene' had emerged as a specialized medical discipline that attempted to control every aspect of the human environment—air, diet, sleep, work, exercise, the evacuations, passions of the mind—and to incorporate them into a 'sanitary' or wholesome way of life. It was a rational approach to bodily function that made no reference at all to the old cosmetic toilette.

Demographics

The incoming Greek tribes were relatively poor. They had come south to colonize a fertile peninsula and archipelago of volcanic islands on the north-eastern Mediterranean coast that had suffered a cataclysmic decline of population from c.1200 to 1051 BCE at the end of the Mycenaean era. This was not a centralized imperial courtly society like those of Babylonia, Persia, or Egypt, but one ruled by loose oligarchies of merchant and farming families. We have no evidence of a wealthy theocracy; instead there was a lively cultic revival of deities who lived in various wild holy places scattered patriotically throughout Greater Greece. As early as c.1200 BCE the Greeks had adopted and adapted the alphabet of their Phoenician trading rivals, in order to write down, preserve, and extend their own language. Greek wealth lay not in land, but solely in their people and their ability to trade. Hence their development of trade-friendly hinterland and port towns; 200,000 people (twice the size of the present town) are believed to have inhabited the Sicilian port city of Akragas (founded 581 BCE), built in the fertile crater of an extinct volcano; and there were other trading towns with populations of over a quarter of a million.

They were hugely successful colonists. Between c.1000 and 400 BCE the Greek population around the Aegean Sea tripled to 3 million inhabitants (with a particularly steep rise between c.800 and c.600 BCE). Steadily rising incomes, rudimentary sanitary and health services, and some educational provision, all supported an ancient standard of living that would have scored highly on the modern World Health Organization Human Development Index. By c.400 BCE such evidence as we have suggests that the health of the Greeks had been in a 'rarely attained state of equilibrium' for about 200 years, and that longevity was an average 38.1 years at death—or more precisely, 42.6 years for men, 33.7 years for women—from an average Neolithic figure of 32.1 years. Their towns contained a wide range of communal public institutions that were totally new to Eurasia; and arguably these ambitious and lavish civic policies started to exert a benign influence on the growth and physical health of the population from around the eighth century onwards.[1] The Greek demographic boom was also sustained by strong bonding and social discipline—discipline meaning knowledge, as well as regulation. The Greeks enjoyed exercising their brains, as well as their bodies. Four mental and physical disciplines in particular—balneology, religion, sport, and medicine—formed the social milieu of early Greek hygiene.

Water, Water, Water

Skin care, nudity, and water go together; and water evidently mattered a lot to the Greeks. They paid particular attention to water in their new-built settlements. For the Greeks a pure water supply was an important part of public policy and a very visible sign of civic growth and prosperity. They collected rainwater in stone cisterns and drew from springs and wells; but from the sixth century BCE, impressive new public water supplies were created from artificial conduits. The tyrants of Samos, Athens, and Piraeus all built water conduits to supply their towns; and the same hydraulic knowledge was going into harnessing the source at new water sanctuaries and temples. Most long-distance conduits were underground, but from at least the fifth century there were some above-ground aqueducts.[2]

Even before the ninth century BCE a unique balneological story was emerging, fully documented in Homer and suggesting technologies and behaviour patterns already hundreds of years old.

Greek water culture was also promoted by the indigenous experience of bathing in the region's own natural springs, grottoes, and hot waters, all of which were included in the divine plan. According to Greek mythology, Apollo and Artemis were the gods most frequently associated with sacred cold springs. The virile and fiery superhero Hercules supposedly created the first hot springs by being thrown into the pool at Thermopylae, and it was his name that was usually associated with all thermal springs, neatly slotting in alongside his reputation for the pleasures of the bed.[3] But it is the trophy-vase water scenes appearing on the earliest Greek pottery that give us much more specific detail, and incidentally demonstrate what the Greeks saw as the three most popular reasons for bathing (and thus for buying the vase)— beauty, religious ritual, and athletic training.

Greek water technology was probably of Mesopotamian, Egyptian, and/or Mycenaean origin, but with a typically Greek social twist. One classic historical survey of Greek *balaneutike* (balneology) starts with the popular Mycenaean-style seated or hip bath, but moves swiftly on to the significance of the early Greek public fountains. Public fountains may seem a small step in the uphill struggle for demographic survival, but they were significant because they were essentially democratic. They mutually aided and bonded the community around them. In this the early Greeks differed greatly from their later rivals the Carthaginians, who provided large water tanks under the floor of every middle-class street tenement in Carthage, with wells at the threshold, and had individual stone baths built inside on the ground floor, near to the heat source—but few public facilities.[4] The new public fountains, or public wells, provided by the Greek tyrants brought free water, running day and night, available to everyone, without distinction, in nobly built surroundings. The few surviving artworks show open-fronted buildings with stone columns and floors, and water gushing inside from bronze lion-head spouts, set at shoulder height,

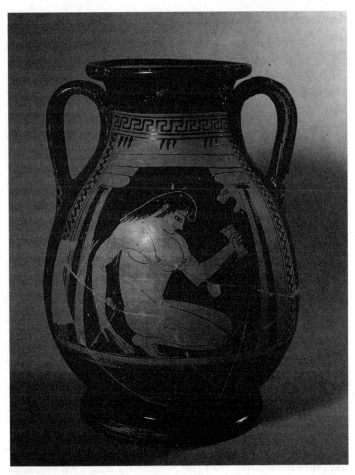

5 A woman showers under the distinctive lion-head water-spout of the Greek public fountain, scourer in hand.

falling into stone basins. Whether there were further pools and laundering involved, as there were at so many later European village wells, we do not know; but we can see that these shoulder-height douches not only would have filled buckets but were also specifically designed to shower the body. The monumental public fountains were of such local importance that special magistrates, of high standing, were appointed to take care of them.

By the fifth century, affluent middle-class Greeks clearly also enjoyed the luxury of a warm bath in the home. Domestic house remains at Olynthus (destroyed c.432 BCE) show bathrooms in one-third of the houses, built at the back of the kitchen fire. As the Roman architect Vitruvius noted 400 years later (and the method continued long after that), by using water piped through the hot kitchen flue 'it will not take long to get a bath ready in the country'. The small 2.25 × 1.5 metre rooms had plastered walls and a terracotta seated bath-tank built into a corner of the room.[5] This same shallow seated bath, very similar to those 400 years earlier, was also the one most frequently found in temples and gymnasiums—rows of them set side by side along the walls, often round a circular space, drained by a single channel below. This half-length bath, or hip bath, did not allow full immersion: the water had to be poured over the upper body, like a shower or a fountain. It was the same with the famous outdoor washbasin, or *louteron*, that was the central feature of so many decorative vase scenes, particularly female grooming scenes.

Vigorous sluicing was what the Greeks preferred, and the longer, deeper immersion bath was slow to develop, though never quite abandoned for the sick or the aged (it was fragile, too, in pottery form). Far more ubiquitous was the wide, shallow, half-metre basin, made of light metal, that could be used for every domestic purpose including washing—for a full strip wash, for washing the hair or hands, or (as seen frequently on the vases) for washing the feet. The metal could be easily cleaned, and heated water quickly. From this basic design evolved, from around the fifth century BCE onwards, a popular domestic three-legged metal foot-basin; a three-quarter basin (in cement mortar or stoneware) designed to hang on walls;

and the elegant free-standing stone pedestal *louteron*. Three particular things stand out at this point. Firstly, this was a society that was actually proud of washing, and not ashamed to show it properly, in the nude. Secondly, anybody could shower or strip wash, and probably did. Thirdly, as demand rose, technology followed it. As the centuries wore on, the rich householder could have treated himself to a new hypocaust and sweat room, as well as an outdoor plunge pool—all of which were pretty superfluous to grooming, in the strict sense. But by that time the rich householder would have perfectly understood that what made you feel well also made you look good.

The archaeological evidence shows how much the Greeks valued washing as a small domestic luxury: eventually their hydraulic engineers managed to bring waters of different temperatures under one monumental public roof. The Greek *balaneion*, or public bathhouse, was yet one more of those grand public entertainments provided for the fortunate Greek citizen (though not for the many poor non-citizens—slaves and immigrants).[6] The first literary evidence of public bath complexes comes from the fifth century BCE, but the archaeological evidence peaks in the third and second centuries BCE, when they began to be built in the towns. The usual bathhouse pattern was of a large rectangular hall with seated baths in recesses, and domed hot sweat baths at one end; the domes circulated and moderated the heat given off by a brazier in the middle. Dry heat in other rooms was provided by the brick hypocaust system of ducted hot air under the floor, later copied and used by the Romans (as were the domes). Larger swimming pools could be put outside the building. This was bathing on a grand scale; but there were also smaller commercial hot baths that used the waste heat from local industries such as potteries or bakeries, and these local enterprises were so well patronized by women that, in the early years, going to the public baths was satirized as an exclusively female occupation (though the bathhouse keepers and attendants were exclusively male, and the baths gradually became segregated).[7] But there were other factors involved in creating this apparently overwhelming demand for water.

Some of the earliest and most sophisticated hydraulic projects were not in the towns but in the religious sanctuaries, specifically the healing sanctuaries of Apollo, the god who brought—or warded off—disease. In the sixth century a new healing cult of the god Asclepius, deemed to be the son of Apollo, took over many of these old sanctuaries, and he became the god of the Hippocratic healers and the giver of divine advice through prayer, divination, personal incubation, and dream therapy.[8] It was his daughter Hygieia who was supposedly handmaiden to Athene the goddess of wisdom, together with her sister Panacea ('Cure-all'), and the two therapeutic goddesses supervised the healing process that the prayers to Asclepius had started, like two nurses round a doctor. Hygieia represented intelligent wholesomeness, purity, and well-being and must have been entirely virtuous, since so little is known of her; but she had her own statue alongside that of her father at Epidaurus.

The earlier religious revival had led to the building of many small stone shrines and larger stone sanctuaries, usually not far away—a short country walk—from the nearby town.[9] Shrines close to mineral springs were usually graced by a temple later, as happened at the old healing shrine of Apollo at Epidaurus, where during the sixth century the cult of Asclepius took over and moved the healing sanctuary and temple up into the valley nearer to the sacred springs. By the third century BCE, a 172-metre conduit had been driven from the source through solid rock into a vast underground cistern 14 metres high, holding 1,000 cubic metres of water, which supplied the sanctuary's basins, fountains, and baths. At the springs in Corinth, the story was very similar. Apollo was in residence in the seventh century, but by the fifth century Asclepius had occupied the site

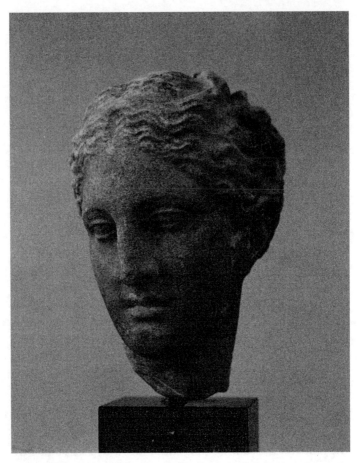

6 The steady gaze and calm matronly placidity of Hygieia, goddess of health.

and a monumental temple complex was built. A small stone fountain-house at the entrance faced the main temple, the incubation rooms (for meditation and dream therapies), smaller therapy rooms, and eating halls, with a spring house containing one deep pool with four smaller pools attached. To the south was the special outdoor fountain-tank that several healing sanctuaries seem to have had, where the patient walked down a flight of steps to immerse in a dark pool, 2 metres deep, built round with rough craggy stones, as if they were descending into the earth to experience the raw mystic powers of the water. At Cos the redevelopment of the Apollo sanctuary happened later, in the third century, but by the first century a large swimming pool and a suite of thermal baths had been built. Best of all, perhaps, were the springs of Asclepius at Gortys in Arcadia, where by the end of the fourth century a veritable 'thermal establishment' had been built with a cold swimming pool, seated baths and immersion baths, and a stove which heated a rotunda sweat room, hot fountains, and hot immersion baths. Add a beautiful site, clean mountain air, simple accommodation and you have—Arcadia. (Or possibly a hydro.)

Greeks were used to thinking holistically about the universe. The Greek natural philosophers who started to divide, or separate off, the material from the immaterial universe only became active and famed during the sixth century. But spoken Greek words commonly described several different layers of existence. At temple healing sites the common noun *katharsis* (meaning purifying, cleansing) could be used to describe the cleansing of blood, or disease from the body, or emotions from the mind, or the stain of ritual pollution. Water was a primordial thing that flowed across all the social and semantic boundaries: it cooled, cleaned, refreshed, comforted, and soothed the body and the soul; and it was, as we know, the focal point of most purification ceremonies, when it took on a simultaneously divine form. Greek purification ceremonies were intrinsic to Greek culture; they also help to explain two other key sites in the history of *hygieia*: Greek religious sports, and the Greek gymnasiums.

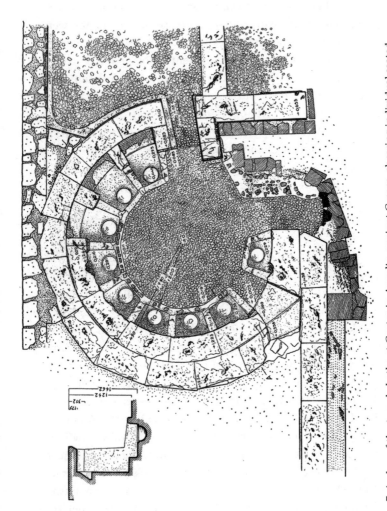

7 A plan of the temple baths at Gortys in Arcadia, ancient Greece, showing individual seated bathing–basins set round a domed circular hall.

The Superstitious Man

There is a famous character of Greek literature, satirized by the poet Theophrastus, called 'the superstitious man':

> The danger of pollution is never far from his thoughts. First thing in the morning he washes his hands (perhaps from three springs), and sprinkles his body with lustral water; for the rest of the day he protects himself by chewing laurel. He constantly has his home purified . . . he declines all contact with birth, death or tombs. He seeks out the *Orphotelestai* every month, and repeatedly undergoes ablutions in the sea. The mere sight of some poor wretch eating the meals of Hecate [suffering death, disease, destruction] requires an elaborate ritual washing; nor is this enough, but a priestess must be summoned to perform a blood purification.

And all this from a man, Theophrastus, who was himself a Pythagorean vegetarian who must have abhorred meat-eating (and animal clothing), at the very least.[10]

Greek literature is soaked in purity rules and purifications. Such intensity of information certainly makes it look very much as though a 'cloud of purity rules' descended on Greece in the fourth and fifth centuries, and subsequent investigations have suggested that new words, and new temple equipment, were indeed imported into Greek culture just prior to this time; but we know that the ancient cosmology of purification was already well established throughout Eurasia, and it is perhaps better to see not an intensification but a fragmentation of this tradition in Greece.[11]

This hypothetical superstitious man was certainly caught up in Orphism, a fifth-century Greek sect known for its onerous ascetic requirements. The followers of Orpheus formed what is known as a 'mantic' cult, deriving from the prophetic traditions of seers and shamans, and their wandering seers or healing priests (*telestai*) would sing beautiful hymns and incantations over the sufferer, prescribing herbs, charms, and a pure new way of life through chastity, vegetarianism, white garments, and the ecstatic worship of Dionysus–Bacchus. Theophrastus meant to imply that the purifications of the superstitious man were excessive, or at least extremely scrupulous by average standards—sufficient even for a sanctified priest. Presumably they lacked the intellectual rigour of Greek Pythagoreanism, which also had ascetic dietary regulations and dress codes but performed no miracle cures over unbelievers. Followers of Pythagoras (581–497 BCE) were committed to living together in cosmic harmony, seeking out eternal cosmic truths, especially those contained in music and mathematics, and their personal purity was also a way of cleansing and fortifying the mind.

But these sects were a minority preoccupation. A glance at the Cyrene Cathartic Law, also from the sixth century BCE, brings one up sharply. This stone fragment was once a large block inscribed with the 'purifications and abstinences' for the citizens of Cyrene from the priests of Cyrene, and is a quasi-legal document reciting the correct purificatory rituals, temple tithes, and other 'payments to the gods', in a way that would not be unfamiliar to a modern church warden; namely,

> Wood growing in a sacred area. If you pay the god the price, you can use the wood for sacred, profane and unclean purposes ... If a grown man is subject to a tithe [a tax or rent] having purified himself with blood, he shall purify the shrine ... Everyone who sacrifices shall bring a vessel ... If property is subject to a tithe, he [the owner] shall assess the value of the property, purify the shrine and the property separately, and then sacrifice first as a penalty a fully grown [animal] victim, not from the tithe, and then sacrifice the tithe and carry it away to a pure spot.... From the property, as long as it is subject to a tithe, no one shall make funerary offerings nor shall he bring libations until he pays a tithe to the gods ... [12]

Tithes and taxes would be much more familiar territory for the Greek citizen, and returns to the idea of religion as a form of insurance, a social contract. The gods protected this citified, or civilized, way of life by demanding from each inhabitant a moral code based on strict religious discipline and personal honesty or piety (*hosia*)—carved above the threshold of the temple of Asclepius at Epidaurus: 'He who goes inside the sweet-smelling temple must be pure. Purity is to have an honest mind.'[13] The ancient communal purificatory ceremonies in Greece, as elsewhere, were built into the solstices of the year, the lunar cycles of the month, the hours of the day and night, and, on a personal level, into the cycles of life. Town boundary purification rituals protected the citizens; and special purification ceremonies for exceptional cases of pollution or sacrilege, of a town or by a person, often required the whole community to pay the price. Of course purity not only defeated death, it also implicitly renewed life. On many if not most of these public ceremonial occasions, the ritual price to pay was not very arduous at all, and simply meant celebrating with the gods in a pleasurable and joyous fashion (*aphrodisia*), and treating them with parties, feasts, plays, music, games, and sports. Religious catharsis could come in many shapes and forms. The first Olympic Games was originally a military thanksgiving and purification ceremony dedicated to Zeus, and became a site of mass catharsis. In fact this festival was an event of such importance to the ruling elites of Hellas that formal political truces were declared throughout its duration. No person could go armed or unclean to the Games.

The Olympic Games

The festive Olympic Games were formally instituted in 776 BCE and were held once every four years until AD 520.[14] They inspired a 'Crown Games' super-league that included the regional Isthmian, Nemean, and Pythian Games, to which all local villages would have sent their champions. Largely owing to their urgent need for strong military muscle, the Greek upper classes vigorously supported popular competitive sports and gradually turned them into a central tenet of society—a sort of patriotic test of Greekness. A convincing case has been made that these Games may originally have had something to do with hunting skills and hunting rituals: the running training, the wrestling, the deodorizing, and other purificatory preparations made before the hunt. They also bonded and graded the young males and kept the warrior instincts alert.[15] But the purity law forbidding the wearing of weapons at the Games fundamentally underlined their serious, peaceful, and civilized purpose:

We seek a certain greater good ... a wreath that is not made of pine or olive or parsley, but contains in itself all human felicity—that is to say, freedom for each individual singly and for the state in general, wealth, glory, enjoyment of ancestral feast-days, safety for one's family, and in short all the blessings that one could pray to receive from the gods. All these things are interwoven in the wreath that I speak of and accrue from the contest to which these exercises and hardships lead.[16]

The Games themselves were structured around a long series of religious rituals. Well before the period of the peaceful truce, all the athletes had already been kept separated from the world for a month on a special purificatory and strengthening regime (diet, exercise, chaste sexual regimen) which had rendered them completely unpolluted, and worthy to compete in the sacred precincts. No women were allowed to enter or participate.[17] The male sports ranged from the *ephebates* (12–18) the *andres* (19–30), to mature males (30-plus), and took five days. The Games started with a sacred procession winding its way from the city of Elis along the Sacred Way towards a great sacrifice to Zeus at Olympia, stopping to purify at the sacred fountain at Pieva. After four days of the music contests, charioteering, and junior sports came the finale: the 200-metre, 400-metre, and long-distance running races, the pentathlon, throwing and wrestling events, and military combat (armed fighting, archery, the race in armour). The day ended with the crowning of the victors in the temple of Zeus, followed by the banquet for the victors in the Prytaneum: a convivial evening of *aphrodisia* for the men, and a rousing confirmation of their physical strength.[18]

Parks and Gymnasiums

It was during the booming sixth century that sports facilities became institutionalized in Greek public parks. Without these public parks there would have been no Socrates, Plato, or Aristotle—or Greek expertise in hygiene. Even before the sixth century local communities had shown themselves dedicated to sport, by starting to clear small levelled running tracks, or stadiums (*stadia*), for local foot races, built along the bottom and sides of nearby valleys. Public shrines and walks were gradually laid out around them. During the sixth century Greek tribal elders decided their young sons, or *ephebes*, should be physically trained and educated in these parks, and built schools, or gymnasiums, (*gymnasia*), next to the original stadiums, with new sports facilities based around a central exercise yard called the *palaestra*. Athens had three early and venerated gymnasiums (and later acquired several others) each of which became the home of a philosophical school.[19] The impetus that sporting athletics gave to Greek social and intellectual life is made evident by the archaeological remains of at least sixty known academic gymnasiums, with their palaestras, in towns throughout later ancient Greece from the third century BCE. In later centuries stadiums for games were built everywhere, in all sizes, throughout the Hellenic empire; later evidence from Egypt shows that in a colonial situation membership of the gymnasiums was an important indication of high social status.[20] Large cities had two or more, often taking up several blocks of city streets—urban 'peristyle gymnasiums' with magnificently colonnaded courts, reading rooms and libraries, lecture rooms, sculpture galleries, and covered pillared shopping arcades backing onto the outer walls, that the Romans later found so attractive.

Gymnos was the Greek word for 'naked': *gymnazo* was the word for 'exercise'. Naked exercise was the ethos of all Greek games and gymnastic training, and led naturally to the aesthetic veneration of the naked human physique. Unique and strange to Eurasia at the time (the neighbouring Persians, for example, disapproved), pure nakedness became symbolic of European hygienic culture and embedded in European art. This purist approach to sports performance supposedly came about by accident, when the Olympic runner Orsippus of Megara (724–652 BCE) supposedly shed his loincloth and won the race naked. Vase painting evidence substantiates the dates: nude athletes appear in archaic art by at least 650 BCE, with over 800 extant representations from the sixth century alone.[21]

Various additional explanations have been given over the years, including ritual catharsis and the homosexual idealization of male beauty. The male cult of Eros was certainly strongly represented in the vase scenes; female nudity, however, was equally often represented through the erotic cult of the Naiades (naiads), or water nymphs. Meanwhile, in their quest for a higher form of gymnosophy, the ethics of love and the perfect education of the perfectly formed male was earnestly discussed by philosophers in the gymnasiums next door. But military fitness would have been a far more urgent public concern. It was stadium training that turned out the archetypal Greek hard man.

Training and Gymnastics

From the eighth century BCE onwards the stadiums and palaestras probably functioned like an experimental laboratory for the therapeutics of hygiene, taking on the challenge to bring and keep a single body in perfect condition through exact training and regimen. Behind the scenes stadiums were lively medical meeting-places, used for viewing both routine and unusual surgical cases. Physical therapies were constantly being devised especially for the athletes during intensive physiotherapy sessions, tried and tested by competitive results.[22] The ebb and flow of therapeutics in the history of medicine and health care is fascinating, and the story of the gymnastic trainers and their well-honed physical methods is little understood; but this period marked their early ascendancy. In a very real sense, they were the first practical hygienists.

In the fifth century BCE the gymnast Herodicus had gained a wide reputation. Herodicus was famed for his command of the training regimen, especially his heroic methods (as practised on himself) of prescribing 40-mile walks, long runs, deep massage, and hot baths. He seemingly tried most things, but what he was most notorious for (according to Plato) was his carefully crafted approach to long-term health care. He was accused by Plato of inventing a longevity health regime for the older male called 'valetudinarianism', or the 'lingering death'—an idea to which Plato was scornfully opposed. Plato thought that an honourable life should be quick and natural, rather than slow and artificially prolonged. Hard training was considered necessary for the defence of the state, but unsuitable for the normal, moderate, or temperate life. Normally the most punishing training regimes were reserved for the fit athlete.[23] Regular training consisted of set routines of running, ball games, jumping, kicking, punching, and wrestling. Wrestling in sand in particular had 'a certain usefulness, not unattended by pleasure, and it gives much strength to their bodies... the continual somersaults in the mud and the open-air struggles in the sand give us our immunity from shafts of the sun, and we have no further need of a cap to keep its rays from striking our heads'.[24] The object was to harden and toughen the body, giving it a much-prized, tanned, leathery skin, and inuring the warrior to all external conditions. After the bout was

over, and after the bath, a second massage and oiling transformed the hardened athlete or warrior 'into something dark
and gleaming, a bronze that breathed'.[25] As in sports medicine
today, an athlete's diet was carefully controlled to build up bulk
and strength. At one extreme the starvation technique, also
known as fasting, was considered to be painful but beneficial.
The opposite therapy, fattening up or body-building, were two
different arts combined; it was done not only with certain rich
foods, but also with certain 'thickening' and 'firming' massages
and manipulations. Massage and baths together produced a
supple, pliable body, unstringing tired and knotted muscles.

Baths had become essential fixtures in the palaestra. The sweating and dusty athletes needed a drink and a wash after their
efforts, but cold immersion also helped to minimize body damage
and aid the self-healing process.[26] There was no particular order of
bathing, no special procedures (except under the watchful eye of
your trainer)—only the basic passage from wet to dry, hot to cold.
Sporting tradition had it that the Laconian Greeks first introduced
the use of the hot sweat baths into athletics to relieve muscular
cramps and exhaustion. Thus a Greek gymnasium might have a
small *pyriaterion* (sweat room) in an annexe alongside its cold
baths. The pedestal washbasin, with a good Delos sponge, was
the basic cold-water shower equipment; but for serious training, a
cold plunge pool or even a swimming pool was a necessity. The
earliest swimming pool is a large rectangular one dating from
*c.*400 BC at Olympia itself, though other pools (such as the one
found at Delphi) were round. The Greeks invented words for the
swimming pool (*kolymbetha*) and pool (*piscine*), and they prided
themselves on their swimming and diving abilities, but swimming was not strictly considered a sport—it was merely a form
of therapeutic exercise. There were no swimming races in the
Greek games, nor were there subsequently in Roman athletics,
though the Romans too were expert swimmers, skilled at breast-
stroke and crawl.[27]

But the population pressure on resources was beginning to tell. A subtle demographic change occurred in Greece after *c.*400 BC. Although the population continued to rise, longevity started to dip—a trend that continued broadly downwards, dropping to an average 36.8 years during the Roman period. Palaeopathology suggests that the nutritional regime had worsened and reveals some already entrenched and stark social divisions, notably the markedly lesser longevity of women, and the extra height and healthiness of skeletons from high-rank graves, as well as a new range of diseases. In fact, as the historian Mirko Grmek carefully notes, scientific Greek medicine arose at the time when the epidemiological equilibrium was disintegrating and the health of the Greeks was deteriorating—'some might consider that a paradox'.[28] The real paradox was that much of scientific Greek medicine was essentially a health discourse for the wealthy—for the top 10 per cent who already lived longer, and better, than the rest.

Scientific Hygiene

COBS grooming and medical first aid had by this time turned into a greatly expanded repertoire of interventionist medical techniques. External practical therapy was supplemented by new disciplines of internal practical therapy, experimenting with special foods, drinks, simple herbs, and rare pharmaceutical ingredients. In the Egyptian, Chinese, Indian, and Greek medical systems, philosophical observations that linked the innards to the outer parts led to the pan-Eurasian medical lore we call humoralism—based variously on three-, four-, and five-element metaphysical cosmologies. Greek natural philosophy (later called 'science', from the Latin *scientia*, to know) eventually, via Aristotle, produced an extremely dualistic cosmography based on four elements (hot, cold, wet, dry) with four matching seasons, four types of internal 'humours', four 'ages of man', and four physical 'temperaments'. The linking of the humours with the seasons proved to be the major step in promoting humoral diagnostics, which started to be widely adopted during the fourth century BCE.[29]

The very latest form of Bronze Age medical lore (as used by Herodicus) was the *techne* that came to be called 'longevity-knowledge'—a premeditated, predictive medical strategy for guiding the body away from crisis situations towards a ripe old age. Between *c.*800 and *c.*400 BC longevity-knowledge for wealthy elites was finding its way into collections of papyrus, skin, and cloth scrolls, or scratched onto tablets or bones, in civilizations at both ends of Eurasia. The Aryans had developed the longevity-knowledge of the ayurveda, while the imperial courtiers of the Han dynasty practised their daily *yangshen* exercises for the 'Cultivation of the Body'. The Greeks named it *hygieia*.[30] Since the activities of the early gymnastic trainers were largely undocumented, most of what we know about Greek longevity-knowledge comes from the famous collection of sixty-three medical texts composed over a long period in Kos, Knidus, and elsewhere, strongly influenced by the famous Koan physician Hippocrates. The Greek science of hygiene emerged gradually over the succeeding centuries—a fragile association of opinions emanating from an increasingly literate and 'educated' cadre of skilled and independent craftsmen, united by their strong belief in the material existence of a rational physio-logos.

One thing that Eurasian healers were all agreed on was that 'the sick body was an impure body'. In India this alone made the healer an outcast; although in bustling commercial Greece, purity rules were evidently slacker and the healer practised his trade without stigma. The Greek language, moreover, was full of overlapping meanings and 'semantic stretch' that blurred any strict cultural or religious categories. The word *hygieia* (from *hygies*, meaning 'healthy') originally meant 'soundness' or 'wholeness' as applied to anything—food, the soul, politics, or

even groups of things like statues or ships.[31] The medical definition of *hygieia* that described the whole and sound (or perfect)
human body, set within a whole and sound (or perfect)
environment, eventually took over the whole meaning. Greek
physicians used the new rational principles of hygienic wholesomeness to extend and enrich artificially the lives of their
patients, with particular success. If this was not biodetermin-
ism, then *hygieia* imitated it very well.

Greek personal hygiene was just that—personal. In Hippocratic medicine long life and carefully planned personal health
care for the individual was categorized under the name of 'dietetics', from the word *diaita*, meaning 'daily way of life'. (Only
later was 'diet' reduced to its current usage, meaning only food
and drink.)[32] Your 'diet' was you: what you did, where you lived,
who you were. A 'regimen' was the correct rule or ordering of
your diet. The Hippocratic doctor was not particularly inter-
ested in your immortal soul; he was a detective who turned
over your life. He checked out the physical location of your
house (damp or dry, hot or cold), sniffed the air, tasted the
water, peered into rooms, felt people's bodies, looked at their
evacuations, displayed (and presumably sold) his personal
choice of *pharmaka*, instructed the household on exactly what
to cook and when to cook it, and reeled off a list of gymnastic
exercises. All of this must have amply satisfied the psychological
needs of the patient (many of whom may have also been on a
steep learning curve). Very much later the various environmental and behavioural factors were simplified into an authoritative
but rule-of-thumb list of dietetic rules called 'the regimen of the
six non-naturals'. These governed (1) the surrounding air, (2)
bodily work and exercise, (3) food and drink, (4) sleep and
wakefulness, (5) the internal evacuations, and (6) passions of
the mind. Armed with this basic information, the body's vital
functions could be monitored and moderated in its immediate
surroundings, on every occasion. The resulting personal

regimen for hygiene that the doctor gave you after the consultation was prescriptive: it told you what to do and when to do it.
It was always the six non-naturals—not the four humours—that
were used to define and explain hygiene in later centuries.

Ever since the eighth century the competitive Greeks had
been extracting extra strength and vitality from the body, and
storing up this knowledge. Compared to the Chinese *Seasonal
Regimen of Ancestor Peng*, the Greek *Regimen of Health* from the
Hippocratic corpus is professionally confident, more than twice
the length, and full of technical expertise. It overflows with
advice on food and exercise, but (unlike the Chinese text) has
absolutely nothing on morning grooming routines, or any spiritual life force; and underlying it all is a solid belief in gymnastic
training. It is also addressed to 'the ordinary man', rather than a
nobleman who lives in a palace:

> 1. The ordinary man should adopt the following regimen. During
> the winter, he should eat as much as possible, drink as little as
> possible and this drink should be wine as undiluted as possible . . .
> 2. . . . Diets then must be conditioned by age, the time of year, habit,
> country, and constitution. They should be opposite in character to
> the prevailing climate, whether winter or summer. Such is the best
> road to health . . . 3. In winter a man should walk quickly, in sum-
> mer more leisurely fashion unless he is walking in the hot sun. More
> baths should be taken in summer than in winter; firm people
> should bathe more than the fleshy ones . . . 7. Those who enjoy
> gymnastics should run and wrestle during the winter; in summer
> wrestling should be restricted and running forbidden, but long
> walks in the cool part of the day should take place . . . 9. A wise
> man ought to realise that health is his most valuable possession and
> learn how to treat his illnesses by his own judgement.[33]

All the ancient Asian medical systems enshrined the principle of
balance and harmony with nature in some form, and instead of
karma or *qi*, the Greeks came to use the doctrine of Temperance
to harmonize the fractious universe (rarely mentioned in the

Hippocratic corpus but developed in contemporary moral philosophy by Aristotle and Plato). Temperance always sought the
perfect balance, the perfect mid-position on the polarity, the
arithmetical golden mean between extremes, in order to reach
the desired state of 'well-being' (*eudaimonia*).[34] Like the *Regimen*,
the popular Hippocratic *Aphorisms* preached the general
method of 'moderation in all things' and the balancing of
opposing elements: 'it is dangerous to disturb the body violently whether it be by starvation or feeding, by making it hot
or cold, or in any way whatsoever... All excesses are inimical to
nature... It is safer to proceed a little at a time, especially when
changing from one regimen to another...'. But sometimes
good psychology improved the medicine: 'it is better to take
something less suitable but pleasing than something which is
more suitable but less pleasing...'.[35]

It was only common sense that all substances entering the
body should be clean and sound throughout; but empirical
observation showed that it was equally essential not to let
these substances linger too long in that warm, damp environment, to rot and become poisonous inside. In Greek humoral
theory, good strong bowel movements were a sign of a healthy
body getting rid of its dangerous wastes, and might save you
from the ubiquitous herbal or mineral purges and emetics.
Failing this, there was the equally ancient method of bloodletting (venesection), and in desperate cases, cauterization with
hot irons, the shock of which was supposed to stop the poisonous disease from migrating through the body: 'two beside the
ears, two on the temples, two in the back of the head, two on
the nose near the corner of the eyes'. Menstruation in women
was carefully described, and treated, as a special form of bloodletting, one which cleansed and purged the ill humours.[36] But
the one form of pollution that most families would have genuinely feared was that of the malign urban disease epidemics
that circulated the Mediterranean—the famous Plague of

Athens took place in the fifth century, with precursors rumbling in the sixth.

Greek healers became expert at classifying and collecting data on different incoming disease types, a process first started in Egypt. The word for the dirt that caused disease was *miasma* (from *miaino*, to pollute, via the root *mia-* meaning defilement or destruction); and miasma could be generated in any place at any time, for whatever divine reason. When it reached the earthly world, however, it was specifically associated with foul airs, waters, and places. Greek scientific disease theory suggested that macrocosmic disease pollution came via certain airborne *miasmin*—germlike 'seeds of disease' wafting down from the outer universe in billowing clouds of polluted air that were immanently poisonous and contagious. Whatever the miasma touched on contact with the microcosm it tainted, and then spread itself steadily through the healthy living material 'like the dyeing or staining of a cloth'. There was no obvious distinction made between macrocosmic miasma and microcosmic contagion, although this was a distinction that greatly concerned physical scientists from the seventeenth to the early twentieth centuries.[37]

Cosmetics

In appearance young Greek aristocrats would have looked like the well-groomed warriors they were: glossy and fit, but not ornately or heavily decorated in the southern Eurasian style. Hard and spare, keen and sinewy, was the male bodily ideal.[38] Greek opinions on the cosmetic beauty toilette in the fifth century had changed significantly since Homer's day. The revelation of the pure naked gymnastic physique must have made older cosmetic customs appear outmoded, and foreign ones unpatriotic; they were certainly not considered hygienic. It was from around this time that the word 'cosmetic' ceased to mean simply the care bestowed on dress and adornment, and became a term of abuse and inferiority, literally a dirty word, to Greek male rationalists. It became normal, in later fifth- or fourth-century Greek philosophical prose, to use the word 'cosmetic' to describe something superficial—or feminine.[39] In plays, flamboyantly dressed and carefully painted cosmetic beauty had become the mark of a disreputable woman, whose lavish ornamentation separated her from the chastely dressed 'respectable' woman. (And the same went for the men.) Plutarch considered it 'whorish' for a wife to wear rouge and perfumes and 'play with her husband'; in his world, that was the job of the *hetera*. Women were considered (among other things) to be creatures of darkness, the moon, the left side, and water— polluted, pale, wet, cool, pliable, weak, changeable by nature, materially impure, and metaphysically 'unbounded'—'she swells, she shrinks, she leaks, she is penetrated, she suffers metamorphosis'. She was the exact opposite of the firm, clean-cut 'Apollonian' male.[40] To the disapproving male philosopher, women were personified in the beautiful, seductive, but ultimately deceiving goddess Pandora, who 'made evil so beautiful'.

Set alongside this type of new misogyny was the new physiology of the dominant-male body, written up by the philosophers, but taken straight from the palaestra. In a fine burst of male virtue, Plato denounced the two evil 'counterfeit' (female) domestic activities which (he claimed) were currently masquerading as health care:

> Cookery then, as I say, is the form of pandering which corresponds to medicine, and in the same way physical training has its counterfeit in beauty-culture, a mischievous, swindling, base, servile trade, which creates an illusion by the use of artificial adjuncts and make-up and depilatories and costume, and makes people assume a borrowed beauty to the neglect of the true beauty which is the product of training.[41]

It is very noticeable that, in theory, none of the physical training in the palaestra applied to 'white-armed' women (as Homer always called them). Young girls could run and play outdoors, but following the arrival of the menses, respectable young women were virtually confined to barracks and shut away from the sun. Those white arms were necessary for perfect female cosmetic beauty. The attacks on 'feminine' cosmetics could have been motivated by any number of things: a patriotic revulsion against foreign toilettes, an aversion to masculine weakness, an incipient ascetic puritanism; or (equally likely) a tightening of family control over its female assets, as female prosperity and rule-breaking opportunities increased; or over its male assets, to ensure the continuation of the family line. They were probably only empty words and mere exhortations; as far as we can tell, grooming was still indispensable, but in later classical Greece it probably had to be discreet (at least while at home, or in front of the parents). But then the Greek toilette was probably like that anyway—modest care rather than urban glamour. In the poet Hesiod, the farmer's daughter bathes and oils herself in front of the kitchen fire while her father works in the winter winds outside. For summer the family probably had a *louteron* outdoors.[42] In the urbane Roman Empire, cosmetics had a very different public profile.

The practical Greeks pioneered collective facilities for the hygienic or healthy way of life—parks, baths, sports, theatres, and temples—that were a pretty comprehensive provision for the body and soul. For the philosophers, however, brain counted more than brawn. In Plato's *Republic* the aim of higher Pythagorean gymnastics was not the training of the body but the training of the senses, the true pathways into the inner soul:

> Let us search for artists who are gifted to discern the true nature of the beautiful and graceful; then will our youth dwell in a land of health, amid fair sights and sounds, and receive the good in

everything; and beauty, the effluence of fair works, shall flow into the eye and ear, like a health-giving breeze from a purer region, and insensibly draw the soul from earliest years into likeness and sympathy with the beauty of reason...

Plato put personal self-control at the heart of all gymnastic training. There was, he said,

within a man's soul a better and also a worse principle; and when the better has the worse under control, then he is said to be master of himself... but when, owing to evil education or association, the better principle, which is also the smaller, is overwhelmed by the greater mass of the worse—in this case he is blamed and is called a slave of self and dissolute.[43]

Set firmly within its materialist framework, the Greek educational doctrine of personal self-control and hygienic self-cultivation became steadily more complex, leading to the Stoic and Christian doctrines of self-examination, personal meditation, prayer, and confession. Most Romans took the practical arts of Greek 'self-cultivation' extremely seriously. They perfected the arts of medical attendance and cosmetic care, applied their fullest resources to the arts of water engineering, and supported the largest numbers of health-conscious leisured classes that western Eurasia had ever known.

chapter 4
roman baths

The Roman baths and aqueducts cleansed and scoured more people in western Eurasia than any previous civilization—over 12 million bodies, if even only a quarter of the imperial population lived in cities and were regular bathers; and historians have rightly viewed them as one of the linchpins of Roman life. The only viable conclusion from Roman baths is that cleanliness was an integral part of the Roman 'civilizing process', and that an ultra-clean, well-groomed body was their badge and symbol of citizenship. But bathing was only one part of a whole regime of grooming and hygienic self-care for which expert written advice was now given by, among others, Ovid, Celsus, and Galen. When the booming Roman economy finally fell apart in the sixth century, a great many things from this extensive body culture were physically destroyed and could not be replaced, while other knowledges or lore strangely survived, or were refashioned.

Most ancient empires took some note of social welfare as part of their governing duties, none more so than the Greeks. The Romans had Greek hygienic statecraft directly in front of them, and were strongly inspired by the Greek concept of 'the managed life'. The Roman state and its richer citizens also invested in social welfare projects from an early date, thereafter erratically spending (as far as we can tell) a varying proportion of gross income on an almost identical range of 'healthy services': pure water supplies, public baths, parks, stadiums, state-sponsored games and sports, and town doctors. The Roman imperial population in and around the Mediterranean, Europe, and Africa was, however, far larger—46 million in AD 200—meaning that their communal treasure chest was wider and deeper than the Greeks'.[1] Urban Roman life would have been inconceivable, and a lot more fetid and visibly filthy, without the various public baths, latrines, fountains, and taps served by the Roman aqueducts.

The Aqueducts

As in Greece, the building of aqueducts quickly became a political tool. The first public aqueduct serving Rome, the Aqua Appia, was built by an ambitious early Roman politician, Appius Claudius, and was constructed at the same time and alongside the very first stone road leading out of Rome, the Via Appia, in 312 BC. As a further flourish of Greek modernity, the first Roman public swimming bath, the Piscina Publica, was built next to it, outside the Porta Capena.[2] The Appian projects were immensely popular and successful, and Roman engineering never looked back. Imperial wealth was used quite blatantly to beautify the major Roman towns and cities, and secure mass support from their ever-growing populations. Successive rulers found that public engineering projects soaked up the surplus workforce, involving millions of people labouring by hand, and much political patronage for senators and salaried officials; as the Roman chronicler Polybius remarked, public building was the chief expense regularly incurred by the state.[3]

Aqueducts had a publicity value at least equal to the job they were built to do. Pliny the Elder (AD 23–79) said boastfully, if anyone will note the abundance of waters skilfully brought into the city for public purposes, for baths, for public basins, for houses, runnels, suburban gardens and villas; if he will note the high aqueducts required for maintaining the proper elevation; the mountains which had to be pierced for the same reason; the valleys it was necessary to fill up; he will conclude that the whole terrestrial globe offers nothing more marvellous.[4]

In first-century Rome the aqueducts flowed into three central tanks that distributed the water strictly according to public priority: 10 per cent to the emperor, 50 per cent to private customers paying water tax, 40 per cent for tax-free public use, including four military camps, fifteen sets of baths and latrines, twelve public fountains, and 133 public troughs, basins, and 'springers'—small taps running day and night. Generation by generation new aqueducts were added: eleven by AD 226, with 1,000 public baths.

There was another sanitary engineering glory in ancient Rome—though not when they backed up after storms and high tides. The *cloacae* were the underground sewers flowing down to the Tiber, a black-water drainage system begun in the sixth century BC, but replaced in the first century BC by Agrippa.[5] The *cloacae* also served the monumental public latrines (*forica*) that were one of the sights of Rome, often heated in winter by a hypocaust, and always good for a gossip:

The Roman *forica* was public in the full sense of the term, like soldiers' latrines in wartime. People met there, conversed, and exchanged invitations to dinner without embarrassment... [it was] decorated with a lavishness we are not wont to spend on such a spot. All round the semicircle or rectangle which it formed, water flowed continuously in little channels, in front of which a score of seats were fixed. The seats were of marble, and the opening was framed with sculpted brackets in the form of dolphins... above the seats it was not unusual to see niches containing statues of gods or heroes . . . and not infrequently the room was cheered by the gay sound of a playing fountain.[6]

Roman latrines evidently met a communal need—or a need for communality—in the same way as the Greek fountains. Archaeologists routinely find villas where three-, five-, seven-, or ten-seater latrines were normal, while even the latrines of the imperial palace 'as majestic and ornate as a sanctuary beneath its dome' contained three seats side by side. You were nothing in Rome without your expensively plumbed latrines, courtyard fountain, pool, or private baths; but for most other people who did not live in Rome (or other well-plumbed cities or forts), water supplies were still dependent on local rivers, springs, wells, and rainwater cisterns, where such effects were more difficult to achieve. In a rapidly growing city like Rome, all the aqueducts did was to maintain a precarious demographic balance, as they were laboriously brought through each new shanty district in turn, creating at least a semblance of the luxuriously paved, watered, and drained city centre.

Public Baths and Spas

The public baths (*balnea*) were a clear barometer of the healthiness of civic life in the Roman world. So vital were they, archaeologists say, that the gradual decline of urban life was quickly manifested in the baths: if the town neglected the baths, it meant there were problems with its economy. Outside Rome itself, the imperial administration really only built the military and political necessities. The all-important 'civic designation', the political rank of a settlement, depended largely upon the extent of its monumental architecture and engineering projects: the more the better. It is not clear how many settlements were actually bath-ranked—400 major baths sites around the Empire have been excavated so far, with many more still beneath the earth, sea, or sand—but the inscription evidence suggests that public bath building was fairly near the top of the list for serious political contenders: 'Julianus built these baths—and the whole town enjoys their charm—with his wife Domna. He gave immense joy, glorifying his hometown.'[7] The Romans were at first suspicious of the intellectual status given to the Greek gymnasiums, and refused to build training and social facilities into their early *balnea*. But modernity won through, and the Greek style was adopted in Rome, around 29–19 BC.

The public baths mainly existed for reasons of pleasure, politics, and propaganda, not disease prevention. In the long term, the hygienic impact of the public bath system was probably marginal—though even that tiny margin may perhaps have tipped the balance towards health for many people. The baths were difficult to maintain and keep clean, and there was also the dubious practice of allowing the sick to bathe with the well, until Hadrian (76 BC–AD 138) attempted to legislate against it.[8] But the military loved and needed them. Gymnasium baths (baths with exercise yards attached) spread throughout the provinces, particularly where there was a garrison, or a garrison town. Like the clubhouses of later European colonists, the baths were the centre of social life for all expatriate soldiers, administrators, and businessmen. New hydropathic fashions, and new architectural styles, spread through the Empire quickly and seamlessly. Medium-sized Londinium (population 50,000–100,000) had one full public bath suite erected in around AD 100, but had ended up with two by the end of the Empire.[9]

The south-eastern imperial provinces had a long history of Graeco-Roman involvement, and baths were an early cultural arrival. Many of the north African Roman baths built later in the Empire were in the grandest style, almost rivalling Rome. There were also many Judaic bath sites in Roman Egypt and Palestine, and women's baths for Judaic purity rituals. The palaces of the thoroughly Hellenized King Herod the Great of

Judaea (74–4 BC) all contained baths and large water tanks; he also started public games, built an aqueduct, public baths, and a promenade by the sea at Laodicea, and regularly visited different mineral spas for his health—dying at 70, a valetudinarian to the end. But ever since the Bar Kochba Revolt in AD 135, when Hadrian pulled down Jerusalem and transformed it into the Roman city of Aelia Capitolina (complete with drainage, baths, etc.) most of the Jewish rabbis were hostile or ambivalent to Roman civic life: 'all that they made, they made for themselves', one rabbi commented sourly.[10]

It is obvious that there was a pre-existing baths culture on their Italic peninsula that predisposed the Romans to a certain type of balneology. The Romans were much more lavish with their hot water. Like the earlier Etruscans, they enjoyed using the volcanic hot springs (*thermae*) encircling ancient volcanic cones sitting on a volcanic fault line stretching down the western seaboard from Vesuvius and the volcanic Phlegrean Fields immediately north-west of the Bay of Naples, down to Etna in Sicily. There were and are dozens of small rustic springs all over this area, flowing into open-air pools and streams fed from thermal sources; and this indigenous experience was presently followed by the social and commercial development of the Roman spa.

The most famous hot springs of all were on the fault line at Baiae, where large quantities of heated volcanic water rose on the coast of the Bay of Naples. Baiae was an ancient shrine dedicated to the cult of Venus, a small sanctuary carved out of the soft tufa rock inside the steaming grottoes and caves. In the first century BC Julius Caesar improved the facilities and widened the range of gods and votaries by building an impressive Thermae of Mercury, enclosing the main hot spring with one of the first domed rotundas in Roman architecture (borrowed from the Greek apse) surrounded by three large stone barrel-vaulted halls.[11] With its mild climate, lush vegetation,

sea views, and hot springs, the bay of Baiae became Rome's most
fashionable holiday retreat, a natural playground which spurred
on the development of a resort coastline that became celebrated
(or notorious) for the unrestrained enjoyment of sensuous
delights; the better-known Pompeii was a pale reflection of
Roman resort life at Baiae. Tiberius (AD 14–37), one of the
most louche of the early emperors, established the new office
of Master of the Imperial Pleasures, and the orgies in his private
villa on the nearby island of Capri were legendary.[12]

By the end of the imperial period, the Thermae of Mercury
were at the centre of a huge hillside complex at Baiae which has
been likened to a grand hotel-cum-sanatorium or a 'thermal
city'.[13] There were rows of large thermal halls; residential and
sightseeing quarters; hillside promenades of stairs, ramps, fountains, basins, and walkways; a coastal parade of colonnades,
statuary, shops, villas, warehousing, and man-made spits into
the sea (which has now covered the lower half of ancient Baiae).
Pliny mentions a hot sea-bathing establishment run by a mineral baths owner, M. Crassus Frugi of Pompeii, that was apparently built in the sea (like an offshore oil platform) around or
over a natural hot spring which came from the seabed and
forced itself up in spectacular clouds of steam.[14] In summer
the beaches would have been crowded with swimmers, since
Romans enjoyed swimming, and believed seawater to be healthful. The Stoic Seneca visited and fled the place, speaking of
'drunk men wandering along the beach, banquets in boats,
the lakes echoing with the voices of singers, and other acts of
debauchery displayed as though the laws had ceased to bind
them'.[15] The resort sprawl continued further down the road
near Naples, where there was another thermal city laid out at
Agnano; and another at Stabiae. There would probably have
been a mix of development at these satellite resorts, ranging
from cheaper rates at communal public pools, to more expensive subscriptions at private, exclusive, bath suites. Moreover,

thermal cities did not have to be beside the sea. They could be inland resort hot-water *thermae*, such as those at Badenweiler, Aix, or Aquae Sulis (Bath). And as interest in balneology spread, the indigenous cold mineral waters were also enthusiastically 'discovered' by the invading Romans and classified for health purposes—Pliny's *Natural History* lists the main mineral-water groups as sulphur, alum, bitumen, alkaline, and acid—leaving a legacy of spa knowledge and spa use that later inspired the spa revival in early modern Europe.

Most urban thermal baths, though, were not connected to special springs; they owed more to Greek technology. This new expertise in heating and hydraulic technology led to the old small half-baths of the Etruscans being replaced by large communal pools—thus relaxing traditional Etruscan disapproval of communal bathing, even for members of the same family. In the new Rome, the imperial *thermae* became masterpieces of the art: the Baths of Agrippa (25 BC) were among the first large baths in Rome, serving 170 bathers. According to Pliny, it was Agrippa who turned them into free public baths for both sexes, in 33 BC, starting a philanthropic tradition. There followed the Baths of Titus (AD 80), the Baths of Trajan (AD 104–9); and finally, the two massive Baths of Caracalla (AD 215) and the Baths of Diocletian (AD 284–305), for which almost all of the Aqua Marcia had to be overhauled to supply enough water. All of these baths displayed the two-storey, grand, symmetrical style that had become typical of Roman bath architecture, through which the customer could wander at will, sampling each cold, hot, tepid, or steam bath (*calidarium, frigidarium, tepidarium, laconicum*) as he or she chose. The Caracalla Baths provided full sports facilities (with marble seats for 1,600 spectators), a large tree-lined courtyard, an *exedrae* arena for philosophical debating, and places for 2,000 bathers at a time. The Diocletian Baths were reputed to hold 18,000 bathers, and were encrusted with mosaics and marble. Women, children, servants, and slave-girls poured in and out of the portals during the women's hours in the morning until noon, the first shift after the baths had got up their heat. The men's hours were from midday to the 'second hour of night', which allowed plenty of time for a little light exercise before bathing and the subsequent grooming–robing session, before hitting the streets, bars, and dinner parties later on.

The discerning Roman, or curious Roman traveller, could also have used one of the many smaller private bathing establishments, almost everywhere, that were a little more discreet, but equally luxurious, and very similar to the modern health club. By luck we have one writer's graceful compliment to one of the favourites in second-century Rome, the clearly fashionable Baths of Hippias, built by the discerning engineer, scientist, and astronomer Hippias in the new high, light style of design, with immaculate attention to architectural detail:

The entrance is high, with a flight of broad steps of which the tread is greater than the pitch, to make them easy to ascend. On entering, one is received into a public hall of good size, with ample accommodations for servants and attendants. On the left are the lounging rooms, also of just the right sort for a bath, brightly lighted retreats. Then, beside them, larger than need be for the purposes of a bath, but necessary for the reception of the rich. Next, capacious locker-rooms to undress in, on each side, with a very high and brilliantly lighted hall between them, in which are three swimming pools of cold water; it is finished in Laconian marble, and has two statues of white marble in the ancient technique, one of Hygieia, the other of Aesculapius.

On leaving the hall you come into another which is slightly warmed instead of meeting you at once with fierce heat; it is oblong, and has a large apse at each side. Next to it, on the right, is a very bright hall, nicely fitted up for massage, which has on each side an entrance decorated with Phrygian marble, and receives those who come from the exercise floor. Near this is another hall, the most beautiful in the world, in which one can sit or stand with comfort. It is also refulgent with Phrygian marble clear to the roof. Next comes the hot corridor, faced with Numidian marble. Beyond it is a very beautiful hall, full of abundant light and aglow with colour like that of purple hangings. It contains three hot tubs. When you have bathed, you need not go back through the same rooms, but can go directly to the cold room through a slightly warmed apartment. Everywhere there is copious illumination . . . furthermore, the height of each room is just, and the breadth proportionate to the length; and everywhere great beauty and loveliness prevail . . . [16]

The difference between these light, glittering interiors and the original cavelike conditions was described by Seneca while staying in the former home of the old warrior Scipio Africanus (d. 182 BC), where he observed the primitive, hardy routines of a much older system, with

a tank beneath the house and garden, big enough to water an army; and a narrow bath, dark as they usually were in ancient times—our fathers did not think a bath was warm unless it was dark . . . He the terror of Carthage . . . stood beneath this mean roof, this cheap pavement felt his footsteps. Nowadays who could bear to take a bath in such a place? Every man thinks himself poor and miserly unless his walls glitter with great costly plaques . . . we will not walk on pavements that are not bejewelled . . . Nowadays we call a bath a cockroach-covert, unless it is arranged to let in sunlight all day by extensive windows, unless we can sunbathe while we are still in the water, unless the country and the sea can be seen from the pool. [17]

Ovid's Grooming

In the new frescoed Roman art and portraiture set up for permanent public display on their household walls and floors, there were no lice, smells, wrinkles, disfigurements, or blemishes— just delicately pencilled oval faces and graceful bodies, as neat and as perfect as their owners had intended themselves to be.

Egypt had formerly dominated the western Asian cosmetics trade; now Rome was becoming the main consumer and entrepôt for powders, oils, perfumes, incense, silk, shawls, artificial flowers, rare woods, gems, jade, porcelain, gold, and silverware flooding in from all over Asia. Rome was also the main entrepôt for the large trade in raw materials and finished products sent back in return; and for the further distribution of the Eastern luxury goods into its northern and western European hinterlands.[18] Social grooming and cleansing had the same purpose then as now. In a rapidly expanding and competitive commercial society, where your outward appearance could propel you up (or down) the social ladder, even cheap perfumes and cosmetics were better than none: they indicated that you had at least made the attempt. Of course there were fine social gradations in cosmetic care, which the poet Ovid was at pains to describe.

P. Ovidius Naso (43 BC–AD 17), the fashionable poet, wit, and scandalous man-about-town, is one of our best sources on Roman cosmetics. His renowned work *Metamorphoses* includes a much-quoted speech on the moral purity of vegetarianism, and was an Orphic ode to love in all its forms. He also produced the only known cosmetic receipt book in verse, while his famous *Ars Amatoria* ('The Art of Love') set new standards of refined courtship and seduction which later made him the idol of aristocratic boudoirs in Renaissance Europe. *Ars Amatoria* showed him to be a close observer and cheerleader of this newly affluent society:

> The good old days indeed! I am, thanks be,
> This age's child: it's just the age for me;
> Not because pliant gold from earth is wrought,
> Nor because pearls from distant coasts are brought,
> Not that from hills their marble hearts we hew,
> While piles encroach upon the ocean's blue:
> It's that we've learnt refinement, and our days
> Inherit not our grandsire's boorish ways.[19]

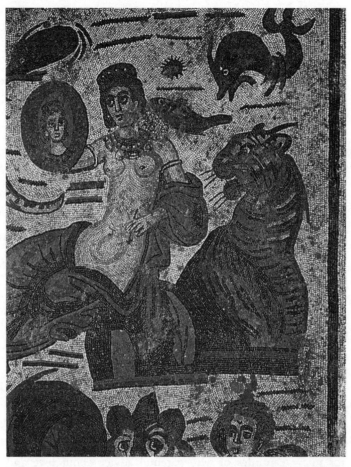

8 A well-dressed naiad reclining in the Hall of the poet Arion, in the late
fourth-century AD Roman villa at Piazza Armerina, Sicily.

Ars Amatoria was in fact a passionate text on the civil arts of grooming. For the male citizen there were masterly instructions on how to dress and woo the fair, with sensitive treatment of the problems of female rejection. For women—'my scholars fair, Pupils of Ovid'—there was comprehensive and *ganika*-like advice on the essential rules of beauty, dress, deportment, hair-styling, music, poetry, manners, and character. By all accounts heavy resources were thrown into the morning regime of the average Roman male and female, and long hours were spent at the toilette table. Fully costumed Roman women were particu-larly splendid and ornate compared to their Greek or Egyptian counterparts, wearing more colour in their clothing, more paint, and far more elaborate jewellery and hairdressing.[20]

Ovid saw cosmetics as a philosophy for life, and his basic message was self-cultivation: look after yourself, make the most of your self. The morality was unabashed hedonism; women should grab beauty with both hands, in the face of ravaging time:

> Looks come by art: looks vanish with neglect...
> While yet you can, while life is at its spring
> —Years fleet like running water—have your fling...
> Pluck then the flower, which left will merely rot...[21]

A more sober tone was adopted in Ovid's cosmetic poem 'Med-icamina Faciei Feminae' ('Cosmetics for Ladies'), the prototype for many centuries of wise parental advice about love and beauty: 'A face will please when character is fine...Love lasts for character: age ruins beauty...Goodness suffices and endures forever; on this throughout its years true love depends.'[22] But Ovid's philosophy of cosmetics was also practical, even polit-ical: it was a social duty to use the cosmetic arts. He saw cos-metics as part of an honourable craft tradition, and endlessly praised human ingenuity. All culture originated from cloacal nature, but the glory was to perfect and tame it: 'To make a ring, first crush the shining ore; that frock of yours was a dirty fleece before.' It was human artifice that produced beauty: 'cultivation sweetens fruit that's bitter... marble hides black soil below'. Hence his technical interest in 'Medicamina Faciei Femina'—'a little guide to make-up I have writ, though small in bulk, in labour infinite'—which consisted of his personal collection of 'cures for damaged looks' (with receipts now mostly lost) using rouge, saffron eye make-up, kohl, patches, wigs, washes, skin lotions, and who knows what else. In large Roman households the making of cosmetics was traditionally supervised by one of the older women (the dresser, or *ornatrix*) with her team of slave girls (*cosmetae*), and was a serious and seasonal business, like all food-preserving.[23]

Ovid knew his world well: 'hair's curled deep in the country; though they're hidden on Athos, they'll be smart on Athos too'. Wealth was not absolutely essential for careful grooming; and Ovid warned his pupils against vulgar ostentation. The idea was to be subtle and restrained and, above all, clean and trim. Use colour artistically, don't overdo the display of jewellery or 'stagger forth in cloth of gold'; neatness was enough: 'By chic we're charmed: no rebel curl should show: A finger's touch, and looks will come or go.'[24] And finally—as if any one would actually need to know about cleanliness!—Ovid laughs off intimate personal hygiene as a joke:

> How nearly had I warned you to beware
> Lest armpits smell or legs be rough with hair!
> But it's no squaws from Vaucasus I teach
> Or Mysian dwellers on Caicus beach;
> As well to bid you wash your face each day,
> Nor leave your teeth to blacken with decay...
> Nor cleaning teeth in public I advise...
> Make sparing gestures while you chat
> Whose nails are scrubby or whose fingers fat.
> Talk not when empty if your breath offend,
> And always keep your distance from your friend.

> ... Beauty's aids should ne'er be shown.
> A face besmeared with [cosmetic] dregs, whose drippings light
> On the warm bosom, is a loathsome sight ...
> All this gives beauty, but it's ugly viewing,
> Much that delights when done disgusts when doing.[25]

Ovid is too discreet to mention the cleaning of that other part or orifice the anus, though archaeology has shown that the Romans were evidently quite fastidious in this respect, using the little sponges, wedged into short sticks, which have been found in debris of their latrines. Sponges and rag cloths were used during female menstruation, with basin-washing, and baths where available.

Roman male fashions were in theory extremely hostile to the painted cosmetics, coloured cloths, and long hair favoured by women, or any other perceived effeminacy or 'dandification'. The fashionable Ovidian ideal was the sober, military, Greek, clean-limbed look:

> Man's beauty needs no varnish ...
> Limbs clean and tanned by exercise delight,
> And spotless clothes that match the figure right ...
> Nor sprawling feet in floppy hides encased.
> Nor wear an ill-kempt crop ineptly sheared,
> Have expert hands to trim both hair and beard.
> Well pared and clean the finger-nails should be,
> The nostrils kept from lurking bristles free.
> Nor by foul breath from unclean lips exhaled ... [26]

Roman men were weaned from their original beards by the arrival of the clean-cut Greek fashion around the first century BCE, and the Roman barber (*tonsor*) was a man with a respected skill. From then on, says the historian Jerome Carcopino, 'nothing but the gravest and most painful crisis would have induced the great men of the day to omit a formality which for them had become a state duty'. Most of the emperors were clean-shaven, and used simple warrior haircuts suitable for a quick, manly 'stroke of the comb'. Perfumes were allowed, and simple rings or other tokens, but the main beauty was muscular, gained in the gymnasium—with 'the swift ball, the hoop, the lance', or by swimming in 'Calm Tiber's streams or Maiden's icy flow'.[27] Training and regimen were not exactly high on Ovid's agenda— they merely helped to produce a pleasing effect. Cosmetics existed to give a final civilized polish to the appearance, smartening up bodies that had already been prepared by all possible means. He left the medical preparations to others.

Physical Methodists

The arts and crafts of Greek hygiene had continued to evolve in the hands of later Greek physicians within the Empire. Many Romans patriotically disliked the modern type of Greek 'butcher' who purged humoral 'plethora' by bloodletting— usually doctors trained in anatomy and humoral theory at the great Alexandrian Library in Egypt, which became the centre of Aristotelian medical learning between 323 BCE and AD 395.[28] But they warmly welcomed the arrival in Rome of one mild-mannered Greek physician, trained in Athens, called Asclepiades of Bithynia (d. *c*.91 BC?), who devised a popular therapeutic system called Methodism, which mostly consisted in doing what the patient naturally liked best, without bloodletting, using a simple regimen and cheap ingredients. The medical author Celsus (who wrote not long after Asclepiades died) thought that he had improved domestic medicine: 'no one troubled about anything except what tradition had handed down to him until Asclepiades changed in large measure the way of curing'.[29] Despite his apparent fame and popularity no copies of his book *Common Aids* have survived; his easy-to-follow Methodist medical theory was vehemently opposed by the Alexandrian and Galenic Rationalists, then and later.

Asclepiades was born in a small Greek coastal resort in northern Asia Minor called Prusias-on-Sea, and was a baths doctor by
trade. With water arriving in Rome in increasing quantities and
the indigenous bath culture developing, he was in the right place
at the right time. He was also an expert manipulator of bodies.
The art of physical massage apparently took up much of his book:
'rubbing if strenuous, hardens the body, if gentle, relaxes; if
much, diminishes; if moderate, fills out'.[30] As might perhaps
be expected from a masseur, he thought of the all-important
humoral evacuations mainly in muscular and corpuscular terms,
later called the 'mechanical' theory of physiology: an unhealthy
body was either too 'constricted' for the humours to flow out, or
too 'relaxed' so that they flowed too much—and the cure was to
do the opposite. Too relaxed, and you were sent out walking,
with cold showers. Too constricted, too tense, and you were
given hot baths and massage. By elevating it into a Methodical
'system', Asclepiades made medical balneology respectable. He
paid careful attention to water temperature and type, using both
hot and cold mineral spa waters, and started the fashion for
drinking large quantities of these as diuretics. He even invented
a new air bath—a suspended 'hanging bath'—but also developed
the old immersion bath, and his patients spent long hours soak-
ing in the hot spas. He tried to avoid bloodletting: since life and
art were so uncertain he believed in doing the least possible
harm; his motto was 'swiftly, safely, sweetly'.[31] Reassuring and
relaxing the patient was essentially part of the Method, which
made it invaluable in gynaecology and childbirth and very popular with women; he was also sympathetic to mental problems
and their cure. The sceptical Methodist beliefs that rejected elaborate drugs, celebrated exercise, and frequently asserted the
rights of the patient and the virtues of empiricism, were all issues
dear to later European hygiene movements.

The awkward difference between theory and practice in
hygienic health care had been discovered by the Greeks fairly

early on. Did you bow to complete professional control? Or were
you the sort of person who just did not have the time (or was not
wealthy enough) to live a life wholly governed by concern for his
or her body?[32] Careful health care required good organization
and practical help, preferably at no great cost, and the Roman
author Celsus (*fl. c.*AD 30) was there to provide it. His work *De
Medicina* later became the classic model for some of the most
famous and widely circulated European medical advice books.
Blunt and conversational, a health educator to his fingertips, he
was far more readable than Galen. Being a well-educated aristo-
crat and not a professional doctor, he was able to take a temperate
view of hygiene—neither of 'one opinion or another, nor exceed-
ingly at variance with both, but hold[ing] a sort of intermediate
place between divers sentiments'—and he opened with some
common-sense general advice on 'The Regimen of Health':

> A man in health, who is both vigorous and his own master, should
> be under no obligatory rules, and have no need, either for a medical
> attendant, or for a rubber and anointer. His kind of life should
> be now in the country, now in the town, and more often about
> the farm; he should sail, hunt, rest sometimes, but more often take
> exercise; for whilst inaction weakens the body, work strengthens it;
> the former brings on premature old age, the latter prolongs youth.
>
> It is well also at times to go to the bath, at times to make use of
> the cold waters... to avoid no kind of food in common use; to
> attend at times a banquet, at times to hold aloof... Such are the
> precautions to be observed by the strong, and they should take care
> that whilst in health their defences against ill-health are not
> used up.

All things considered, Celsus believed that it was 'more useful to
have in the practitioner a friend rather than a stranger'. The art
of medicine ought to be rational and explorative, but draw
instruction from obvious natural causes, 'all obscure ones
being rejected from the practice of the Art, though not from
the practitioner's study'.[33] A hundred years later Galen based

his physiology on anatomical knowledge taken straight from the practitioner's study, and ultimately removed the art of medicine from untutored hands.

Galen's Hygiene

Galen's epic contribution to Western medicine came in the confident days of the mid-Empire. He was born in the reign of Hadrian in AD 129, lived his mature life under the great philosopher–emperor Marcus Aurelius (161–80), and died several emperors later in c.216. His professional influence from writing a corpus of over 350 titles cannot be underestimated—in total about as much as all other Greek medical writings put together. As he said, Hippocrates 'staked the way, but I made it passable'. He was an expert anatomist who left a continuing legacy of heroic bloodletting in Western medicine; but he was equally concerned to make his mark as a dietitian. Galen's long-lasting influence on hygiene came largely from his famous work *De Sanitate Tuenda* ('On the Healthy Life'); but also, from the way in which he extended and dominated the field of hygienic medical classification in general, as a teacher of 'the best of the young physicians'.[34] It was Galen who absorbed Plato's dualist philosophy of *psyche et soma* (soul and body), and always took *mens sana in corpore sano* ('a healthy mind in a healthy body') fully into account. He extended the hygienic regimen of the psyche—passions of the mind—by joining the humours with the elements; this eventually resulted in the four famous mental and physical 'temperaments' (choleric, sanguine, phlegmatic, and melancholic).[35] He also laid down a new set of medical 'means' (things to be administered, things to be removed, things to be done, and things to be applied) and a much more comprehensive list of 'neutrals' (food, drink, 'some kinds of drugs', air, massage, walking, exercise 'and all motor activity', baths, sleep, sexual activity, and the emotions). Thus, from being entirely unclassified, environmental hygienic interventions had been called Aids,

Means, Things—and were now Neutrals. Galen's 'Neutrals' were later turned into the famous 'Non-Naturals' owing to a translation error in the *Isagoge*, or Introduction, to medicine by Johannitius, which became the primary text for medical schools from the twelfth century onwards. For a fairly long period the actual number of non-naturals was not fixed, but in the end they stayed at six.[36]

De Sanitate Tuenda was ostensibly the main work through which classical hygiene was transferred to the later West. Unfortunately, it was only a fragment from a much larger œuvre:

> And especially I wish him who would study these writings to read the book in which I consider of what art hygiene is (it is inscribed Thrasybulus), and likewise the one about the best condition of the body and the one about good health. Both are short books, and whoever reads them before coming to this discussion will easily follow what is now being said. And it has previously been said that my book about the elements according to Hippocrates is essential for the present discussion, and it is followed by the one about the optimum constitution and the one about good health.[37]

So really all we have in *De Sanitate Tuenda* is an introductory lecture course: most of the rest is missing. But those who preserved it obviously thought it sufficiently comprehensive. It contains many pithy definitions and generalizations on Graeco-Roman hygiene: health is 'a sort of harmony', 'a mean between extremes', a 'due proportion', a 'slight deviation from perfection'.

A good half of *De Sanitate Tuenda* was on the ideal methods of training the youth, 'placed under the art of hygiene' from birth, and raising him into a perfect constitution in peak condition, starting with the hygiene of the newborn and children up to 7 years. It then went on to a large section on 'training the lad', and for this Galen made extensive use of Theon's *Gymnastics* (another entirely lost work). He casually mentions the contemporary existence of 'so many varieties of rubbing, that you could not readily enumerate them', but at the same time warns students that it is difficult to learn such practices from 'the old books' alone.[38] He also gives general advice on dealing with the typical patient—the busy middle-aged man. Roman businessmen apparently suffered from the perennial 'diseases of civilization'—a rich diet, lack of time, lack of exercise, headaches, piles, kidney stones, obesity, and stomach and bowel disorders.

Late Antique Baths

Two hundred years after his death, Galen's Rome no longer existed; it was a spent political force. The Empire was split and beleaguered, and outside the small world of medicine life had moved on. The baths yet again prove to be a sensitive barometer of social and economic change. For generations of fascinated historians, Roman baths have appeared as an extraordinary exercise in communal sensuality on a grand and public scale, and then—like the dinosaurs—they suddenly disappeared. At least it was thought they did: but the cataclysmic decline, it seems, only occurred in the western parts of the Empire, while the post-imperial period of Late Antiquity in the southern and eastern regions of the Empire remained, internally, a very old and fixed world.[39]

The aqueducts were the most obvious casualties during war. They were costly, difficult to maintain, and vulnerable. Very few remained intact in the western Empire. Many of the arched sections of the aqueducts supplying Rome were cut when the Goths laid full siege to the city in AD 537—some by the Goths to cut off water supply, some by the defenders to stop the Goths from using them to march into the city. Despite this, the favourites were almost always patched up or rebuilt. The real crunch came later, with the general failure of the aqueducts from the ninth century: 'it is not likely that any of them continued to be

used in anything like their original form later than sometime
between 900 and 1000'.[40] Some of them came back: the Virgo
aqueduct ceased operation in the tenth century, but was restored
again after 1453, while the old conduits of the Marcia never
dried up, and continue to send water into Rome. Elsewhere the
infrastructural decline was more gradual. Londinium struggled
to sustain its two public baths through the troubled 300–400s
after the Roman retreat, but in the end the problems of maintenance were too great, and when the tiled roofs collapsed in AD
430, they were not rebuilt. The same story could be told in
countless western provincial towns. Occupying a central site,
the baths at Londinium were later covered by a growing town,
and their stone reused for other purposes. The next time
stone-built public baths reappeared in London was in the mid-
nineteenth century.

In the eastern Empire it was a different story. Further east, and
in the southern provinces, the baths habit had taken a much
stronger hold, and the public baths were maintained or taken
over by others. In Late Antiquity the most impressive baths were
at Constantinople, which had almost as many baths as Rome, as
well as the longest aqueduct. Throughout the Byzantine Empire
the larger *thermae* ceased to be built after the fourth century, but
were maintained until about the ninth century. Smaller local
baths changed when the lives of their patrons changed, and
they were maintained because they had become valued. Practical and inconspicuous, small baths were the bedrock of popular bathing culture, and in Spain, France, Germany, Italy, Egypt,
Asia Minor, Syria, Judaea, and Arabia, town baths continued in
use for many centuries. More generally, however, the Graeco-
Roman influence was retreating in the face of the mass religious
movements of Christianity and Islam. The early Christian
Church was ambivalent towards the public baths; but it
was the breakdown of the ephebate Roman educational system
in the mid-fourth century that helped destroy the classical

gymnasiums and palaestras. The nudity and the public games were deemed offensive by ascetic clerics of all persuasions; for Romano-Christians especially the gymnasiums were a hated symbol of pagan ideals. Within a few decades of Constantine's official Christian conversion in AD 330, the gymnasiums had begun to disappear; the Olympic Games at Antioch struggled on until AD 520, the end of a thousand-year tradition.

The exercise yard did not feature in the magnificent bathhouses built by Islamic engineers who carried on where Rome left off following the Muslim conquests from the seventh century onwards. The town baths of the growing Islamic empire were turned into a very different type of social centre and grooming arena; in AD 900 there were 1,500 bathhouses in Baghdad. They contained eating and drinking areas, massage halls, and semi-private bath suites containing small baths in small annexes, where the Roman cold-water *frigidarium* was reduced to a fountain playing prettily in the hall while the occupants chatted—as in the eighth-century civic bath at Qasi al-Hayr, in Syria. More spectacularly they built large baths for the sporting aristocracy, like the luxurious painted and bejewelled hunting-lodge bath halls, way out in the desert, at eighth-century Qasr al-Amra in Jordan. The sultans also built more great bath halls in the desert for the caravanserai and other travellers to rest in and perform their devotions. Such desert baths literally became an oasis of talk and refreshment, cool and reviving in daytime yet warm in the cold desert nights; desert travellers used the baths like an inn or a hostel.[41]

Not long after the magnificent Roman buildings and engineering works had caved in, were pilfered, had crumbled and rotted or become covered by undergrowth, silt, or sand, the remnants of Greek and Roman classical learning were being absorbed into the eastern Byzantine and southern Arabic empires, while western Europe struggled to preserve precious scrolls from marauders in remote monastic and aristocratic libraries. During this same period the ancient culture of the desert was playing yet another historic role, as the solitary home of the ascetic hermit or holy man, and of the Christian Desert Fathers. The surge of personal asceticism in Late Antiquity is particularly crucial to the history of Christian cleanliness in Europe: it was a turning point—a change in the metaphysics. The sensual and simple pleasures of cleanliness that the Greeks and Romans so enjoyed were about to be condemned as a sin.

chapter 5
asceticism

Religious asceticism played a large part in reconfiguring European culture after the fall of Rome. So much of Christian history flows from this ascetic philosophy of purity; and so many bodies were subsequently constrained, cleansed, or physically altered because of it—especially those of monks, nuns, and many other devout men and women. In order to appreciate the milieu of cleanliness in medieval and early modern Europe, we need at least some grasp of the seismic events that occurred in that crucial 500-year period of religious upheaval in the Late Empire. The basic outlines are fairly clear. There was a religious revolution in which the moral duty to 'know thyself' became infinitely more important than the secular hygienic duty to 'look after yourself'.[1] As a result, the ideology of cleanliness was turned upside down and inside out. Judaeo-Christian asceticism insisted that the cleansing of the inner soul was absolutely imperative, whereas the cleansing of the outer body was a worldly distraction, and its ornamentation a positive sin. In effect the extreme religious devotion that was previously reserved for the sanctified few was now being urged by ascetics as daily practice for the masses.

Eurasian Asceticism

Asceticism itself was an ancient phenomenon. The effect of severe privation on the human body suggests that ascetic practices were connected to earlier psychic, ecstatic, trance-like, or otherwise 'magical' religious states that demanded exceptional physical self-control; and various ascetic regimes—including celibacy and virginity—are practised worldwide.[2] In ancient Eurasia formal theologies gradually evolved at both ends of the continent as the tide of institutional priesthoods and wealthy, temple-based gods swept over earlier local pantheons; as we have seen, the discipline of purification was well entrenched, with many types of physical and sensory privations enforced on temple servants. Throughout later ancient Eurasia, highly specialized mind–body training regimes for the selected few were being practised in religious communities from an early age by young priests (novices), leading by degrees and stages to full wisdom and perfect spiritual attainment. Among the earliest of these 'religious virtuosi' was Pythagoras (581–497 BCE); another was the young aristocratic ascetic Sakyamuni, later known as Buddha (c.560–480 BCE), whose Vinaya rules of self-discipline became canonical in eastern Eurasia in the centuries after his death (and almost certainly reached western Eurasia via the trade routes).[3]

Advanced Eurasian asceticism included the physical techniques of isolated meditation, trance and breath control, gymnastics, music, and dance: the whole object of Taoist tai chi, Vedic yoga, Kerala martial arts, or the Kathakali dance form, is to spiritually 'centre' and fortify the spirit–body through physically controlling and training it. In China the earlier traditions of self-cultivation through the myth of Ancestor Peng gave way to the highly theological Xian cult, which concentrated on training the body for transcendent spiritual immortality, obviously a much more glamorous prospect than mere healthfulness. Greek meditations on the soul were a pale echo of the innumerable steps of Tantric initiation into the superconscious state of the Vedic *samadhi*; or the four stages of Buddhist *dhyana*.[4] The Greek word *askesis* was derived from the word for 'athletic training': an ascetic was a spiritual athlete. A preliminary *paraskeuazo* ('getting prepared') ascertained the true state of the soul, but there were no set gymnosophic rules or craft techniques; Greek ethics proceeded by logic and dialogue. By the first and second centuries AD the Stoic philosophy had become fashionable among educated imperial classes, requiring a daily meditation and a thorough *exagorusis* (from *exagmen*, or 'tongue of balance') of your soul; as the emperor Marcus Aurelius (AD 121–80) wrote in his *Meditations*, 'a man who values a soul . . . no longer cares for anything else, but aims solely at keeping the temper of his own soul and all its activities rational and social, and works together with his fellows to this end'.[5]

Without increasing mass literacy, none of the new utopian prophetic religions that emerged in Eurasia between *c*.500 BCE and AD 500 would have survived, or spread so quickly. Asceticism played a large part in driving those literacy rates up. Ascetic prose supplemented the earlier holy scriptures—all the ceremonial instructions, calendrical mathematics, sacrificial duties, purification rules, and prophetic utterances that had begun to find their way into collective 'holy' books, alongside theological myths and courtly sagas of gods and human heroes (like the Mesopotamian *Epic of Gilgamesh*, the Greek Homer, or the Hindu *Ramayana* and *Mahabharata*). As the knowledge and habit of reading and writing spread, ascetic sermons, letters, and rules came in a deluge. There were increasing numbers of narrative stories of heroic personal asceticism from lone hermits, sages, and 'disciples' of ascetic prophets such as Buddha, Confucius, Jesus, or Muhammad. The ascetic lives of the early Christian saints and martyrs in particular were written up in highly literate style by the early Christian commentators, the Fathers of the Church, in reams of critical, passionate, and effortless Roman rhetorical prose.

As group bonds and state security disintegrated in the western Eurasian lands, maybe the mass of the people did not feel so well guarded as before—or so the Roman Christian author Arnobius thought: 'Since the nature of the future is such that it cannot be grasped or comprehended by any anticipation, is it not more rational rather to believe that which carries with it some hopes, than that which brings none at all?'[6] Scores of ecstatic religious movements, guided by charismatic leaders and aimed at the rural and urban poor, were moving away from the older rites and ceremonies of ancient civic life and demanding more onerous religious duties. In a single thirty-year period in Babylonia, c.AD 220–50, in a region only 200 miles long and 50 miles wide, there were followers of Mazdeism, Manichaeism, Mithraism, Judaism, and Christianity.[7] The so-called 'locus of the supernatural' was shifting away from the temple and towards the sacred holiness of self-selected, highly trained ascetic individuals, or groups of individuals, in constant communication with their god.

Christian Purity

Cleanness was innate to the Holy Spirit. According to the early theology of Jesus Christ, Jesus carried his holiness within and about him, in incorruptible flesh. Like any sacred priest, anything he touched made it holy. When Jesus washed the leper's feet, or embraced other untouchables, such as the poor, the sick, or the prostitute Mary Magdalene, he was not thereby rendered unclean. On the contrary, his holiness, his cleanness, healed them and made them whole. For Christians, full purity was only achievable through the act of baptism into the faith, which enabled the Holy Spirit to enter the individual converted soul: 'Then will I sprinkle clean water upon you, and ye shall be clean from all your filthiness and from all your idols will I cleanse you. And a new heart also will I give you, and a new spirit will I put within you . . . '.[8] It was for this reason that the Christian Church was sometimes called a *balaneion*; at the same time, baptism recalled old lustral rites. It poses the crucial problem of how far the new Christians were prepared to go in breaking away from their old Judaic faith and customs, and how much they retained.

Asceticism was firmly planted in Judaism. The wandering holy man was an ancient religious type, a solitary 'scapegoat' who took on the sins of the community by cutting himself off from the world—a living human sacrifice; while the ancient tradition of desert retreat in Egypt (the right of being able to move away from your neighbour) was strongly linked to the nomadic herder's ancient distrust of settled life. The radical Judaic shepherd–prophet Amos spoke for the masses living beyond the town and temple gates, expounding a trenchant form of anti-urban, anti-capitalist puritanism that became central to the ideology of Christian religious fundamentalists:

> They hateth him that rebuketh in the gate . . . Forasmuch therefore as your treading is upon the poor, and ye take from him burdens of wheat: ye have built houses of hewn stone, but ye shall not dwell in them . . . woe to them that are at ease in Zion . . . that lie upon beds of ivory, and stretch themselves upon their couches . . . drink wine in bowls, and anoint themselves with the chief ointments . . . [9]

But for the Judaic scribes who wrote the holy books, mere ignorance did not let any sinner off the hook: the population had to be taught the rituals of cleanness and uncleanness. Hence the book of Leviticus (and hundreds of other Old Testament passages) in which the defilements, abominations, and uncleannesses of cursing, copulation, unclean women, plague, leprosy, the menses, sperm, blood, nakedness, physical blemishes, clean foods, and correct ritual sacrifices were fully written out. But genuine faith counted most. A single God spoke directly to the heart, mind, and soul. As the later medieval Jewish theologian Maimonides put it in his commentary on the 'Book of Cleanness' in the sacred *Mishneh torah*, even though the temple rules laid down in Scripture were 'not matters about which human understanding is capable of forming a judgement', nevertheless, 'he who has set his heart on cleansing himself . . . becomes clean as soon as he consents in his heart . . . and brings his soul to the waters of pure reason'. Judaism was a religion of the heart; and so was Judaic Christianity.[10]

Nothing could have been more different from the shaven heads of Egyptian priests than the wild, flowing, uncut beards and hair of the Jewish prophets; they had clearly set themselves against this aspect of Egyptian purification ritual. Their particular type of asceticism rejected the worldly vanity of close body care. In this regard we should note especially the lesser-known grooming prohibitions of Leviticus: 'Ye shall not round the corners of your heads, neither shalt thou mar the corners of thy beard. Ye shall not make any cuttings in your flesh for the dead, nor print any marks upon you'; and 'They shall not make baldness upon their head, neither shall they shave off the corner of their beard, nor make any cuttings in the flesh.'[11] This was mild rebuke against ancient body culture compared to other testament writers. The prophet Isaiah's blistering attack on women and cosmetic beauty was an explicit reference to sexual disease, and a withering description of urban fashions:

> Therefore the Lord will smite with a scab the crown of the head of the daughters of Zion, and the Lord will discover their secret parts. In that day the Lord will take away the bravery of their tinkling ornaments about their feet, and their cauls, and their round tires [headdresses] like the moon, the chains and the bracelets . . . And it shall come to pass, that instead of a sweet smell there shall be a stink; and instead of a girdle a rent; and instead of well-set hair baldness; and instead of a stomacher, a girding of sackcloth; and burning instead of beauty.[12]

The Essenes from Engeddi, by the Red Sea, were a celibate, ascetic Jewish group known for their sober ways, rites of baptism, vegetarianism, and white robes—Jesus is thought to have had Essene family connections, through John the Baptist. The ascetic renunciations required by Jesus and his wandering followers were severe enough—'Go, sell all that you have and give to the poor'— but they were benevolent. They were not extreme, exclusive, or hermetic. After all, Jesus himself had deliberately broken almost all the purity laws of the Torah by associating with unclean people all his life, telling the priests: 'They that are whole need not a physician; but they that are sick. I come not to call the righteous, but sinners to repentance.' The proselytizing Apostles of Jesus, like Paul of Tarsus, were resolutely inclusive. They did not insist on circumcision for non-Jews, or on making a division between clean or unclean food, or clean or unclean women, or other customary matters: while they were spreading the word, no one was to be excluded. The Apostles were thus emphatically not priests, but radical ecstatic mystics in the Judaic tradition.[13]

Neoplatonism

Most of the Church Fathers were soaked in the classics of Roman scholarship: St Jerome had to put himself under a special penance to stop himself from reading them. The pagan philosophies themselves were still strong and active. The Alexandrian philosopher Plotinus (AD 205–70) had inspired an ascetic, Neoplatonic, or 'gnostic' tradition within the early Christian Church, and his prolific writings on the joys of con- templation lived long after him.[14] Plotinus believed that all physical matter was inherently evil. It clogged up the soul and kept it earthbound, when its true celestial existence depended on weightlessness, mingling with the universe above to attain the state of the pure absolute Being, the One. The pure soul had minimal bodily needs, and had to renounce all sexual desire; chastity was an essential qualification. Neoplatonic asceticism was widespread among intellectuals of the small farm or villa population, and among poor but spiritually ambitious civic scholars such as St Augustine (354–430), who was converted to contemplative asceticism by Plotinus, and later turned to his mother's religion, Christianity, to help him sublimate his strong sexual urges by adopting celibacy, or chastity.[15] Chastity had always been an attribute of priesthood but was now the ultimate ascetic challenge for the Christian believer.

Thanks to the Neoplatonic–Manichaean 'twofold' philosophy of the outer body and inner soul, ordinary Christians now had two bodies to look after—and one of them was inherently evil, full of burning lust, and a mere mortal shell. As St Paul described it, 'Though our outer person is wasting away, the inner is being renewed.' St Athanasius explained this 'two-body' early Christian physiology in a sermon *On Sickness and Health*: 'In short, one must know that the body is composed of members, but the inner person is not composed of bodily members, but rather possesses the significance of the member's action . . . so too the intellectual substance of the soul accomplishes the entire work of the commandments with the five senses.'[16] The duty of the Christian ascetic anchorite (*anakhoretes*, from *anakhoreo*, 'retire') was to subdue the natural sensory impulses that threatened the inner person, by literally starving them into submission, sense by sense. The shrivelled bodies of the anchorites told this tale precisely: sleep deprivation, semi-starvation, minimal water, no comforts, hard labour, coarse clothing, and unwashed skin. Jesus' asceticism was moderate compared to some of his followers. He went into the desert and fasted for forty days and forty nights; but Saint Anthony (AD 251–356) spent twenty years there. The penances of the holiest ascetic (male or female) were the most severe; the monk St Pachomius only ate every third day, though lesser anchorites were allowed a meagre daily ration of bread with salt, and water.[17] Like the actions of the Vedic yogi, anchorite asceticism contained pathological self-wounding elements deliberately designed to test the will and train the soul to a point just short of suicide. Many, many anchorites underwent sufficient suffering to attain sainthood in later centuries.[18]

During the first four centuries the Christian debate on spiritual virtues of continence and celibacy was urgent and highly charged. A wave of self-mortifying sects arose after Jesus' death, experimenting with every form of bodily abasement.[19] The burning fires of lust were the worst of evils—and so difficult to put out. Commentators such as St John Cassian, St Augustine, and St Benedict regarded male nocturnal emissions as a special challenge, especially when male members were gathered together under one roof. St Pachomius' monastic Rules on celibacy included covering knees when sitting together; not bending down or pulling tunics up too high when doing laundering; keeping the eyes lowered, avoiding direct glances, never performing 'intimacies' such as bathing or oiling one another, or removing thorns from the skin; never talking in the dark or holding hands, and always keeping a distance. Nudity was forbidden, even when alone, and for this reason bathing was discouraged, except for the sick or aged; under St Benedict's Rules, even washing was a complicated procedure that involved keeping the body concealed at all times with different bits of clothing.[20]

Asceticism was either highly democratic or highly anarchic, and was not easily controlled.[21] St Athanasius' *Life of Anthony* (published only a year after Anthony's death) became the inspiration for a surge of Christian rock-dwelling anchorites pursuing 'the myth of the desert' in Egypt. Pachomius (AD 290–347) founded the first disciplined monastic settlement of anchorites in order to house them, which had quickly multiplied to thousands of monks during his lifetime (and became worryingly wealthy from their daily labours). By the time St Simeon Stylites (387–459) drew crowds from nearby Antioch to see him perched on top of his 70-foot rock pillar, Pachomine monasteries were being visited by a constantly increasing stream of devout pilgrims from all over newly Christianized Europe—the 'Egyptomania' of the age.[22] Despite certain reservations, the Catholic Church was being inexorably shaped and moulded by popular religious asceticism, both in the desert and in the towns.

The Apostles—including St Paul—had always carefully distinguished between 'moderate' asceticism for most of their flock and 'advanced' asceticism for the 'ardent'; and were careful never to impugn sex in marriage (though strictly for the purposes of procreation). From the third and fourth centuries AD onwards, with the numbers of ardent ascetics increasing, the politics of the Church swung constantly between the moderate and radical ascetic camps. Radical ascetics were at first removed from bishoprics, but then returned; or moved to activism in Corinth, or Jerusalem, or Gaul. One significant purity law that was resurrected after the Council of Laodicea in AD 352 forbade women to serve as priests or preside over churches; but ordaining the sexual celibacy of the male clergy was evidently a tougher proposition. Ever since Nicaea internal debates had raged, with married priests at first defended (in 362) so long as they had married before ordination and their wife had been a virgin—not a widow, a divorced woman, or a concubine. But the Church puritans were not to be denied. In AD 385–6 Pope Siricius, pressured by ascetic propagandists centred on Jerome and his circle in Rome and Bethlehem, finally persuaded the bishops to bind the higher clergy to 'inviolate celibacy' and offered the promise of a pure priesthood vowed to chastity. Thus another ancient purity law was reinstated.

Virginity

It was the excesses of Roman urban life that really repelled the ascetics—food, clothing, and public baths especially. 'Why do you gorge your body with excess?' asked St John Chrysostom (c.AD 347–407). 'Consider what comes of food and into what it is changed. Are you not disgusted at it? The increase of luxury is but

the multiplication of filth.'[23] Most early Christians were city
dwellers. Lacking a synagogue or a legal meeting place, they had
turned their households into churches; some went further and
turned them into ascetic cells; and many of these ascetics were
women. After AD 352 hermetic virginity was almost the only route
left to the ardent female. The Virgins of Alexandria, Rome, and
Jerusalem were impressive individuals and a crucial support to the
early Church.[24] Virgins were among the first martyrs; they joined
the early Christian communities in large numbers, and played
host to them; they also played a large part in funding the early
Church, and later hospitals, abbeys, and convents, out of the
proceeds of their relinquished estates. When later gathered together in institutional convents, they were called nuns.

The Christian virgins first appeared among the educated or
wealthy female elites: people who had plenty of material goods
to give up, but who would normally be under the complete
control of their families, such as widows or heiresses, but who
now openly and rebelliously vowed themselves to celibacy,
sackcloth, and ashes. Early Christians were exhorted to see the
advantages of having a virgin in the household, like an amulet,
insurance policy, or shrine: 'The virgin is an offering for her
mother, by whose daily sacrifice divine power is appeased.
A virgin is the inseparable pledge of her parents, who neither
troubles them for a dowry, nor forsakes them, nor injures them
in word or deed.' Many centuries later the notorious virgins of
Venice, the unwanted daughters of aristocratic families who
could not afford their dowry payments, were locked away in
large numbers for precisely these reasons.[25]

The ascetic virgin was designated the 'Bride of Christ', eternally betrothed to Jesus, and the virgin's special role was that of
the chief female mourner. The great rhetorical theme of virginity was penance, and weeping for the sins of the world. Weeping
real and constant tears, it was said, 'cleanses and prepares a
person for purification'. The physical dirt on the holy body

was both potent (in the sense of an inverted pollution) and a sign of faith. The redoubtable virgin Paula, the platonic friend and companion of St Jerome, 'subdued' him with her lachrymose behaviour and fetid appearance: 'She mourned, she fasted, she was squalid with dirt, her eyes were dim with weeping.' When the widow Fabiola became a Christian penitent, she put on sackcloth and publicly confessed her sins, standing in the Basilica in Rome 'with dishevelled hair, pale features, soiled hands and unwashed neck...she took the millstone and ground meal, she passed bare-footed through rivers of tears ... That face by which she once pleased her second husband she now smote with blows, and she hated jewels, shunned ornaments and could not bear to look upon fine linen.'[26]

Because they inevitably lived in towns, and at the centre of their households, female virgins had an extra set of sensory deprivations to undertake. Spiritual seclusion could be achieved through the self-imposed purdah that Churchmen called 'modesty'—anonymity, silence, and guarded movements, gestures, and gait: 'Thus the movement of the body is a sort of voice of the soul...That virgin is not sufficiently worthy of approval who has to be enquired about when seen.' As well as penitential fasting, praying, and weeping, virgins should veil the head, cover themselves down to their fingertips, walk with 'sober gait', talk in a low voice, look at the floor with 'bashful countenance', stay silent and speechless, avoid visits and visitors, keep company with no men, attend no feasts, and keep a distance from all strangers 'lest your foot ever stumble against a stone'.[27]

Washing and Bathing

Instead of perfumes, a holy virgin gave off the true odour of sanctity: 'Thy first odour is above all spices, which were used in the burying of the Saviour, and the fragrance arises from the mortified motions of the body, and the perishing of the delights

of the members. Thy second odour, like the odour of Lebanon,
exhales the incorruption of the Lord's body, the flower of virginal chastity.'[28] The pungent fragrance of bodily perishing and
mortification was not only a sign of genuine hermeticism but
was all the more likely when that body was heavily clothed
(closely covered) but rarely washed. In the early days of the
virginity movement desperate times had clearly called for desperate measures, and washing—or rather not washing—became
a symbolic act of public defiance. When the virgin Melania
began her long campaign to persuade her reluctant husband,
Pinian, to make a joint vow of chastity, her first act was to stop
bathing (she eventually succeeded). Rather less amusing, and
less common, was the fate of the early virgin martyr Thecla,
condemned to death for defending herself against a noble
suitor, who claimed Christian baptism as she leapt into a tank
full of sharks in the Antioch arena, crying out 'now is the time
for me to wash!'[29]

Later virgins did not have persecution to contend with, but
washing was still fraught with religious implications. St Augustine thought that holy dirt was 'ostentatious' and washed daily;
St Anthony never washed at all. Somewhere in between was a
range of personal preferences and personal solutions. The
wealthy virgin Olympias lived like a nun at the centre of a
large palace, with a luxurious bath suite, but always took her
baths covered in a voluminous black robe.[30] Modesty was natural, said the theologians, and the private parts shameful: 'those
parts in which there is a compliance with the necessities of
nature, she has partly put away and hidden in the body itself,
lest they should present a disgusting appearance, and partly,
too, she has taught and persuaded us to cover them. Is not
nature herself a teacher of modesty?' Many people covered
themselves in the baths, St Ambrose continued, so 'that part
of it at least may be covered', and recommended loincloths or
breeches 'as it was told Moses by the Lord: "And thou shalt

make them linen breeches to cover their shame: from the loins
even to the thighs they shall reach".'[31] St Jerome regarded daily
bathing as an 'over-niceness' and a refinement, and constantly
cited 'frequenting the public baths' as an evil in his Letters—
especially by those he regarded as loose public women, who
'allow themselves more liberty than ever, frequenting the
baths, flitting through the streets, showing their harlot faces
everywhere'.[32] Perfumes, paints, hairstyles, golden jewellery,
open litters, music, drink, dancing, costly clothes 'dragging'
on the ground, were all anathema. They belonged to what St
Athanasius contemptuously called 'the adorned class'.

By contrast, Athanasius' silent, gentle, dovelike virgin had no
need whatsoever of the noise and commotion of the public
baths, or to be mingling with the daughters of Babylon parading
their nudity. A passage from his chapter on the 'dangers of the
public bath' in his Second Letter to Virgins gives us a just a
breath of that virginal air—and also tells us that small basins,
not large baths, were to be the Christian bathing implements of
the future:

The dove is acquainted with the bath in the ordinary waters in the
basin; she does not take off her garment or reveal her nudity.
Observe her appearance: see how her appearance is pure, without
force or cleansings, how she is adorned by her insight and not from
the adornment that enters from outside. . . . A basin is sufficient for
you to wash away your dirt. Ask and learn how Sarah washed
herself while living in a tent; how Rachel followed the flock; how
Miriam sojourned in the desert without water. . . Have you not
heard that the apostles and disciples of our Lord ate food without
washing their hands (Matt. 15: 1–20) and St Peter declined to have
his feet washed by the Lord (John 13: 3–11)? And who is purer than
the aforementioned people? For they who were pure on the inside
were also completely pure on the outside (Matt. 23: 26). But learn
how the women who bathe have been injured and have dragged
others down into corruption. The first is Bathsheba, the wife of

Uriah, who, when she stripped, instantly stripped such a great man of holiness and rule (2 Sam. 11).... Was it not by the greatness of his repentance that he returned to power? Did he not eat ashes like bread and mix his drink with tears (Ps. 101 (102): 10)? Was it not with tears he dampened the defiled bed (Ps. 6: 7)? Did not his knees become weak with fasting and his flesh lean from anointing (Ps. 108 (109): 24)? Did he not make sack-cloth his garment (Ps. 68 (69): 12)? Did he not also take off his pure linen garment? You see how she who wanted to bathe poured out filth on such a man; for because she washed her body, she defiled another man's soul.[33]

Where Athanasius led, many others followed then and in later centuries. The public liking for public baths survived the fall of the Roman Empire, but a vociferous minority of religious puritans always opposed them.

Early Christians evidently had a rooted aversion to baths and nakedness, but in this they were strangely alone, compared to their neighbours: even the northern Eurasian pagans had their weekly Saturday 'washing day'. From the unique Christian perspective, baths and cosmetic care were dangerous, if not an abomination. It was therefore quite impossible for them to adopt any religious code of washing or cosmetic practices, such as those laid down later (and further south) by the prophet Muhammad in the Qur'ān from *c.*AD 625, in which cleanliness was commended as 'one half of the faith'. As in ancient Egypt, and in Persian Zoroastrianism, Islamic washing practices were no light undertaking. First and foremost were the *wudu*, the minor ablutions of the appendages of the body. The *ghusl* (total ablution of the whole body) was performed at certain times and in a certain minimum amount of water that must touch every part and every hair of the body, and usually took place in the *hamam* (plunge pool). The minor *wudu* of the parts was performed five times daily before each of the five prayer sessions, from a water tank or tap. Various other natural practices (*fitrah*) of personal cleanliness were also sanctioned by the Prophet: 'It would seem that filth in

any form was repugnant to Muhammad, particularly to his olfactory sense . . . tradition is insistent in ascribing them to Muhammad.' These *fitrah* included the use of the toothpick, cleansing the
nose and gargling the mouth with water, clipping the ends of
the moustaches, clipping fingernails, cleaning the finger joints,
depilation of the armpits, shaving of the pubic hair, cleaning
with water or dry earth or a piece of stone after evacuation and
urination, washing hands before and after meals, and circumcision (nowhere mentioned in the Qur'ān, but a *fitrah* which
appears in other writings).[34]

In Christian Europe later popes never revised the Church's
somewhat ambiguous teachings on personal cleanliness, with
their prejudices no doubt revived by the diametrically opposed
practices of Islam. They merely discouraged what they saw as
empty bodily rituals—Pope Gregory I ('the Great') was indiffer-
ent as to whether or not menstruating women or unclean men
should be allowed sacrament in church—and focused on inner
mental strength instead, and the cleansing power of the confessional. Nevertheless, most Christians clearly believed in, and
wanted, some liturgical purification rituals; so the Church did
not disallow them, but left them to individual discretion.
A simplified liturgical discipline was maintained through baptism, 'churching' (a month's exclusion from the Church after
birth), not eating meat on Fridays, fasting at Lent, clothing,
feeding, and cleansing the poor on Maundy Thursday; and
diverting the pre-existing rituals of house and body-cleansing
towards the Lord's day (moved from the Judaic Saturday to the
Christian Sunday).

The Healing Mission
But the true mark of Christian self-denial was to give help
continually to others; and, especially, voluntarily to touch and
treat the foul bodies of the sick poor. Jesus had taken up a

healing mission as evidence of his care for all others, even those
beyond his religion's sacred boundaries, while noticeably not
taking a great deal of care of himself, in defiance of Roman
fashion. St Augustine had also felt a charitable Christian love
for the poor and dispossessed. The rising numbers of sick poor,
and those without kin or homes to help them in need—slaves,
soldiers, travellers—were increasingly visible all around the
remotely administered Empire. From these new if barely perceived needs came the development of the last major public
building of the classical world, the only one specifically devoted
to medicine itself, the Roman hospital. The first Roman military
hospitals (*valetudinarium*) started in the first century AD, and set
high standards of medical equipment and architectural design;
but most civilians (and slaves) were treated at home. The first
civilian hospitals appeared after Christianization in the mid-
fourth century AD; there was one in Rome but far more in the
eastern Empire, and in the great Christian capital of Constantinople in the eastern Empire. In Constantinople in AD 388
Olympias turned her wealth over to the Church, and her palace
over to sick poor relief—gardens, bakery, baths and all; while
St John Chrysostom, the charismatic Patriarch of Constantinople, spent most of his revenues on the city's hospitals, thus
earning his later title as one of the Doctors of the Church. By AD
500 a sixteen-volume Galenic canon had been adopted, probably
used in the civic hospitals and monastic infirmaries, with further
well-written compilations in the sixth and seventh centuries
showing evidence of continuing research. By AD 600 Constantinople and Antioch had large hospitals with a total of 600 beds,
divided into male and female wards; three centuries later the
hospital movement continued to flourish within the Islamic
Empire, with hospitals sponsored by wealthy rulers, pious
women, and local citizens.[35] The healing mission was perhaps
the greatest single legacy of the late Roman ascetic Christian
faith.

The monastic Church therefore nurtured the classical medical traditions in western Europe and kept them alive. The Holy Roman Church itself was also very much alive and growing— the barbarian invasions of Roman Europa were closely followed by an evangelical and military campaign of Christian religious conversion. Meanwhile, the Catholic Church of Rome was steadily accruing wealth through its growing monastic lands and labour, at the same time as the well-endowed Orthodox Church based in Constantinople emerged as the standard-bearer of the ancient civilized life. When barbarian or pagan leaders were converted or submitted to Christianity in Europe, what the Church represented to them, above all, was the potential for economic and social development.[36] Later on, they settled down and started producing great artistic and cultural icons of their own. Asceticism was eventually tamed: nowhere had such excellent baths and latrines as the grand medieval monasteries.

chapter 6
medieval morals

From now on we move northwards into western and central Europe to investigate patterns of personal health and hygiene from the medieval period onwards through to what later Europeans triumphantly called the early modern and modern world—finally putting the economic and demographic disasters of the fall of Rome well behind them. The 'civilizing process' that seeped through cash-strapped Europe in these medieval and early modern centuries was in effect the slow escalation of domestic luxuries, spread thinly over more ancient ways of subsistence life—hut life—that endured well into the twentieth century. Apart from the economy, the Church, education, and baths, the greatest single difference in the physical regime of medieval personal hygiene (whether because of tribal history, northern geography, or Christianity) was probably the development of underlinen and the close-fitting tailored garment, either of which can trap the body's evacuations in a layer above the skin, allowing fetid bacterial decomposition to take place; elsewhere in subtropical Eurasia robes and loose clothing remained the norm.

On the face of it, there is every justification for the old-style textbook descriptions of swarming lice and manure-like stenches in medieval life, but the closer you look, the more it seems an exaggeration. Like their biological ancestors medieval people certainly groomed themselves, and—so it seems—a great number of them tried to be as well groomed and clean as it was individually possible to be. They improved their houses and their manners, dressed well, knew their medical regimens, and used baths and cosmetic care. To say that medieval faces, hands, and bodies were always dirty, their clothes tattered and evil-smelling, or that the rushes on the floor were always greasy would be to condemn generations of careful and hardworking medieval housewives, and the honour and dignity of their households.

Using the many available sources from the highly visible European upper ranks to reconstruct post-Roman European domestic life is rather like trying to reconstruct a whole society from 'society' magazines in c.AD 2000—you miss 90 per cent of the population.[1] But even if the very rich were the tip of the iceberg, what they did and had many others would have aspired to. So far as the rich were concerned in c.AD 800, the long 'Romanesque' party had only just begun.

Charlemagne's Courtesie

The manners and customs of Charlemagne's court were part-Frankish, part-Christian, and part-Roman. The strongest influence on the dress and manners of his courtiers was wealthy Christian Byzantium, where ceremonial dress and court etiquette held the eastern Empire together. Charlemagne himself liked to fight and feast with his bards and his family gathered around him, but also relaxed in Roman style. He wore Frankish costume with underlinen, bound leggings, a knee-length tunic, fur jerkin, a long military cloak, and was bearded and moustached; but definitely rejected any tattooing on his body 'like the pagans who obey the notions of the Devil'. Nor did he wear gilded boots with laces 'more than four feet long', scarlet wrappings round his legs, floor-length embroidered tunics, or the new style of bright blue or white (or striped) short cloaks to the waist: 'what is the use of these little napkins? I can't cover myself with them in bed. When I am on horseback I can't protect myself from the winds and the rain. When I go off to empty my bowels, I catch cold because my backside is frozen.' When Charlemagne died in 816, his tutor and lifelong friend Einhard wrote an insider's account of the reign. Among other things he especially noted his great fondness for thermal baths:

> He took delight in steam-baths at the thermal springs, and loved to exercise himself in the water whenever he could. He was an extremely strong swimmer and in this sport no one could surpass him. It was for this reason that he built his palace at Aachen and remained continuously in residence there during the last years of his life and indeed until the moment of his death. He would invite not only his sons to bathe with him, but his nobles and friends as well, and occasionally even a crowd of his attendants and body-guards, so that sometimes a hundred men or more would be in the water together.[2]

Einhard was the architect of Charlemagne's new Romanesque villa palace in Aachen, built next to his Byzantine chapel, and had presumably engineered the link between the palace and the hot springs that archaeologists found later, providing the luxury of heating throughout the building.

A new courtly honour system known as *courtesie* (courtesy) spread rapidly via the Frankish courts throughout northern and southern Europe. Clerical courtly tutors had from the beginning used the Roman canon of educational self-discipline (notably Cicero) to persuade the young offspring of the nobility to curb their barbaric ways, and to inculcate propriety, decorum, temperance, and all the other noble virtues—listed in one medieval encyclopedia as: 'shamefastnesse...trouth...confidence...

suffereance ... stablenesse ... pacience ... devotion ... truthfulness
... benignity ... wisdom ... chastity ... faire speech'. Being 'suave
of speech and manner, courtly in love-making' (with the
accompanying natty dress code) became the fashionable hallmark
of medieval nobility and rank, especially among the young.[3]

Along with courtliness came physical refinement. Early manuscript books on household duties and manners, used for training
table and body servants, covered every possible embarrassing
social situation and breaches of social etiquette; this is where all
the well-known 'abominations' of the medieval body—farting,
sweating, spitting, gobbling, sneezing, slurping, burping, etc.—
are listed.[4] Guest honour rituals like handwashing (*donner à laver*,
offering a wash) at all meals were scrupulously observed; also the
washing of the feet of guests on arrival (practised in both abbeys
and palaces). A whole raft of complex rituals of courteous etiquette (eating etiquette, linen tablecloths, and napkins) radiated
out from the meal table—including the development and use of
cutlery. For many centuries metal and glass was expensive and
utensils were scarce or made of wood. The metal table fork was
introduced into Europe by a Byzantine princess at her wedding in
Venice in 955; everyone else ate with their hands. By the 1500s
only peasants ate with their hands.[5]

The Southern Lands

The Roman Catholic Church's homilies and exhortations on
cleanness were constant throughout these centuries, treading
a fine line between the virtue of civility and the vice of vanity.
Officially, the Church stood as the defender of Roman *civilitas*,
and encouraged civilized ablutions as an obeisance to God; but
excessive grooming 'in the Italian manner' was condemned, as
we see in Notker the Stammerer's cautionary tale for wide-eyed
novice monks of *The Deacon Who Washed Too Much*:

> There was a certain deacon who followed the habits of the Italians
> in that he was perpetually trying to resist nature. He used to take
> baths, he had his head very closely shaved, he polished his skin, he
> cleaned his nails, he had his hair cut short as if it had been turned
> on a lathe, and he wore linen underclothes and a snow-white
> shirt...Just how unclean his heart was became apparent by what
> followed. As he was reading, a spider suddenly came down on its
> thread from the ceiling, touched the deacon's head with its feeler
> and then ran quickly up again...when he came out of the cath-
> edral he began to swell up. Within an hour he was dead.[6]

Nature, in clerical terms, meant your pious inner nature, not your
lowly corporeal self. Baptism and lustral bathing were clerical
duties; and since bathing and cleansing were known to be medically therapeutic, providing hot baths, grooming, and clothes for
the poor was a righteous and pious act.[7] Decent but not lavish
clerical grooming regimens, at fixed hours and at fixed seasons,
were included in all monastic Rules, and laundries were provided,
even though the number of times allowed for 'shifting' the clothing was severely rationed. Most monks were clean-shaven and
carefully tonsured: the wearing of beards was regarded as lowly or
hermit-like. The Church tried very hard to curb public morals and
'the habits of the Italians', but only partially succeeded. The
constant lure of the hot southern lands, and their wicked sensuous ways, was irresistible to the rest of Europe.

Around the Mediterranean, baths, dancing girls, and Roman-
style feasting had continued within Islamic culture. Few northern
courts were as luxurious as the stronghold Norman raiders had
wrested from Arab rulers in southern Italy and Sicily during the
twelfth century, where the energetically self-cultivated Norman
kings Roger I and Roger II spent much of their time enjoying their
Arabic hunting lodges, pleasure pavilions, the hot springs in the
north of the island, and at their new palace at Zisa (meaning
'magnificent' in Arabic). On Christmas Day in 1184 an Arab
observer noted that 'the Christian women all went forth in

robes of gold-embroidered silk, concealed with coloured veils and shod with gilt slippers ... bearing all the adornments of Muslim women, including jewellery, henna on the fingers, and perfumes'.[8] When Roger II conquered Thebes and Corinth in the Peloponnese in 1147, he had carried off all their stock of silk cloth, along with all their craftsmen and looms, to strengthen his conquered Arab cloth industry (which included the silk workshops of the royal harem, the Tiraz, at Palermo—another custom which the Normans had 'appropriated with enthusiasm').[9]

Islam also undoubtedly influenced the twelfth-century courts of Anjou and Aquitaine across the Mediterranean in Provence— a hotbed of 'courtly love' and the sensuous clothing that was the badge of the new romantics. All tribal courts had their poets or bards to entertain them at the feast, and courtly romantic *lais* (lays) from the poets of southern Provence spread northwards and became part of the ideology of chivalry; including the court poets who blossomed in fourteenth-century Middle English.[10] The Middle English poem *Cleanness* conjured up a courtly vision of the Lord of Heaven with his perfectly groomed heavenly hosts, in the form of a long sermon on sexual purity, the 'pearl' of virginity, and keeping the sabbath clean:

> So clean in his court is that king who rules all,
> So upright a householder, so honourably served
> By angels of utter purity without and within,
> Beautifully bright, in brilliant mantles ...

> But watch, if you will, that you wear clean clothes
> To honour the holy day, lest harm come to you
> When you approach the Prince of precious lineage,
> He hates not even hell more hotly than the unclean ...

> They shall see in those shimmering mansions,
> Who are burnished as beryl, bound to be pure,
> Sound on every side, with no seams anywhere,
> Immaculate and moteless like the margery-pearl ...[11]

Beds, sex, baths—and nature—were constantly associated in the literature and imagery of romance. Some of the best-known and best-loved images of medieval art are probably the crimson-embroidered tapestries now at the Musée Cluny, Paris, showing a high-born lady with her unicorn (a symbol of virginal purity) experiensing all the delights of the senses, in a series of flowery woodland glades; and in the same collection, and in the same style, is another tapestry illustrating the sensuous outdoor romanticized courtly bath. Courtly baths frequently made their way into stories and poems in scenes of trickery, transgressions, and lover's trysts. In one French courtly love poem the boiling hot bath prepared for the noble husband was given to the adulterers instead; in the early medieval German poem *Parsival*, the hero was attended by beautiful maidens strewing the floor with rose petals, and given a truly Homeric knightly bath.[12] The twelfth-century Order of the Bath at the Anglo-Norman court was equally romantic and sumptuous: it was created as a lustral bath of purification, signifying their passage into adulthood, for the young elite warriors, the 'companions of the king', and lasted two days with the holy evening vigil, the bath, and the ceremonial knighting, followed by games, sports, and feasts. The English Royal Wardrobe bath accounts in the fourteenth century show large expenditures in which the chivalric bed and clothes cost as much as, if not more than, the chivalric bath. In 1327 King Edward III was knighted, crowned, and bathed at the same time:

> cloth of gold diapered, to cover his Bath for his knighthood, sheets for the same, and washing his feet, a tunic and a cloak of Persian cloth for his vigil, and tunic, cloak, and mantle of purple velvet, with fur lining the same, and red curtains, with shields of his Arms on the corners for ornamenting his chamber on the night before he received the Order of Knighthood.[13]

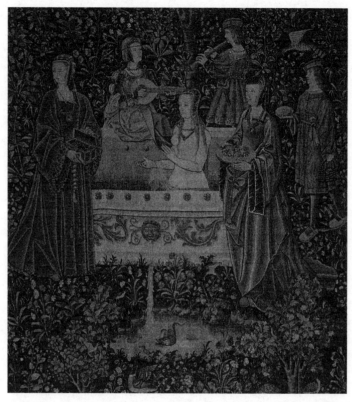

9 Tapestry depicting a heavily romanticized courtly bath in the early 1500s, set in a woodland glade, surrounded by sensuous delights (food, music, sweet smells).

Sicily was an earthly paradise for northerners that did not last. However, the concentration of luxury in the hands of the eager Norman *arrivistes* set off another chain of events that did last. Frankish Palermo had become the foremost centre of Hellenic and Arabic studies and the commercial and cultural clearing house of three continents, drawing traders from around the southern Mediterranean and scholars dispersed from Alexandria. Just across the water on mainland Italy was a small southern spa

town called Salerno, one of Europe's first medical centres of
learning; and the health education that emerged from Salerno
and later universities fully restored the old classical advice on
how to 'take care of yourself'.

The Salerno Regimen

Salerno was originally a Roman coastal health resort and spa,
situated 35 miles south-east of Naples down the coast from
Baiae. In 847 Salerno became the port capital of a new Lombard
principality, and the first Benedictine medical monks arrived.
Over 300 years nine monasteries were established, and Salerno's
three Roman aqueducts were rebuilt, serving a series of public
fountains, the old public bathhouses, and private customers en
route, some with their own private bathhouses; including the
nunnery of San Giorgio, and the bathhouse of the male monastery of Santa Sofia, a large establishment with furnaces and
bronze cauldrons and a cold pool, open to all monks, nuns,
and visiting clergy that might need them.[14] Salerno became
renowned for its healing facilities, and, being a port town,
treated many damaged, health-seeking travellers, traders, and
passing soldiers. By the twelfth century the medical School of
Salerno had reached a peak of literary activity, finding and
translating into Latin the works of Hippocrates, Galen, and
the Alexandrian and Arabic schools, and compiling a new
canon of medical authorities known as the *Articella* ('Little Art
of Medicine'). In addition, the Salerno translation of the plan-
tlore of Dioscorides provided the foundation for later European
herbals; the *Trotula* corpus helped to preserve what remained of
classical cosmetics; while the so-called *Regimen Sanitatis Salernitanum* became the most famous health text of the Middle
Ages. But by the end of the thirteenth century Salerno had
become a backwater. Islamic centres of learning such as those
in Baghdad, Cairo, or Córdoba in Spain, along with university

foundations in Padua, Bologna, Montpellier, Paris, and Oxford, had dispersed intellectual talent throughout Europe.[15]

The new universities fed the early medieval 'Romanesque' enthusiasm for literacy, culture, and self-improvement. The message of the health-conscious regimen was strongly promoted by the new university-trained *medici*, supported by Romano-Islamic classical scholarship such as that of the comprehensive, easy-to-memorize, four-volume *Canon of Medicine* by Ibn Sina (Avicenna; 980–1037). The physicians were eager to get classical preventive medicine on board alongside their other 'cures', and profited well from it: their personally tailored regimens and *consilia* (letters of advice) were available to anyone who could afford them. Throughout Europe there were growing numbers of manuscript tracts and volumes for general readers on all subjects religious and secular—and roughly 3 to 4 per cent of these were medical works.[16] Evidently one had to be 'wise in science' at court. Encyclopedic 'books of secrets' (such as the famous *Aristotle's Secrets*) could be read or memorized in short bursts, as well as being an invitation to further study:

> Therefore it is worth that your mekeness have this present boke in the which of all science some profite is conteyned... and in parcell speke couertly [courtly], he made this boke spekying by apparances, examples and signes, techying outward, by littrature, philosophik and phisick doctrine, pertenying unto lordes for kepying of the helth of their bodies, and unto ineffabill profite in knowlechyng of the hevenly bodies.[17]

In England the earliest medical manuscripts, the old Anglo-Saxon 'leech books', were collections of folkloric receipts overlaid with traces of Graeco-Roman medicine; but from the eleventh century onwards the ancient courtly tradition of wise longevity and medical advice to rulers was revived and repackaged in a genre known to us as 'Mirrors of Princes', with titles such as 'The Mirror of Health' or 'Regiment for Princes', largely

based on Galenic dietary advice. More rare and expensive
were the hand-painted dietary tacuinums derived from Arabic
humoral medicine—medical calendars on large vellum pages,
similar to the well-known 'Books of Hours', painted with
brightly coloured and gilded courtly pictures of the correct
monthly regimes for food, drink, and 'the six non-naturals:
'the six things which are needed by every man for the preservation of his health, about their exact use and effects . . . we shall
insert all these elements into simple tables because the discussions of sages and the discordances of many different books may
bore the reader'.[18]

The *Regimen Sanitatis Salernitanum* typified the genre of small
popular books that became simply known as 'regimens'—the
basis of public health education for the next eight centuries.
With 240 different editions by 1846, the first 'Salerno' Regimen
was written (or copied from Arab sources) in Spain in the late
twelfth century, and was gradually extended into a jocular health
poem, with up to 363 verses. It steadily progressed through the
dietetic imbalances of each Galenic humour, matching them
with their opposite therapies. These consisted almost entirely of
endless varieties of foods (including herbs) and drinks, with their
qualities enhanced by cooking and spicing: light foods versus
heavy foods, hot foods to counter cold diseases, cold foods to
counter hot diseases. All extremes of intake were condemned as
gluttonous and weakening, and any humoral 'plethora' (excess)
was relieved by bleeding, baths, and exercise.

It was via these regimens that the morning grooming session
was institutionalized in medieval life. The morning regimen in
the Salerno Regimen (and all other later regimens) was always
the most elaborate: firstly, wake at the proper hour (not too
much or too little sleep, with more sleep in the winter than in
the summer); secondly, clear the evacuations by getting rid of
the waste products (going to stool), by clearing the nose, throat,
and mouth (sneezing, coughing, spitting, sighing, singing).

Then cleanse the night residue from the eyes, face, hands, and limbs (by washing and sluicing, or dry-rubbing with cloths) and clean the residue from the teeth (by rubbing them with cloth, sage, or other aromatic leaves, or by picking them with resinous wood twigs). Applying scented fumigations and perfumed ointments could also stimulate the body and 'gladden the spirit'—an important point, from the medieval perspective. It was correct to take a little light exercise in the morning until lethargy was dispersed, the heavy vapours released, and the stomach prepared to digest a moderate breakfast (the main meal being shortly after noon, with a second main meal at the end of the day). In the Salerno Regimen itself, 'Grasse, Glasse, and Fountains', seems to be a direct reference to spa therapy:

> Rise early in the morne, and straight remember,
> With water cold to wash your hands and eyes,
> And to refresh your brain when as you rise,
> In heat, in cold, in July and December.
> Both comb your head and rub your teeth likewise:
> If bled you have, keep coole, if bath keepe warm:
> If din'd, to stand or walke will do no harm
> Three things preserve the sight, Grasse, Glasse, & Fountains,
> At eve'n springs, at morning visit mountains.[19]

But even in merrymaking temperance should always prevail: 'wine, women, Baths, by Art of Nature warme, us'd or abus'd do men much good or harme'. After the Black Death in 1348, manuscript health advice poured onto the market, going well beyond the range of the Salerno prototype: 'little books' of health regimens for plague, pregnancy, childcare, travel, sea voyages, or army campaigns.[20] In late medieval England at least six regimens or 'dietaries' were regularly copied out, including *Lydgate's Dietary* and *John of Burgundy's Regimen*, of which there are nearly fifty surviving copies.[21]

Grooming Zones

In the 700 years between *c.*800 and 1500 the urge for constant domestic improvement is visible in the steady separation and multiplication of spaces—something we now recognize as a sign of increased personal refinement. For families that had achieved that extra economic margin, rooms were added, others were divided, second storeys added, window-bays and chimneys invented, and 'dirty' service areas separated and put out of sight, usually in outdoor yards or courts. From the eighth century onwards water engineering had become an architectural essential for the wealthy and self-confident church foundations. Monasteries had rows of latrines, their *lavatoria* (washrooms) were large, and they often handed on their considerable expertise to the local nobility, or town councils.[22] Where money and expensive stonework was no object, external drop-latrines with indoor seating were loved for their convenience and were installed in most newbuilt castles (even the most isolated knightly residence in Wales in the 1450s required an indoor latrine for its guest bedrooms); larger castles had up to twenty latrines, sometimes arranged as threeand four-seaters. England's King Edward III (1327–77) had hot and cold running water installed in two of his palaces.[23] For the rest of the population, stone-built conduits and drop-latrines were rare, and the old dry sewage system sufficed. In the country, cesspits and middens were relatively easy to manage; in town they had to be regularly emptied and scavenged by the local authority.[24]

Inside the medieval bedroom the 'close-stool' discreetly enclosed the evacuations, while the simple 'jerry' was pushed underneath the bed. It was also at this time that the fixed stone washbasin, or *laver*, with a can of water hanging above it and a cloth hanging by, reappeared as a common domestic fixture; along with the portable washstand; and the portable wooden bathtub made from a sawn half-cask, lined with linen cloth, possibly with a richer fabric draped over an iron hoop above, making a draught-free private enclosure, or private grooming zone. The new enclosed bed recesses, or personal *garderobes* (dressing closets), were like the new bay-window recesses that became popular in many chateaux—they both created a separated intimate space. Two chambers, a *garderobe*, a private oratory, a study closet, and a 'generous provision of latrines' was the ideal *logis*, or private suite, in late fourteenth-century France.[25]

Most grooming would have taken place on or near the bed, wherever it was situated. The bed was usually the focal point of the main living room on the ground floor; but if the household was really wealthy, it would be in a chamber above. The bed was easily the largest display piece in the medieval house, a major item of expenditure, and was usually lifted up on a dais, with heavy curtain drapes that were as much to display the cloth as for privacy or keeping out draughts. Following Roman precursors, many types of tall wooden furniture were developed in Europe—stools, benches, chairs, tables, sideboards, and cupboards, in a proliferation of styles—which lifted the body and other objects high off the floor and away from the dirty or dusty surfaces below.[26] Wooden floors in upper storeys and bedchambers could be covered with straw matting or rugs; ground floors were kept strewn with hay, rushes, sand, or other absorbent materials—although with more funds, more resources, you could have a stone, wood, or tiled floor, as many wealthier households did.

Cloth was one of the great new staple trades of Europe, and medieval culture is inconceivable without it. More work now went into one piece of cloth, ornamented with deep dyes, precious stones, and minute embroidery, than ever before. For the housewife pure white linen was one of the most coveted luxury domestic products, requiring yet more careful preserving and cleaning. In Christine de Pizan's sermon for laywomen *The Treasure of the City of Ladies* (1405), virtuous women should have fine wide cloth, tablecloths, napkins and other linen made. She will be most painstaking about this, for it is the natural pleasure of women [to be] not odious and sluttish, but upright and proper... she will have very fine linen—delicate, generously embroidered and well-made... [and] will keep it white and sweet smelling, neatly folded in a chest; she will be most conscientious about this. She will use it to serve the important people that her husband brings home, by whom she will be greatly esteemed, honoured, and praised.[27]

Underlinen was now standard. During the Roman Empire, Tacitus had noted that the 'wild tribes' of Germania thought it 'a mark of great wealth to wear undergarments'; only a few centuries later linen garments were worn more or less regardless of social rank—linen shirts, gowns (cottes), leggings, trousers (braises), caps (coifs), and veils—even if there was no expensive outer cloth to go over them. The only time linen was not worn was at night.[28] If the grooming was good, and the underlinen regularly 'shifted', the vermin and dirt load would be significantly reduced, and could be controlled.

'Shifting' linen was obviously not a problem for anyone of high rank: Edward IV's court accounts show regular money given for the 'lavender-man' (the launderer or washing-man) to obtain 'sweet flowers and roots to make the king's gowns and sheets brethe more wholesomely and delectable'. But shifting his shirt and picking out vermin from the seams of his clothes was a major chore for the poor student Thomas Platter, in Germany in 1499: 'you cannot imagine how the scholars young and old, as well as some of the common people, crawled with vermin... Often, particularly in the summer, I used to go and wash my shirt on the banks of the Oder... whilst it dried I cleaned my clothes. I dug a hole, threw in a pile of vermin, filled it in, and planted a cross on top.' Delousing was more usually done by wives, mothers, and intimates in the slow leisured hours—something that perhaps Platter, like other urban scholars and apprentices, had left behind with his faraway family. A rare description of delousing customs in the French village of Montaillou was fleetingly captured in a fourteenth-century Inquisition testimonial:

> Pierre Clergue had himself deloused by his mistresses . . . the operation might take place in bed, or by the fire, at the window or on a shoemaker's bench . . . Raymonde Guilhou also deloused the priest's mother, wife of old Pons Clergue, in full view of everybody in the doorway of the 'ostal', retailing the latest gossip as she did so. The Clergues, as leading citizens, had no difficulty in finding women to relieve them of their insect life . . . [29]

Delousing was rarely recorded as minutely as that. A single fifteenth-century manuscript shows a well-dressed older woman brushing the downturned head of a young man outside in a garden with a large hand-brush, with the lice flying into a bowl he is holding. In one medieval romance a nobleman enters the damsel's chamber and removes his shirt so that they can scratch him with combs made of wood, bone, and ivory 'with two rows of teeth', and brush his hair with their 'small brooms'. It seems that the privacy of this sort of bedroom activity was well respected; a well-known passage from the fourteenth-century bourgeois classic *The Menagier's Wife* gives some timeless advice:

> Whereof cherish the person of your husband carefully, and, I pray you, keep him in clean linen, for 'tis your business . . . and nothing harms him because he is upheld by the hope he has in his wife's care of him on his return . . . to have his shoes removed before a good fire, his feet washed and to have fresh shoes and stockings, to be given good food and drink, to be well served and well looked after, well bedded in white sheets and nightcaps, well covered with good furs, and assuaged with other joys and amusements, privities, loves, and secrets, concerning which I am silent; and on the next day fresh shirts and garments. Certes, fair sister, such service

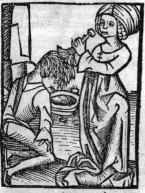

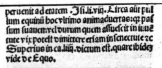

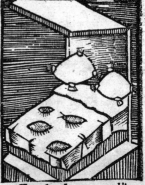

10 Bedbugs and head lice—a rare illustration of these ubiquitous bugs from the medieval encyclopedia *Hortatus Sanitatis*.

maketh a man love and desire to return to his home and to see his goodwife and to be distant with other women.[30]

The Trotula Corpus

It has long been thought that Trotula was a woman physician working in Salerno who wrote a famous book on cosmetics; but recent detective work has proved that this was a myth perpetuated in the 1544 edition by a humanist doctor, Georg Kraut. Like so many medieval popular works, the corpus of work known as *The Trotula* was compiled by many different hands. During the twelfth century in Salerno two scholarly tracts, *Treatise on the Diseases of Women* and *On the Conditions of*

Women, were bound together with a more practical and com-mercial compilation called *Treatments for Women* and what may have been a local Salernitan classic, a detailed tract called *Cos-metics for Women*. Just to clear up a confusion which has long existed, until 1544 the first two were called *Trotula Major* and the second two, *Trotula Minor*; but both were pillaged and adapted in various ways, with a surge of editions in the four-teenth century, including pocket-sized vernacular translations into almost all European languages. Two further treatises (*De Ornatu Mulierum*, and *De Decorationibus Mulierum*) were trans-formed into the highly popular *Ornement des dames* ('Adorn-ment of Women').[31]

The Galenic, Alexandrian, Methodist, and Arab techniques found in European cosmetic literature were pale reflections of the knowledge available in the Arab Empire, where cosmetic treatments were well respected. Al-Razi (Rhazes; 841–924), Ibn Zuhr (Avenzoar; 1091–1161), Avicenna, and many others drew on a technical revolution in Arabic chemistry that included mastering the art of distillation, with obvious uses in per-fumery and medicines, and the incorporation of exotic herbs, vegetables, minerals, and spices from the Middle East, India, China, and South-East Asian trade routes.[32] Women had long practised practical medicine of the sort that kept men and women alive, without benefit of literacy; but from this time onwards, following the introduction of university-based med-ical licensing (and given the Christian injunction for women to 'be silent'), practical domestic medicine goes to ground and the historical record does indeed fall silent—certainly when compared to the new socially stratified public world of the male *medici*.[33] In fact 'women's medicine' was neither particu-larly hidden nor 'impenetrable' to most people in the semi-literate medieval period; indeed it could be said to have been in its heyday. What we have in the *Trotula* manuscripts is a brief snapshot of the private domain of the bedroom, where women traditionally ruled, ministered, and suffered, and men submitted (a truth that Christian male authors were loath to admit). For any historian of dermatology and COBS grooming, they are a bright light shone on previously hidden practices, and the remains of classical cosmetic lore.

It is interesting to see just how thorough COBS practical medicine could be. All of the *Trotula* texts dealt with internal female gynaecological problems (the menses, childbirth obstetrics, womb disorders, infertility) as well as external skin disorders, and skin 'adornments'. Slicing, picking, or abrading the skin to clean out 'simple wounds and apostemes' were part of the cosmetic art; while other, internal complaints were approached through the orifices requiring major and lengthy medical operations, but without any deep cutting through the skin into the body—which was obviously considered far more dangerous and not to be undertaken lightly, i.e. not without sufficient knowledge. One example from *On the Conditions of Women*, showing what could be done manually for the wandering or 'dropped' womb after childbirth, suggests fumigation of the nose and vagina with aromatic spices, giving warm bitter drinks, oiling and warming the navel prior to manipulating the womb 'to the place from which it was shaken', followed by baths and steam baths:

> Afterward, let the woman enter water in which there have been cooked pomegranates, roses, oak apples, sumac, bilberries, the fruit, leaves and bark of oak, and juniper nuts, and lentils. Then let there be made a steambath, which works very well. For Dioscorides prescribes that there be made for them a steambath of boxwood placed in a pot upon live coals, and let the woman, covered on top, sit on it, and let her receive the smoke inside.[34]

A dropped womb was a medical emergency; but even begetting a child could be a severe personal problem, for which infertile women traditionally sought treatment at temples, holy wells, and spas. Enhanced attractiveness, using 'beauty' recipes for seduction, was a tried and test method; but intimate knowledge of the workings of the womb, vagina, and genitalia led naturally to treatment of the problems of intercourse—including sexual hygiene. One particular *Trotula* treatment (suppressed in later editions) dealt with severe and unpleasant vaginal odours: 'There are some women who because of the magnitude of their instrument and its severe odour are sometimes found unpleasant and unsuitable for intercourse.' The practical remedy was to constrict the vagina with a scented astringent wash, prior to intercourse, and to apply a sweet powder to her chest, breasts, and genitalia, as well as washing her partner's genitals and drying them with a cloth sprinkled with the same powder.[35] For women 'in whom pieces of flesh hang from the womb... note that this happens to them from semen retained inside and congealed, because they do not clean themselves after intercourse. These women we always foment with a decoction of hot herbs.' It is probable that this type of practical sex-medicine went into the barber's (and surgeon's) trade, but no higher; in the eighteenth century the treatment of sexual disease (venereology) was a hidden or 'quack' male medical specialism, albeit with a high-class clientele.[36]

Note the assumption that women should clean themselves after intercourse. Note too the application of complementary remedies to men. There was no apparent gender divide in the treatment of external skin disorders on the other, more neutral parts—the hair, face, hands, eyes, ears, feet, breath ('stench of the mouth'), or underarms:

> For lice which arise in the pubic area and armpits, we mix ashes with oil and anoint. And for lice which are around the eyes, we should make an ointment suitable for expelling them and for swelling of the eyes and soothing them... For scabies of the hips and other parts, a very good ointment. Take elecampane, vinegar, quicksilver, as much oil as you like, and animal grease....[37]

Bad breath, bad odours, lice, spots, swellings, or genital problems were of course never gender-specific; and skin salves were
urgently required for the victims of the endemic and epidemic
outbreaks of diseases that gathered pace from the twelfth century onwards. Vast quantities of herbs, oils, minerals, and spices
were thrown at the very visible symptoms, making barbers and
apothecaries rich in the process. A whole battery of cosmetic
medicaments anointed King Edward I of England's body the
year before his death in 1307: '282 lbs of electuaries; 106 lbs of
white powder; ointments, gums, oils, turpentine; aromatics for
the bath; a special electuary containing ambergris, musk, pearls,
gums. Gold and silver medicated wines; a plaster for the king's
neck; a drying ointment for his legs and more for anointing his
body'.[38]

The *Trotula* texts made the basic assumption that women
readers would wish to 'cleanse themselves of all impurities'
and were repulsed by all sordidness, and gave large numbers of
recipes for the 'clarification' of the skin, especially the face,
neck, hands, and breasts. The ideal complexion was red and
white, with healthy red gums and lips, white teeth and skin,
and clear eyes; the hair could be dyed black or blonde, and was
combed through frequently with perfumed powders or waters.
But *On Women's Cosmetics*, which had a very authentic southern
classical Arab flavour, started with the old full-body make-
over—total depilation:

> In order that a woman might become very soft and smooth and
> without hairs from the head down, first of all let her go into the
> baths, and if she is accustomed to do so, let there be made for a
> steambath in this manner, [just like women beyond the Alps]. Take
> burning tiles and stones, and with these placed in the steambath, let
> the woman sit in it. Or... place them in a pit made in the earth. Then
> let hot water be poured in so that steam is produced, and let the
> woman sit upon it well covered with cloths so that she sweats. And
> when she has well sweated, let her enter hot water and wash herself

very well, and thus let her exit from the bath and wipe herself off well with a linen cloth. Afterwards let her also anoint herself all over with this depilatory which is made from well-sifted quick-lime [a cooked recipe of 'leaves of squirting cucumber', almond milk, quicklime, orpiment, galbanum, oil, and quicksilver, perfumed with the powders of mastic, frankincense, cinnamon, nutmeg, and clove] . . . Take care, however, that it is not cooked too much, and that it not stay too long on the skin, because it causes intense heat. But if it happens that the skin is burned from this depilatory, take *populeon* with rose or violet oil or with the juice of houseleek, and mix them until the heat is sedated.

This was followed by a lukewarm bran bath, and another anointment with henna and whites of eggs: 'This smoothes the flesh, and if any burn should happen from the depilatory, this removes it and renders it clear and smooth . . . Then let her rinse herself with warm water, and finally with a very whiten linen cloth wrapped around her, let her go to bed.'[39]

Body depilation was a day-long job; the facial depilatories were put on with a spatula for an hour; the facial compresses overnight. The face-whitening oils with white powders or white lead were for daytime use, with the rouging of lips and cheeks to 'make red a whitened face'. Saracen women often 'dyed their faces' by mixing the two—'a most beautiful colour appears, combining red and white'—to make a pink day cream. This particular tract continued with advice for stinking breath from putrid gums, fissures of the lips, facial abscesses; and a vaginal constrictor 'so that a woman who has been corrupted might be thought to be a virgin', in the form of a powder that also helped check nosebleeds and excessive menstrual flow.

It was a very short step indeed from medical treatment to beauty treatment; from infection to disfigurement—'veins in the face', or 'freckles of the face', or 'removing redness of the face'. It was not one that any Arab (or indeed Indian) physician would have thought worth considering; but Christian Europe had brought its own particular ascetic philosophy to the study of the cosmetic art and craft. The French surgeon Henri de Mondeville (1260–1325) was one of the first to take a high moral tone, in print, about cosmetic care: 'It goes against God and righteousness; it is not ordinarily the treatment of an illness, but something that goes outside of this with the intention of concealment or disguise.' His pupil Guy de Chauliac (1300–68) went further and confined surgical cosmetic care only to serious disorders and defects of the skin, in his influential textbook *Chirurgia Magna* (1363).[40] Post-Black Death medical licensing, followed by development of the medical guild system, formally drew the line between the university-educated surgeons and craft-trained barbers, and the cosmetic corpus itself underwent a subtle transformation. The professional aspects of gynaecology and cosmetics were emphasized—'the address to female readers was one of the first elements to go'—and the later *Trotula* manuscripts, it seems, were more often owned by barber–surgeons, and noble households, than noble women. Gradually, barbering and cosmetic work was taken out of surgery. By the sixteenth century the detailed sections on cosmetics given by earlier medieval authorities were deemed 'unnecessary', and after Kraut no further editions of the *Trotula* were required.[41] It was a long process. The ordinary general-purpose barber–surgeon would not willingly dispense with such a lucrative trade, especially one so close to the domestic hearth; for as even de Mondeville had admitted, 'the favour of women cannot be overestimated. Without it one comes to nothing; without it no one can obtain the goodwill of the men . . . '.

Medical licensing could easily create public resentment if it too severely limited the supply of available healers, or did not reflect the true nature of public demand. Wherever licensing figures are available, it appears that it was the lower-rank practical medical crafts that were highest in public esteem. Licensed medical craftsmen not only had private clients, but could also open up street shops (as in many parts of the world today) that thrived as urban residency increased. In the region of Valencia between 1325 and 1334, just over a half of all practitioners were barbers and apothecaries, in equal numbers; in other cities, all-purpose barber–surgeons made up the bedrock of medical care, and university-trained (theoretical) physicians were always in a distinct minority.[42] Even after the Christian conquest of Spain many Muslim doctors continued to practise, got their licences, and were used by Christian and Muslim families; and among them were the traditional Muslim *metgesses*, women doctors known to be expert at treating eyes, hands, feet, and other parts, presumably in the manner of the *Trotula*. The 1329 Valencian law excluding women from medical practice should have hit them hard; but because of their popularity (and possibly their rich clientele) they frequently appear to have escaped prosecution, at least at first.[43] But the loss of professional prestige eventually affected European cosmetics more permanently. Many of the finer therapeutic details of the classical œuvre must have disappeared at street level—especially, perhaps, the care of the private parts, and the skilful use of massage. Cosmetic care (barbering) became a commercial male craft occupation supported by craft apprenticeship, oral tradition, and random sources of expert knowledge (often tucked at the back of surgeons' handbooks). Women, who had no access to male barber's shops or formal education, eventually resorted to collecting, and often publishing, their own books of receipts and sharing them around their friends and family circle. These became incorporated into the well-known receipt book genre that included all housewifery receipts, which lasted well into the late eighteenth century until it was superseded by mass-produced advice literature.

In practical terms the professional demotion of cosmetics may have had fewer repercussions in domestic medicine than we might think, certainly in the medieval period. For example,

it hardly dented the popularity of baths; indeed the casual
reference to the old Neolithic steam pit shows how easily such
a sweat bath could be set up on a patch of land, and how
ubiquitous they may have been. The great numbers of different
references to baths throughout the medieval sources show they
obviously held a special place in medieval life socially, medically, and spiritually. The public baths, in particular, show even
more clearly how baths still represented all the old antique
pleasures of water, and were genuine communal occasions.
From the ninth to the sixteenth century the public hot bathhouses—the 'stews' and the *thermae*—were a large and well-run
leisure industry.

The Public Baths

We can view the medieval baths culture of northern Europe as
being similar to the bathhouse culture of Japan or Finland: it
was innocent of any shame. No one blushes for their nakedness
in the communal baths and saunas of Japan or Finland. No one
blushed in ancient Germany, where, as Julius Caesar noted,
'both sexes bathe communally in rivers, and display the body
mostly naked under small covers of animal hides'. Nor in
medieval Europe, where communal naked bathing, and the
segregation of the sexes, was only suppressed with difficulty,
if at all. Some purity rules in Church law were apparently
widely observed, but it evidently failed to change earlier tribal,
or customary, laws concerning sexual rights over the body.
Regular puritanical attacks on traditional spring carnivals,
town brothel-keeping, and communal bathing—in other
words against fornication, nakedness, lewd clothing, and
baths—seem to have been largely ignored until the sixteenth
century. The Church edict of Boniface in 745 forbade joint
bathing between the sexes, and a later edict made it a sin to be
confessed. An eleventh-century Church Correction Book states:

'Hast thou washed thyself in the bath with thy wife and other women and seen them nude, and they thee? If thou hast, thou shouldst fast for three days on bread and water.' But it was not a grievous sin. Much more common was the use of the Church fine; a typical fine for bathing infringements (such as coming into church straight from the bath improperly dressed 'with naked legs') could take the form of a pound of wax for the church candles.

Virtually all commentators, approving or disapproving, agreed on the essential innocence of the free manners of the public baths. Some even saw nakedness as a natural right. In one imaginary peasant utopia (bearing some resemblance to the painter Hieronymus Bosch's visionary *Garden of Delights*) every-one would be 'totally free' of all restrictions, including clothes:

> Neither skirts nor cloaks are needed there,
> Nor shirts, nor pants at any time:
> They all go naked, modest maids and stable boys.
> There is neither heat nor cold at any time.
> Everybody sees and touches the others as much as he desires:
> Oh what a happy life, oh what a good time... [44]

Defending communal bathing later in the sixteenth century, Ulrich von Hutten said 'Yes, they touch one another in friendly fashion [but] nowhere can you see women's honour more clearly than with these people who don't regulate it. Nowhere is honour stronger than here... They trust one another and live in good faith free and humbly without deception.' Numer-ous prohibitive regulations in Germany about naked legs in the street were constantly resisted, according to Wilhelm Rudeck's classic *History of Public Morality in Germany* (1905). There was a slow move towards the separation of the sexes in French baths during the fourteenth and fifteenth centuries, with some towns adopting it up to a century later than others, but even then 'it was never in practice universal'. [45]

There were twenty-six guild-run bathhouses in Paris in 1292 (probably an underestimate, just as the supposedly 200 baths in the town of Ulm were probably an overestimate). In Finland, Sweden, Russia, and Germany every village had its bathhouse. The concentration of the old sweat hut tradition in the colder parts of Europe is explained (as in Japan) by their heating qualities: the colder the region, the more their extreme heat thawed out the body (and allowed the wearing of lighter clothes). And the heat that they got up and the fuel that they used (as the Romans also understood) was too valuable to waste on individuals. Family sweat rooms weren't so difficult to achieve. The original bathhouse of central Europe was centred on the house's stove, where the hot bread ovens were tapped by a tube that carried steam into an adjoining room; and in towns, the bakeries performed the same functions.[46] The many sixteenth-century etchings we have of one-room communal baths in Germany seem to show not only a steam but a hot-tub culture, with many little tubs scattered across the floor, used for different purposes; but there must have been a good heat got up in one wood-panelled room illustrated by Dürer, with a tall ceramic stove, and bathers of all ages lounging naked except for their decorative jewellery and their ornate bath caps.[47] Such communal scenes were replicated throughout northern Europe for centuries afterwards, as witnessed by the nineteenth-century French traveller Paul du Chaillu, at a 'Saturday bath' in an isolated village in Finland:

> There was a crowd of visitors, neighbours of different ages, and among them three old fellows—a grandfather, father, and an uncle—who were sitting upon one of the benches minus a particle of clothing, shaving themselves without a looking-glass. Nobody seemed to mind them, for the women were knitting, weaving and chatting... When the men finished shaving, clean shirts were brought, and then they dressed themselves while seated. The men usually shave once a week, and always after the bath [every

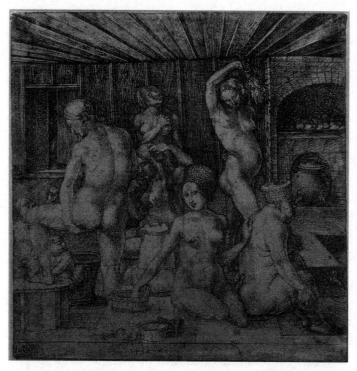

11 *The Women's Bathhouse* (*c*.1496), by Albrecht Dürer, a companion-piece
to his etching *The Men's Bathhouse*—vividly realistic examples from the
fifteenth–century German genre of public bathhouse scenes.

Saturday], for the beard then becomes soft . . . The custom described
has come down from olden times; the Norsemen called Saturday,
Laudag (washing day) . . . at present *Loerdag*, but it is now chiefly
observed in the [northern] regions of Scandinavia . . . [48]

This customary Saturday bath that was so widespread in various regions of Europe cleaned off the sweat and grime once a
week. It was something any respectable Christian citizen might
care to do prior to a holy day, and also fitted the religious calendar of Jewish communities. A seventeenth-century (clerical)

eyewitness account of the Saturday bath from Basel in Switzerland shows just how medieval villagers had brought their
homely habits into the towns:

> In the morning the bath-keeper gave a horn blow, that everything
> is ready. Then the members of the lower classes [and] polite citizens
> undressed in the house and walked naked across the public road to
> the bath-house...Yes, how often the father runs naked from the
> house with a single shirt together with his equally naked wife and
> naked children to the bath. How often I can see (that is why I do
> not go through the town) little girls of 10, 12, 14, 16, 18 years,
> completely undressed, except for a short linen bath-coat (*badehr*)
> often torn...They run along the roads at lunchtime, to the baths.
> And alongside them the totally naked 10, 12, 14, 16, and 18 year-
> old boys, accompanying these respectable young women.[49]

There were other family and kin celebrations that the Church
also found it hard to control or outlaw, despite the fact that
other ancient festivals had been incorporated into the festive
Church 'holidays'. The large numbers of accounts of lying-in
baths, marriage baths, and spring carnival baths seem rather to
fit earlier customs connected with the rites of Venus (or any
other local fertility goddess). They were the bath feasts, the bath
parties that slotted naturally into the bathing calendar.

Bath Feasts

Prenuptial marriage baths and feasts are a worldwide phenomenon, roughly equivalent to our hen nights and stag nights. In
Europe they survived well into the twentieth century in Russia,
Turkey, and elsewhere.[50] In medieval Scandinavia the bridal party
was given in the communal hot bathhouse, to which the bride
and her female friends would walk in procession, preceded by
men carrying jars of ale or wine, bread, sugar, and spices. The
guests wore elaborate clothes and jewellery and received bathing
hats and bathrobes from their hosts, but disrobing was common

among 'the young men who come with naked legs, and dance in that attire'. By the sixteenth century, European marriage baths had become so expensive that some local authorities imposed restrictions, saying that young couples could not afford them. The lying-in bath was supposed to be more modest and intimate—but not if the lying-in was expensive, like the one Christine de Pizan visited in a rich merchant's house in Paris:

> In this bed lay the woman who was going to give birth, dressed in crimson silk cloth and propped up on pillows of the same silk with big pearl buttons, adorned like a young lady. And God knows how much money was wasted on the amusements, bathing and various social gatherings, according to the customs of Paris for women in childbed (some more than others), at this lying-in![51]

The lying-in bath (like the American 'baby shower') would have been hosted by the woman herself, for her female friends, her 'gossips': in fact her bath companions, since (judging from stories and woodcuts) women apparently did a great deal of socializing in the baths, and often held impromptu parties there, bringing their food and drink with them. The Italian, French, Portuguese, English, and Hungarian natural *thermae* were in full swing during this period, and in many if not most of them, the situation would have been similar to those described in the thermal town of Baden in 1416, with its two central public baths and twenty-eight private baths:

> In some of the private baths, the men mix promiscuously with their female relatives and friends. They go into the water three or four times every day; and they spend the greater part of their time in the baths, where they amuse themselves with singing, drinking, and dancing. In the shallower part of the water, they also play upon the harp. It is a pleasant sight to see young lasses tuning their lyres, like nymphs, with their scanty robes floating on the surface of the waters. They look indeed like so many Venuses, emerging from the ocean . . . The men wear only a pair of drawers. The women are clad

in linen vests, which are however slashed in the sides so that they neither cover the neck, the breast, nor the arms of the wearer... every one has free access to all the baths, to see the company, to talk and joke with them. As the ladies go in and out of the water, they expose to view a considerable portion of their persons; yet there are no doorkeepers, nor do they entertain the least idea of any thing approaching to indelicacy.[52]

Diplomatic Baths

The most expensive bath parties of all were held in royal or aristocratic circles, in private bath suites and *thermae*. Charlemagne had held court in the *thermae* at his palace at Aachen, with his advisers and kin sitting around him, up to their necks in hot water. He had deliberately rebuilt the spring for communal bathing; as local legend later had it: 'At his sole expense immense basins were dug... these baths were open to the indiscriminate use of persons of all classes, and he himself frequently displayed his skill in swimming before his court and a numerous concourse of spectators.'[53] Most European hot springs were probably never abandoned locally, regardless of whether or not they attracted the attention of the current rulers, and they began to be developed by local kings in this period, as at Bath, which was supposedly reopened by King Bladud around 800. In Budapest the hot baths were founded by the first king of Hungary, King Stephen, in 1015–27. Aachen (Aquisgranum, now Aix-la-Chapelle) had been developed by the Romans, who had found the hot springs of the area much in use by local tribes such as the Mattiaci, who also settled around the hot springs of Wiesbaden, a few hundred miles down the Rhine valley (a substantial Frankish villa was found in Wiesbaden). In Wiesbaden the hot-water rights were much fought over from 496 onwards, but were eventually claimed by the dukes of Austria. Overlords also of course owned the many cold mineral springs and local holy wells where people were 'dipped' rather than bathed; as overlords even the Church could be the proprietors of locally valued hot springs, as they were in Bad Kreuth in Switzerland, or at the Bagni de Vignoli in Italy, where a papal palace was built. Direct ownership of a town bathhouse was a valuable asset, handed down from father to son; wealthy highborn proprietors usually gave it over to another family to manage on franchise, charging them an annual rent, with strict regulations concerning cleanliness and orderliness.[54]

The overlords were clearly mixing pleasure with politics, and by the early fifteenth century, diplomatic bath feasts were in full swing. In 1446 the bathing arrangements in the Grand Palace of the duke of Burgundy, at Bruges, were overhauled and renewed for the wedding of Charles the Bold and Margaret of York. Steam rooms and barber's shops were provided for the duke and his guests, but the star attraction was a great bathing basin (probably a cauldron made of metal, like the one in the Salerno monastery) brought to Bruges from Valenciennes by canal; this bath was so large that a hole had to be made in the wall of the palace to accommodate it.[55] Essentially, many of these aristocratic bath feasts were used for political purposes, and for the ostentatious display that accompanied them. The accounts of Philip the Good show how he used them to give important guests a good time. Throughout December 1462 the duke gave several banquets in the baths at his palace for most of the local nobility, including one for the ambassadors of the wealthy duke of Bavaria and the count of Württemburg, where he 'had five meat dishes prepared to regale himself at the baths'. Philippe de Bourgogne hired both the bathhouse and its prostitutes at Valenciennes, 'in honour of the English ambassador who was paying him a visit'. Nor were noblewomen excluded: in 1476 a reception was given in Paris to Queen Charlotte of Savoy and her court, where 'they were received and regaled most royally and lavishly, and four beautiful and richly adorned baths had been prepared'.[56] The larger bath feasts also often took place outside in the open air; as they probably did at diplomatic parties in Baden in the 1480s, where the hot springs were now hosting a rather more select clientele, not just the townspeople:

> From the year 1474 the [imperial] confederation held their great assemblies regularly every summer at Baden with many other visitors attending.... In the summer of 1474 the councillor of Halle, Hans von Waldheim, spent four weeks at the baths, and in his report, highly praised the good society of the place, and in the same year, Princess Eleonora of Scotland [attended], and her court.[57]

Spring Baths

There were certain particular times of the year when the baths became the centre for openly erotic mass revelry: spring carnival time, the time of Fleshly Lust. It was also the Galenic time for bleeding and purging: 'Spring (Ver)...good for all animals and for the products that germinate from the earth. Dangers: Bad for unclean bodies. Neutralisation of dangers: by cleaning the body.'[58] The 'bucolic' spring festivals included the wearing of flower garlands and bringing flowers and leaves into the house, and (as in the English May Day) always involved a ritual excursion by youths and maidens into the surrounding countryside. All monthly calendars of scenes from the agricultural year, almost without exception, including the great *Très Riches Heures du duc de Berri*, show spring—the month of May—as a festive time of lovemaking, bathing, boating, swimming, picnicking, and music-making. The general theme is fertility and rejuvenation, and the rites of youth. The so-called 'fountains of youth' scenes, and the outdoor 'love gardens' (*Liebesgarten*) of the German bath houses were favourite etching subjects in fifteenth-century art. So common are these spring calendar scenes that we cannot see them only as scenes of knightly or aristocratic revelry: the local river did just as well if you could not afford the 10 pfennigs it might cost you to enter the most fashionable local baths. Or you might 'bring out your baths' in your own garden, or on the front porch. French carnival records—especially court records—show how the local bath-house featured heavily as a destination for the procession, and as a base for the town or village party to come. It was a natural headquarters for the notorious *société joyeuse*—the groups of young men that organized the communal *charivari*.[59]

Most erotic spring bath evidence stood little chance of sur-vival during the succeeding centuries—such as Count von Edelstein's infamous painted fresco *Of Fleshly Lust*, which he enjoyed in his bathhouse at Wiesbaden in the 1390s, and which was apparently 'shocking through its fleshliness, and soaked in sensual voluptuousness'. It showed scenes from the famous Wiesbaden Festival—which, in a reversal of the urban springtime exodus, was obviously the time when rural inhabit-ants came into town from the countryside to have some carni-val fun. The festival itself was observed with pious horror and sadness by a visiting monk:

> Everyone brings food, drink, money, strange dresses are worn along the way. In anticipation of enjoyment they are already playing, singing, gossiping, as people who would expect the absolute epit-ome of happiness to come. When they arrive at the baths, the food is spread out... In the baths they sit naked, with other naked people, they dance naked with naked people, and I shall keep quiet about what happens in the dark, because everything happens in public anyway...

Of course he made sure he stayed until the bitter end:

> The coming and the going of this ridiculous festival is not the same. When, after everything has been eaten, the cupboards go back empty, the pouches empty of money, they regret having wasted so much money.... Meanwhile they return home, their bodies are washed white, their hearts are black through sin. Those

who went there healthy, come back contaminated. Those who were strong through the virtues of chastity return home wounded by the arrows of Venus... And so they experience through such events, when they return, the truth of the sentence that the end of all fleshly lust ends sadness.[60]

'The Stews'

The salacious bath picture that shows a king and a bishop holding the keys to 'the stews' was not far wide of the mark.[61] Hot baths never lost the taint of the brothel pinned on them by puritans for the good reason that they were the favourite— indeed licensed—places for sexual seduction, sanctioned by the elders of the community. The medieval municipal bath-house shared this job with the medieval municipal brothel (in Germany the *Frauenhaus*, in France the *maison des fillettes*), where the public women based their trade. The town authorities seemed to have regarded both the baths and the brothels as a necessary outlet for the energies of the town's young men, and simply tried to control them. According to one recent history of prostitution: 'Everywhere that their operation can be clearly ascertained, the *étuves* [stoves] served both the honest purpose of bathing and the more "dishonest" one of prostitution. This continued to be true in spite of innumerable regulations against receiving prostitutes in the bathhouses or specifying hours or days...'[62] Bath prostitutes and bath-keepers were thus as firmly regulated as brothels. In medieval London the city's main eighteen hot baths in Southwark were on land owned by the bishop of Winchester, instantly giving the prostitutes who traded there the name Winchester Geese. In 1161 the Southwark stews were newly regulated—not closed (for they were an 'old custom used for times out of mind'), but reorganized to ensure fair trading and orderliness. The women were to be free to come and go; they were not to open on Sundays; no more than 14 shillings' rent for each women's chamber; no nuns; money to be paid for the full night; no women with venereal diseases—and no food on the premises. This last must have been a great blow, precisely calculated to send the party trade elsewhere, but was probably not observed for long.[63]

By the fifteenth century, bath feasting in the many town bathhouses seems to have been as common as going out to a restaurant was to become four centuries later. German bath etchings from the fifteenth century often feature the town bathhouse, with a long row of bathing couples eating a meal naked in bathtubs, often several to a tub, with other couples seen smiling in beds in the mid-distance. In one well-known version, the bathers sit in curtained-off, two-seater baths, being served their food on a cloth-covered table alongside the bath. Guests enter, and waiters scurry to and fro.[64] The illustrations show the high-waisted, low-cut, breast-exposed styles for women that had become fashionable, with the men wearing very short doublets and hose, with buttocks and codpieces exposed. The medieval bathing party was then very nearly at its height. 'Twenty five years ago, nothing was more fashionable in Brabant than the public baths,' said Erasmus in 1526; 'today there are none, the new plague has taught us to avoid them.'

The Failure of the Baths

The etchings and literature of the early 1500s captured a way of life that was just about to go into a steep decline. In England, Henry VIII closed the stews of Southwark and Bankside in 1546; the brothels and stews of Chester were closed in 1542. In France the four steam baths at Dijon were suppressed in 1556; in 1566 they were closed throughout the Duchy of Orléans, while those at Beauvais, Angers, and Sens were gone by the end of the century. In Paris there were 'only a handful by the end of the seventeenth century'.[65]

No single cause is sufficient to account for the disappearance of such deep-rooted customs. Wilhelm Rudeck suggested reasons that were primarily material, and economic, citing syphilis and the rising cost of fuel as the two main factors that put bathhouses out of business in Germany.[66] Recent historians have preferred to emphasize the fear of the plague, poisonously infiltrating steamed-open bodies, and this certainly fits with the reappearance of severe epidemic plague in the sixteenth century; but then why did the baths not disappear earlier, after the Black Death? Rudeck probably underestimated the effect of the general decline of rurally based peasant culture; and the popular urban roots of the moral Reformation, especially in certain areas of growing population. There were changes in the political climate that either put puritanical religious reformers, or activists of the Catholic Counter-Reformation into power, many of whom were ascetics who were likely to view the bathhouses as hotbeds of sexual uncleanness and political dissent.

Pressure from growing urban populations meant that, by the end of the fifteenth century, the bathhouses (like the bawdy houses) were increasingly seen as places of lawlessness and social disorder; they disturbed the regular inhabitants, breaking the fragile trust of the community, and the numbers of arrests and prosecutions grew.[67] But arguably it was the arrival of acute epidemic syphilis in 1493 which achieved what endemic plague, rising costs, religion, or lawlessness had failed to do: it closed them immediately and peremptorily, and when or if they reopened, they were never the same again. The innocence was gone.

Syphilis

Syphilis hit at the heart of the body culture that featured so strongly in the baths and festivals. Grossly disfiguring to the face and private parts, and highly contagious, it created an unprecedented fear of sexuality, and also polluted the act. You had to check, now, that the vessel was 'clean'. Rottenness could be hidden beneath superficial beauty. New ways and new avoidances had to be learnt, and learnt fast:

> Take heed of the perils of lovemaking
> And change your ways accordingly...
> Avoid blotchy folk, and don't despise those who are loyal partners,
> Stick to sweethearts, who are not to be lightly dismissed.
> But make sure you don't start the job
> Without a candle; don't be afraid to
> Take a good look, both high and low,
> And then you may frolic to your heart's content.[68]

Better still, remain chaste until marriage: 'keep thee clene unto the tyme thou be maryed'. The only true surety of cleanness was prenuptial virginity, for both men and women. The printed broadsheet *The Wedding of Youth and Cleanness* (1509) showed how 'Virtue conquers Sensuosity and is rewarded by Love.' For those who had not yet got the disease, they should avoid infected people 'as one avoids contact with a leper'. A good regimen, without Venus, was essential; or if with Venus, a meticulous hygiene of the genital areas was required at all times—bathing with hot water and wine (or vinegar), using herbal washes, dusting with mineral powders, and 'above all, avoid using towels belonging to prostitutes'.[69]

The offspring of an 'ancestral spirochete' (treponematosis) that is now thought to have been endemic worldwide from ancient times, syphilis suddenly mutated into a far more virulent form in the Spanish Atlantic ports in 1492 and reached central Europe by 1502, before travelling on to India, the East Indies, Japan, and all colonial trading islands. Eventually it retreated, and over the succeeding five centuries became endemic, dwindling into a curiosity, then into 'silence and contempt', leaving a huge legacy of syphilitic wives and children throughout the world, before finally dropping off the list of scourges in the mid-twentieth century. In the worst cases, the syphilitic tubercles were followed by a tumour that bored into bone tissue and then liquefied, exposing the bones and eating away at the nose, the lips, the palate, the larynx, and the genitals.

Syphilis (unlike plague) was not a disease of poverty, but raged equally among the nobility, royalty, and clergy, partly due to the wide sexual licence given to aristocratic youth who visited brothels for their education—with the result, said Montaigne (1533–92), that 'we are taught to live when life has already passed us by. A hundred schoolboys have caught the pox before they have studied Aristotle on Temperance.'[70] But anyone was at risk; and syphilis was emotionally described in real-life patient experiences pouring out of the new printing presses, the start of a long tradition of popular self-help medical auto-biographies. In 1498 a young canon, Josephus Grunpeck, wrote a most horrifying and graphic personal account in which he described how he worked his way downwards from fashionable physicians before finally, in desperation, seeking help from 'louts and uneducated folk'—to whom with hindsight he gave due credit:

> These uncouth men, whoever they were, cesspool emptiers, rub-bish collectors, cobblers, reapers and mowers, had to lance the tubercles, those harbingers of countless horrible and incurable wounds, and thus drive away or suppress the consumption with pills, ointments, creams, or some other such medicine; and it is undoubtedly due to the zeal, industry, and application of these men . . . that I, afflicted for the second time, and very severely at that, with this illness, recovered my forces sufficiently to resume my usual activities.[71]

Syphilis had a profound effect on the trades of the barber–tonsors and barber–surgeons. In a tradition probably dating back to classical times, barbers' back rooms and yards (if they had them) were used for minor surgery and baths; the front of the shop dealt with hair-cutting and shaving, and the jovial grooming atmosphere encouraged the sale of books, drinks, and pharmaceuticals on the side. To start with, as Grunpeck's experience shows, long-term venereal treatment could be done by anyone, certainly by any barber; but it was later regulated on the grounds that it was too 'perilous' to keep the (clean) grooming and (unclean) curing activities together. The English 1540 Act that joined the Barbers' and Surgeons' companies gave the educated barber–surgeons (and of course the physicians) the lucrative monopoly on treating venereal disease, and excluded the older general handymen, the barber–tonsors (as also happened in France). But the English Parliament also made it quite clear that the ancient practices of mutual aid and empiric medicine should not be allowed to disappear, by promptly passing the so-called Quacks' Charter in 1542–3 that legally enabled anyone to practise medicine, if they could 'so help their neighbours and the poor'.[72]

Meanwhile the baths, bathsmen, and their guilds disappeared completely, along with the regulated stews. As was realized by many at the time, the closure of these licensed stews concentrated in the central parts of major towns was a public health disaster. In London old leper hospitals isolated some of the syphilitic poor, but the main means of transmission—the public prostitutes—were dispersed, and went 'private': 'Since those common whores were quite put down, a damned crue of private whores are growne . . . '. The prostitutes of London served a town that had one of the fastest-growing populations in Europe, and the bawdy houses quickly spread to the suburbs outside the walls (St Giles, Blackheath, Stepney, Saffron Hill, Petticoat Lane).[73] These were more secretive, and more furtive, establishments that found a new home in small lower-class alehouses, and in upper-class taverns. But the aristocracy did not forgo the illicit pleasures of water for long; a century later the steam bath reappeared in the luxurious upper-class establishments known as bagnios.

In most respects medieval society was not a 'dirty' society—far from it. Alongside intense religiosity, there was intense materialism. Socially speaking, personal freshness actually mattered, and was quite an accomplishment under the circumstances; though perhaps too difficult an accomplishment for many, at least on a regular basis. But the Catholic Church, which as a whole had fought so hard to impose intellectual refinement, physical cleanliness, and sexual cleanness over the centuries, adapting itself to various strategies to win over unwilling populations, suddenly found itself under a bruising attack for its own moral laxities. The Church had unwisely persecuted extreme ascetic Church reformers such as the Albigensian Cathars (Greek *kathari*, the pure ones); but the ascetic movements refused to die away, and asceticism split the Church once more. A renewed programme of ascetic austerity (and celibacy) was reimposed successfully on all Catholic clergy after the Counter-Reformation Council of Trent in 1562–3, but by then the damage had been done.[74] The trend towards decentralized Christianity was irreversible in northern Europe at least, where many Protestant ascetics had come to believe that each sinner held his or her own conscience, and bodily welfare, entirely in his or her own hands.

chapter 7
protestant regimens

TO THE PRESENT AND FUTURE AGES, GREETINGS.

> ...For it is my hope and my desire that [this work] will
> contribute to the common good; that through it the higher
> physicians will somewhat raise their thoughts, and not de-
> vote all their time to common cures, nor be honoured for
> necessity only; but that they will become instruments and
> dispensers of God's power and mercy in prolonging and
> renewing the life of man, the rather because it is effected
> by safe, convenient, and civil, though hitherto unattempted
> methods. For although we Christians ever arrive and pant
> after the land of promise, yet meanwhile it will be a mark of
> God's favour if in our pilgrimage through the wilderness of
> this world, these our shoes and garments (I mean our frail
> bodies) are as little worn out as possible.[1]

Thus in 1623 Francis Bacon opened his 'History of Life and
Death', Part III of his famous *Instauratio Magna*, a rallying cry
for the reform of European science. Three hundred years later
Europeans would be stripping off their heavy clothes and
exposing their naked skin to water, exercise, light, and air, and
often living until they were 80, all in the name of prolongevity
hygiene—truly a triumph for 'safe, convenient and civil'
methods. The early modern period starts the final countdown

to modernity, c.AD 1500–2007. From now on the scene shifts to northern Europe and the interrelationships between the British Isles, France, and Germany (in particular), and their many long-lasting contributions to the modern European hygienic renaissance; and more especially to the story of English Protestantism, with its enthusiastic adherence to ideologies of health and purity.

Throughout the sixteenth and seventeenth centuries the classical discipline of hygiene was the subject of intense speculation and equally intense beliefs, in which humanism played a significant role. The idea of political cleansing or 'purging' entered European discourse with a vengeance between 1500 and 1700, brilliantly and viscerally heralded by the ascetic Dutch scholar Desiderius Erasmus (1466–1536), the godfather of humanism. His extraordinary burlesque on the excesses of late medieval life *Folly's Praise of Folly* (1511) was an instant hit throughout Europe (with forty-three editions in his lifetime); his next manifesto, *Antibarbari* (1514), railed against a corrupt Church, and corrupted Church scholars writing corrupted barbaric texts: 'what disaster it was that had swept away the rich, flourishing, joyful fruits of the finest culture, and why a tragic and terrible deluge had shamefully overwhelmed all the literature of the ancients that used to be so pure'.[2] Reform of the Catholic Church was Erasmus' aim; but the Protestant Reformation in northern Europe became a massive and irreversible social revolution.

In England the break from Rome created a new national identity permeated and defined by both Protestantism and humanism. When Bacon wrote in the 1620s, there was already an army of English Protestant readers and authors ready and willing to accept the Baconian challenge to go out and 'experiment' on the natural world. These efforts created a distinctive school of English science and hygiene, which later evolved into a full-blown scientific project. Following the upheavals of the Civil War and the Restoration, a peaceful religious settlement after 1688 gave English scientists a renewed opportunity to cleanse learning and deliver it from the obscure 'Rubbish of the Schools'. Open experimentation and transparent proof was to provide the new 'clear gaze' of natural science—the light that was to illuminate the next century's Enlightenment. Protestantism itself was thoroughly caught up in the triangular philosophical relationship between Reason, Flesh, and the Soul that we have seen before, in Greece and Late Antiquity—and it was set firmly against the Flesh.[3] The Flesh, however, remained naturally of the most immediate concern to most populations, most of the time. Throughout both of these centuries Flesh was privately pampered, and everywhere on display.

Humanist Princes

The Renaissance continued the love affair with domestic bodily delights begun in the ancient courts and continued throughout the Middle Ages. Between 1500 and 1750 the European population doubled to around 127.5 million, most of this growth occurring before 1625. There was an explosion of ostentatious fine art and architecture as kings, noblemen, and merchant princes spent fortunes in a tidal wave of brick and stone— palaces, town and suburban mansions, with parks furnished with elegant knot gardens, water features, and little pavilions set by lakes. In 1500 only four cities (Paris, Milan, Naples, and Venice) had populations of more than 100,000 inhabitants; by 1700 there were twelve, with London and Paris containing over 500,000 inhabitants.[4] Over the next two centuries in Europe, urban fresh-water and riverine sources were extended, and water-carrying became an important service industry; the public fountain ('conduit' in English) was the basic and most popular public facility, often equipped with large laundering tanks. But the public pipes were also being tapped by increasing numbers of private pipes; in England the medieval prohibition on private tapping of this scarce communal resource had gradually

eroded from the thirteenth century onwards, although generally for privileged persons only.[5]

By the mid-1500s the grander European palaces were installing plumbed water supplies with full drainage, in the neoclassical style. The built-in bath or grooming suite was a luxury
many princes and nobility were eager to acquire, as in Duke
Frederico da Montefeltro's palace at Urbino, which had a fixed
stone bath, latrine, and a small reading closet set in an external
tower adjoining his large bedroom and public antechambers.
Francis I of France had a full suite of baths installed in his
ground floor suite, leading out into the garden, at his new
palace at Fontainebleau; and there is no doubt that bathtubs
held a special place in the sixteenth-century artistic School of
Fontainebleau.[6] Not to be outdone, Henry VIII of England also
built to modern Renaissance standards of convenience at his
new palace at Hampton Court, and in renovations at Whitehall
and other palaces. At Hampton Court he built an extra tower—
the Bayne Tower—with a bath, drop-latrine, and private suite;
he also had cold-water cisterns installed on the roof above the
upper-level suites to give them piped-water facilities, for fixed
stone hand-basins if not fixed baths (though well supplied with
the usual portable, upholstered, hooped bathtub). Another of
his sanitary innovations at Hampton Court was the Great House
of Easement, a four-tier, twenty-eight-seater communal latrine
block set over the west arm of the moat. He also laid out two
tennis courts, two bowling alleys, and a tilt-yard, having a great
humanist passion for sporting exercise.[7]

Italy was the epicentre of the court life until the rise of Paris in
the mid-seventeenth century, and Baldesar Castiglione's famous
etiquette manual *The Book of the Courtier* (1528) was a *courtesie*
for its time—a new type of Ovidian self-cultivation using classical authors instead of Christian ones, foreshadowing the rise
of what historians have called 'affective individualism', or a new
psychology of 'intimacy'.[8] Elizabeth I of England, educated as a

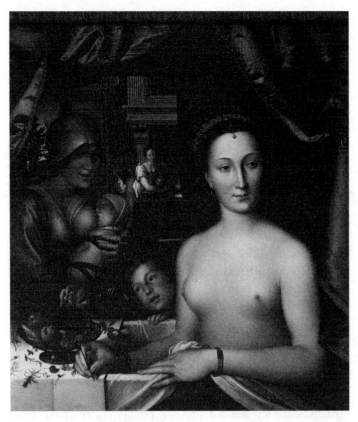

12 The royal courtesan Diane de Poitiers disrobed and relaxing in her bath annexe and living quarters, by the sixteenth-century French court painter François Clouet, of the School of Fontainebleau, where bathing was held in high esteem.

humanist princess, was a perfect exemplar of this new Italian civility (and almost a royal *ganika*).[9] Elizabeth was known to be fussy about her health—she hated being ill. She preserved her health and lived to old age by apparently following a sensible humanist health regimen; she ate and drank abstemiously, took plenty of exercise, and undoubtedly owned a copy of Sir

Thomas Elyot's hugely successful *Castel of Helth* (1539; five editions by 1560), dedicated to her father's chief minister Thomas Cromwell. She always travelled with her bed and hip bath, and had bathing facilities in all of her palaces, including a sweat bath—her 'warm box' or 'warm nest'—inherited from her father at Richmond, her favourite palace. At Richmond she also installed a prototype of the water closet, the invention of her godson 'Boy Jack', Sir John Harington (translator of the Salerno Regimen). At Whitehall, Elizabeth also had a hot room with a ceramic tiled stove, as well as a large bath and grooming suite, both inherited from her father, in which to spend time with her intimate companions. This suite was effectively her Cabinet of the Morning. It contained her bedroom, and next to it 'a fine bathroom ... [where] the water pours from oyster shells and different kinds of rock'. Next to the bathroom was a room with an organ 'on which two people can play duets, also a large chest completely covered in silk, and a clock which plays times by striking a bell'. Next to this was a room 'where the Queen keeps her books'.[10] Indeed royal baths were so *à la mode* that a bathhouse was specially built for Mary, Queen of Scots, at Holyrood Palace in the late 1560s; so there is no reason to think that Queen Elizabeth I did not thoroughly enjoy her monthly bath 'whether she needed it or no' (probably at the time of the menses) and was certainly likely to have taken them more often than that, when returning to Richmond or Whitehall after a long cold journey or a dusty ride on a hot afternoon.

In any case she would have known all about baths, being well versed in the 'arts of adornment' and having a passionate interest in Italian cosmetics. The whole edifice of practical therapeutics stood firm during this very late phase of medieval culture. Galenic traditions were firmly built into domestic medicine—as seen especially in early modern descriptions of childbirth, where the mother was supplied with a battery of hot relaxing foods, drinks, washes, and anointments, in a heated chamber,

by her family, female neighbours, and friends.[11] 'Social' grooming affected rich and poor alike. At the lower end of society, the
political hierarchy of a village was as complex as any court, and
it imposed its own rules and festivities on its participants on all
important occasions—at birth, marriage, and death—when
grooming would have been lengthy, giving great attention to
all the parts (hair, face, hands, feet) and using whatever simple
cosmetics could be made, gathered, or borrowed. Daily grooming with basins, combs, and cloths may have been more limited,
and was probably non-existent among vagrants or the lowest
ranks of the 'shame-faced poor' (except for the most ancient
basic manual actions); but family sickness would have been the
time when such old cosmetic and herbal skills of 'kitchen phy-
sik' as the household had were brought into play. The symbolic
division between long periods of work and short periods of
play was marked by the now near-universal habit of having
(wherever possible, and certainly among the godly) two sets of
clothing: dirty work clothing, and Sunday or festive best.

But it was the luxury trades that set the pace of popular
consumerism, and aristocratic fashions were again the driving
force in creating markets. At the beginning of Elizabeth's reign
in 1558, the Venetian ambassador noted the court ladies' 'fresh'
complexions and general lack of paint, at a time when Venetian
beauty boxes were large and elaborate affairs, with waters,
paints, patches, and 'even preparations for tinting the teeth
and eyelids'. Fifty years later the whole of the English court
and aristocracy were 'very Italianate' and cosmetics-mad, with
paints, beauty patches, wigs (blonde and henna-auburn), and
bejewelled hair. The trade of the barbers themselves was now
situated well beyond the professional ramparts; but despite this
the barbers and apothecaries were doing a flourishing trade in
this period, servicing a needy population from their small street
shops. Down at street level, customers were not looking for
moral judgements, but were involved in a more 'desperate or

cynical search for the means of personal definition and social acceptability'. In London generally, it was 'a rare face if it be not painted', according to one satirical broadside:

> Waters she hath to make her face to shine,
> Confections, eke, to clarify her skin;
> Lip salve and cloths of a rich scarlet dye...
> Ointment, wherewith she sprinkles oe'r her face,
> And lustrifies her beauty's dying grace...
> Storax and spikenard, she burns in her chamber,
> And daubs herself with civet, musk, and amber.[12]

More careful skin care went into the later sixteenth-century fashion for low-cut necklines, and even bared breasts, a throwback to the fashions of the late fifteenth century: 'Your garments must be so worne always, that your white pappes may be seene...'. But male fashion was equally sensuous. Young Elizabethan courtiers were peacocking dandies like their medieval counterparts; the courtly English 'Cavalier' of the seventeenth century (albeit often armed for battle) has been described as an 'ornament of conversation, personal beauty and erotic attraction', and his loose flowing locks mirrored the curls and tresses of the courtly women.[13] Sixteenth- and seventeenth-century European male and female fashions were ornamented with ribbons and lace and garnished with quantities of important accessories such as fans, pomanders, gloves, and handkerchiefs. These fashion accessories were all objects of refinement (like forks): they defended the user against external dirt. Gloves kept the hands white, clean, and soft, handkerchiefs wiped away dirt; fans and pomanders wafted away bad air. (Interestingly, some of these accessories also defended against extremes of heat and cold; another refinement—or retraining—of the senses.)

Fortunes were made by barbers, apothecaries, wig-makers, perfumiers, clothiers, and stay-makers—and soap-boilers. High-quality hard-soap imports began to rise steadily in England from the late sixteenth century, and increasingly wealthy local manufacturers such as the London wholesaler Henry Bradstreet manufactured perfumed toilet soaps as well as soft soap for clothes and household cleaning. By 1643 English soap production and consumption had risen so steadily that soap was designated one of the eight staple domestic 'necessities' (namely, soap, beer, spirits, cloth, salt, glass, leather, and candles) that were to be taxed under a new Commonwealth Excise system borrowed from the Dutch Republic; this marked the start of an extensive and long-running 'black market' soap-smuggling trade between England and the northern coast of France.[14]

Linen was the hallmark of the courtier and the man of distinction: 'It is enough if he always has fine linen, and very white.' According to the historian Georges Vigarello, a daily change of shirt had become normal for men in French court circles by the late sixteenth century, while French probate inventories show a steep rise in numbers of gentlemen's shirts (up to an average of thirty) by the end of the seventeenth century. French court correspondence from women in the seventeenth century show an almost nunlike attention to clean linen, and the word 'clean' (*propre*) became a significant term of praise: Mme de Maintenon had a 'noble and clean' appearance; Mme de Contie had 'extreme cleanliness'; Mme Seguier 'was never beautiful, but she was clean' (the modest epitaph of many a gentlewoman for centuries to come).

White underlinen displayed every trace of dirt, absorbed the waste juices from the pores, protected the skin, and was increasingly seen as a cleansing agent in its own right. So far had the theory of underlinen progressed by 1626 that a fashionable French architect could confidently denounce the necessity for building domestic baths: 'We can more easily do without them than the ancients, because of our use of linen, which today serves to keep the body clean, more conveniently than could the steam-baths and baths of the ancients, who were denied the use and convenience of linen.'[15] This was to some extent a self-fulfilling prophecy, as French architects stopped building the old palatial *appartements de bains* in towers, but replaced them by much smaller and more intimate *cabinets de bains* next to the bedchamber.[16] Two marble-built bath suites went into Louis XIV's own and his mistress's chambers at Versailles, and six *cabinets de bains* were built in other bedroom suites; but Louis did not like bathing, and rarely took one: 'The King was never pleased to become accustomed to bathing in his chamber.' On the other hand, he was kept perfectly clean by his attendants, who continually rubbed him down with scented linen cloths, changed sweaty shirts at night, and changed his complete costume two or three times a day at least—'the consequence of the king's love of comfort, and fear of being uncomfortable'.[17]

It is worth noting, however, in comparison to all this courtly daintiness, that for much of the population, one or two rough hemp (rather than soft linen) undershirts or shifts were enough to get by with, for bare necessity. But the peasant economy was also expanding. Linen wares sold by pedlars and packmen to English rural farming households showed a steady rise 'from at least the 1680s'; while the French and German peasantry, too, were beginning to accumulate household linen (if not much underwear) for their marriage trousseaus. Linen was a major European commodity, and new cloth industries such as lace-making, or weaving fustian (a new linen–wool mix) brought vital work to many villages, as well as cloth for their backs. But it was the people in the towns who bought most of the mercer's wares.[18]

The (English) Middling Classes

Compared to Paris, Venice, or Florence, up until the sixteenth century London had been a European cultural backwater; all this was to change over the next hundred years, during the course of the English Reformation, as London slowly became a major European port—especially after the East India Company was founded in 1600. Money talked to money, and the City and the court literally grew towards each other along the north bank of the Thames; both joined in grief when the London Stock Exchange burned down in the Great Fire of London in 1666 (it was quickly rebuilt on an even larger and grander scale). The English population was roughly 3 million in 1541, and 5 million by 1700. As trade and manufacturing grew, the rural population flocked to a new life in the market towns, provincial capitals, and above all London, an upwardly mobile emigration which sharpened their 'horizontal' sense of rank and respectability while increasing the social distance they set between themselves and the poor—an ongoing 'civilizing process' now extending into the middle ranks.[19] In late seventeenth-century London the middling classes formed an estimated 25 per cent of the population—less than half of the 70 per cent of the labouring classes, but far more numerous than the 5 per cent of the nobility; and far more numerous than in any rural parish. The elite squires, doctors, lawyers, or merchants at the top of their trade—the 'plums' (those earning over £10,000 a year)—had everything that money could buy. In their new tall urban houses they had spacious saloons for public display and private parlours for conversation, while the old bedroom-cum-meeting-place was transferred upstairs to new private suites of bed and dressing chambers. But the majority of the English middling classes were not rich. As the decades went by they could increasingly afford little luxuries here and there—a new clock, a piece of new furniture, a few books, more clothes, white bread instead of brown, candles instead of oil, bought soap instead of homemade. 'An income of £50 was some three, four, or even five times the annual income of a labourer, and would allow a family to eat well, employ a servant and live comfortably.'[20]

The real social stresses occurred towards the bottom of the social scale, where any population increase battled with scarce local resources, seasonal employment, and subsistence wages—all traditional causes of peasant revolt and urban disorder. It was in these groups that radical English Protestantism took deep root and later supplied the muscle and the democratic fervour of the Commonwealth Revolution. But the real revolution among the English middling classes had already occurred when John Wyclif (1329–84) translated the Bible into vernacular English for the common reader, opening up all the endless possibilities of the Word.[21] Wyclif's English followers, the Lollards, were early precursors of the flood of religious protestation in Europe that led to Calvin in Geneva, Zwingli in Zurich, and the Lutherans in Saxony; and eventually to a solidly Protestant 'rim' emerging around the North Sea—in Scandinavia, Denmark, Germany, the Netherlands, England, and Scotland—which later extended across the North Atlantic to the east coast of North America.[22] The map of Protestantism within the British Isles shows reform and radicalism strong among the lower-middle classes in towns and semi-industrial rural areas, among independent craftsmen, textile workers, smallholders, and provincial retailers. They found a secure footing at local level, forming small cells of local Saints, congregations, magistrates, and preaching ministers. They took their new 'seriousness' into all walks of professional life, including law, medicine, trade, and the universities; in London they inhabited the coffee-houses, scoured the newspapers, and formed the bedrock of a new breed of industrious civil servants (of whom Samuel Pepys was one).[23]

English Protestant puritans led a fierce spiritual and intellectual life. Above all (and this was a strong appeal for migrant families who had left old social ties behind them) their religion promised an entirely new start: 'New minds, new memories, new judgements, new affects...new love, new joy...new food, new raiment, new language, new company...new ends and aims... [This is] the Excellence, Amiableness, Comfort and Content which is to be found in the ways of Purity and Holiness.'[24] Yet again there were profound historical consequences from the revival of asceticism, especially one that was noted long ago in the monasteries, and which had worked well for the Catholic Church: if you worked hard and lived soberly, you were almost bound to accumulate money. You could also give that money away, in good works. Money obviously had its attractions for fellow-travellers, backsliders, and the disillusioned; but for the moment, English puritan movements relished their attacks on filthy Lucre and the privileges of the rich, in their attempt to capture and purify society and the state.

They also embraced the healing mission. The democratic political content of the early Protestant health message was a particularly powerful one: God made everyone equal, and the means of cure were apparently open to all. This message liberated individuals, and put the care of their health firmly in their own hands. Many English sectarians were staunch popular empiricists who (like Gerrard Winstanley) asserted the moral right to judge the world and see things 'by the material eyes of this flesh'; and also, increasingly, the right to experiment on their own bodies.

Printed Advice and the Sober Life
The renewed sixteenth- and seventeenth-century plague outbreaks, unlike syphilis, struck the innocents of all classes and terrified everyone equally. They concentrated everybody's mind on self-help and self-preservation. Daniel Defoe later described the ravaged silence of empty London streets, with green grass growing between the cobbles outside, and people locked indoors living quietly and soberly like himself, sticking rigidly to all the health instructions they could find. In the early days of an attack the quacks were out in force selling magical

elixirs, amulets, charms, potions, pamphlets, and broadsides, but public disillusion soon set in.[25] The deeply rooted belief in internal potions and purges continued, but as the severity of the plague visitations increased, there must have been many people who heard recommendations on regimen, or opened a printed advice book or pamphlet for the first time during an epidemic, and thereafter found a way to order not only their health, but their whole life: 'This boke techyng al people to governe them in helthe...is as profitable as needeful to be had...' announced the title page of the printed *Regimen Sanitatis Salerni*, translated by Thomas Paynell (first edition 1528; five more editions by 1617). The very first printed English medical advice book, *The Gouernayle [Governor] of Helthe*, was taken from an older manuscript and published by William Caxton in 1489. The early printed medical advice market in England was not large (possibly 3 per cent of all titles, reaching roughly one in twenty book owners), but it grew steadily and was mostly in readable English; the number of English medical works actually published in Latin between *c.*1500 and 1640, remarks one historian, 'was paltry'.[26] Thomas Phayre's *The Book of Children* (1544), Thomas Moulton's *The Myrrour or Glasse of Helth* (1545), and Andrew Boorde's *Compendious Regiment or a Dyetary of Helth* (1562), to name but a few, were sold alongside the growing numbers of do-it-yourself herbals, almanacs, receipt books, and surgical manuals.

Many early small books and pamphlets for poor, defenceless, and suffering households were written out of Christian charity and fellow feeling. Charitable Protestant authors found themselves not only grappling with 'barbarous' medical terminology, but having to defend themselves against their abuse of medical privileges—laying open all those craft 'secrets' and breaking the conventional monopolies of medical knowledge. It was a difficult task they managed with some aplomb, as in Humphrey

Lloyd's *The Treasuri of Helth contayning Many Profitable Medicines* (*c*.1556):

> [I do not do this] to maintayne thru filthy lucre and blind bold-ness...but...I hold that it should be for the use and profyte of such honeste persons as might modestly and discreetly (either in tyme of necessitye when no lerned physicion is at hande, or els conferring wyth some lerned man and usynge hys councel) myn-ister the thynges herein conteyned to go about the practyse thereof, and upon these most honest and godly consideracions, I take upon me this heavy burthen and hard province... [Do not] despise this symple work because it is not garnished wyth colours of rhetoricke and fine polished termes, but rather consider that physicke is an arte certaine only to be plainly and distinctly taught...Wherefore I, trusting to the sincere and indifferent judgement of the reader, do entirely desire him to pray wyth me and to him that created the physicks of the earth, and commended that we should honour the Physician, to preserve this Realme of England in most prosperous and contiynuall health, and to endow the inhabitants thereof, with perfect understanding and the most desired knowledge of his holy word. Amen.[27]

Temperance and moderation—'how to govern and preserve thy-self'—were godly virtues that came into their own in these des-perate times, and was popularly known as 'the Sober Life'. The increased emphasis on the absolutely correct balance of the bod-ily humours, and a greater emphasis on the environmental rules of the non-naturals (newly rediscovered from the Greek texts), suggest that full hygienic regimen was considered to be the latest, most modern, weapon against the plague. The doctors were unswerving in their recommendation of hygienic temperance and moderation during plague outbreaks—the body should not be pushed to any extremes whatsoever: '[neither] all manner of excess and outrage of meat and drink...no hot foods...no lechery...Also use no baths or stoves; nor swet not too much, for all openeth the pores of a manne's body and maketh the

venemous ayre to enter and for to infecte the bloude...'.[28]
Covering up and keeping clean in every other way but that was
considered safer. The plague regimens were insistent on clean
streets and clean rooms, fresh air and sweet odours, a sober diet,
good grooming and clean skin, and well-kept clothing.

Many English authors embraced the idea of a reformed
'humane' classical medicine with enthusiasm, and Thomas
Elyot's *Castel of Helth* was their benchmark for over a century.
His conversational prose was modelled on Celsus (whom he
cites constantly) and Galen's *De Sanitate Tuenda*, 'newly translated' from corrupted texts. In the true style of humanist intimacy he pours out his autobiography onto the page, to explain
why he 'is become a physician, and writeth in publick, which
beseemeth not a knight, he mought have been much better
occupied', and then describing his four-year health crisis (his
diacrasie) in detail, concluding he had been 'long in error' with
an over-hot Galenic regimen—'wherefore first I did throw away
my quilted cappe, & my other close bonnets, & only did lye in a
thinne capes, which I have after used both winter and summer'.[29] In Elyot each section on the six 'Thynges not Natural'
is carefully laid out according to the correct complexions, seasons, diet, and evacuations—but with a scattering of new moral
prohibitions. The artificial evacuations, for example (vomit,
letting of blood, scarifying or cupping, and purging) are dealt
with at length; whereas the natural evacuations (sweating,
provocation of urine, spitting, and 'naturall purgations'—the
bowels, the menses) are considered too shameful to mention:
'I do purposely omit to write of them in this place, for as much
as in this realme it has been accompted not honest, to declare
them in the vulgar tongue, but only secretly.' Baths are briefly
mentioned, as a good evacuation, but only if they are temperate; whereas exercise is enthused about at length—exercise 'for
them that desire to remayne long in helthe, is most diligently,
and as I must say, most scrupulously to be observed'.

Exercise was to become a strong 'localized' feature of English hygienic regimen over the next few centuries, in part because the customary sports and older Church festivities (known as 'Church ales') had been early targets for sober ascetic reformers—'some Puritaines and precise people', as King James I described them. Humanist princes had augmented their hunting and dancing with new courtly sports, such as indoor tennis and outdoor bowling, which could be played in their new pleasure parks, and Everard Digby's famous manual and treatise on swimming, *De Arte Natande*, was published in 1587.[30] Elyot's exercise regimen was taken directly from the Greek texts—including even some of the old Methodist 'passive' exercise therapies such as being carried by chair, sitting in a boat or barge, or riding on an ambling horse. In the morning there should if possible be vigorous rubbing of the limbs and loud 'vociferous' singing; and in the afternoon, outdoor games and sports.[31] The popular sporting revival of the sixteenth century was only temporarily crushed by Commonwealth decree in the mid-seventeenth century, and was enthusiastically revived after the Restoration.

One major effect of the humanist neoclassical hygiene revival was the spur it gave to empirical experimentation—and the widespread publicity these efforts now received through mass printing. The first and most famous European experimenter in hygienic health care was Luigi Cornaro, whose *Discorsi della Vita Sobria* ('Discourses on the Sober Life', 1558) seemed to provide proof that a disciplined regimen actually worked. The Discourses were published in sections over a number of years, translated into many European languages, and were effectively health diaries describing Cornaro's many years of moderate diet and simple regimen, up to the age of 83. A eulogy of Cornaro translated into English in a work entitled *Hygiasticon: or, The Right Cause of Preserving Life and Health unto Extream Old Age* (1636)—an early and rare use of the Greek word 'hygiene' in English—described a sober Life or diet, [as that] which sets stint not only in drink but also in meat; so that a man must neither eat not drink any more, than the constitution of his bodie allows, with reference to the services of his mind ... It expells diseases, preserves the body agil, healthful, pure and clean from noysomeness and filthinesse, causeth long life, breeds quiet sleep, makes ordinary fare equall in sweetness to the greatest dainties and moreover keeps the senses sound, and the memories fresh, quiets the passions, drives away Wrath and Melancholie, and breaks the fire of Lust; in a word, replenesheth both soul and body with exceeding good things, so that it may well be termed, the mother of Health, of cheerfulnesse, of Wisdom, and in summe, of all Vertues ... [32]

The self-experiments of Cornaro were the inspiration for another landmark hygienist author, the early seventeenth-century Italian experimenter and friend of Galileo, Sanctorius Sanctorius (1561–1636), whose deeply mathematical and atomistic work *Medicina Statica* (1614) was an early contribution to iatro-mechanism in European physiology. In the cause of purified classicism, Sanctorius set out to revive the neglected philosophy of Asclepiades, in particular the mechanical Methodist theory of *strictum et laxum*—the relaxing or tightening of the atoms, corpuscles, pores, or ducts—which was also attracting interest in other quarters. Sanctorius tested the Sober Diet by gradually reducing his food (and his excrement) to exact and minute portions, and then weighing himself daily in his famous 'balance chair' (always illustrated on the frontispiece).[33] By measuring the shortfall between his intake and outgo, Sanctorius thought he had experimentally exposed the action of something classical authors had called the 'insensible perspiration', an involuntary evacuation which apparently wafted waste products away through the pores of the skin; and thus he concluded that it was vital that the pores were not closed up or 'obstructed', in order to let the poisonous waste matter vaporize freely. This was certainly modern mechanical science to seventeenth-century eyes, and set off a popular craze for

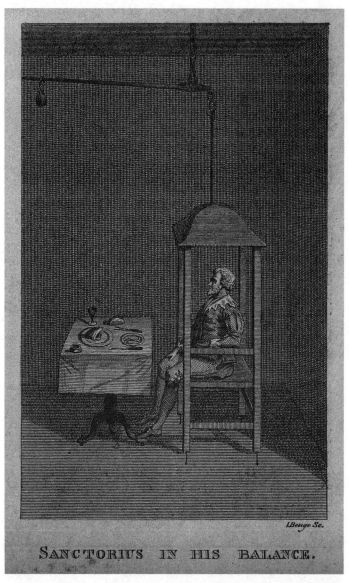

SANCTORIUS IN HIS BALANCE.

13 The weighing-scales, or balance-chair, from Sanctorius' *Medicina Statica* (1614).

weighing and measuring one's own body—forerunner to the precise 'weight-watching' regimes of the modern slimming diet. Thanks to Sanctorius, the doctrine of cleansing 'insensible perspiration' became one of the earliest popularly known hard facts of the physiological sciences, and did not lose its persuasive hold on the European public mind until the late nineteenth century; in the eighteenth century it played a particularly large part in all hygienic rhetoric.[34]

Spas and Public Baths

In 1553 yet another trickle of humanist medical thought joined the main flow when a Venetian publisher, Thomas Junta, took it upon himself to compile a definitive description of all the major European mineral and thermal waters, *De Balneis Omnia* (1553), which primed yet another revival of European mineral-water balneology.[35] Disciples of the iconoclastic Protestant chemist Paracelsus (1493–1542) turned up at mineral springs everywhere, with all their equipment, eagerly checking the mineral content and its supposed effects, carrying on the classification process started by the Romans. The doctors were given a professional springboard via Paracelsian chemistry, and their enthusiasm transmitted itself both to their clients and to baths builders. The English medical author Dr William Turner visited Italy, translated Junta, and produced England's first spa guide, *A Book of the Natures and properties as well as of the Bathes in England as of Other Bathes in Germanye and Italye—very necessary for all those persons that can not be healed without the help of natural bathes* (1562, 1568). As the Anglican dean of Wells Cathedral, he devoutly deplored the still-prevalent custom of mixed bathing, and still more the lack of Christian charity towards 'the poure sicke and diseased people that resort thither... There is money enough spent upon cockfightings, tennys playces, parkes, banquetings, pageants, plays... but I have not heard tell of a rich man hath spent upon these notable Bathes... one grote in [many] years.'[36] He carefully gave directions for cheap and homely domestic medical baths—'certayne rules how that everye man maye make artificiall bathes at home'—with the learned physician supplying the correct brimstone, alum, salt-petre, salt, or copper according to the disease of his patient.

But the new mineral waters were mostly taken internally, as a purge. 'Spa' became the generic word for a new crop of lesser cold mineral springs, after the success of the fashionable late sixteenth-century water resort at Spa in the Ardennes. European spa illustrations from the seventeenth century show stone-built neoclassical-style town squares, with richly and fully clad fig-ures gathered around tall fountains and basins with cups in their hands, testifying to the new craze for drinking the water. The three main categories of chalybeate, sulphurous, and saline ('tart, stinking, and salt') were used as diuretics to 'provoke' the evacuation of very large quantities of stools and urine—'as Soap put to Foul Linnen with Water Pirgeth and Cleanseth all Filth and maketh them to become White again; so these Waters with their Saponary and Detersive Quality clean well the whole Microcosm or Body of Man from all Feculency and Impurities'.[37]

Exposing the external skin to watery ablution and purifica-tion, however, was quite another matter. In Germany the period of hot-bath decline coincided with a rise of increasingly hysterical river-bathing regulations, suggesting that artisanal, merchant, and courtly youth had taken to brothels and cold river-bathing—naked bathing—the old German custom from pre-bathhouse days; while in France, river-bathing became not only popular but fashionable at court.[38] As far as hot water is concerned, there is (so far) little evidence of small local artisa-nal stews or public baths ever existing, in England, to the same extent as in other parts of Europe. For the wealthy few in seventeenth-century London there were private 'bagnios' based on Italian models, but also owing much to the influence of the Turkish 'hummums' imported into Europe from the flourishing Turkish Empire. These later bagnios were discreet private club-like establishments serving an exclusive (usually aristocratic) male and female clientele.[39] We have a rare description of a real but rather special English Royal Bagnio at Charing Cross, London, built into the back of the palace gardens in Charles II's reign, which in 1795 was still a substantial brick-built complex, with a 'large and noble cold bath', sweating rooms, and a suite of upstairs entertaining rooms, with columns, mouldings, and wide staircases, all guarded by a 'massive gate nearly four inches thick [with] a strong iron grating, and in the middle of it a very small iron grating as all such houses had to peep through'.[40] Samuel Pepys's wife famously went once to some public baths 'intending to be very clean' and then reportedly never went again—was she scared of getting into deep water?

In seventeenth-century London public baths were evidently deeply mistrusted. When Dr Peter Chamberlen attempted to open a set of 'Publick Artificiall Baths and Bath-Stoves' in London in 1648, similar to those in 'Germany, Poland, Denmark and Muscovia', and arguing that public hot baths could 'save above 10,000 lives a year', he was firmly rebuffed. The Civil War Parliamentary Committee told him that his baths would be 'hurtful to the Commonwealth' since it was well known that public baths had often been the cause of 'much Physical Prejudice, effeminating bodies and procuring infirmities, and morall in debauching the manners of the people'. There were already enough 'divers Cradles, Tubbs, Boxes, Chairs, Baths and bath-stoves' in private houses.[41] In their eyes, the plague and pox had taught everyone to be vigilant about their health, and to stay sober and clean in every way. Public baths were no longer necessary. The godly could clean themselves at home. The hot bath represented the bad old days and ways, and in England moral prejudice against hot baths continued well into the nine-teenth century.

Puritan Grooming

Each Reformed body was the temple of the soul, kept pure by the familiar practices of asceticism: diet, dress, voice, gait, demeanour, and religious duties. Ascetic doctrines effectively threw a cordon between the true Saints and the rest of the population, so that even the houses of the ungodly were like 'so many filthy cages of unclean Birds, so many styes of all manner of abominations'.[42] Protestant housewifery reached its culmination in Geneva, and particularly in the Netherlands, where even the streets were swept and washed, and domestic manuals were proudly decorated with symbolic brooms and mops; Dutch artists also painted tender scenes of domestic nit-picking, unequalled before or since. The English Protestant housewifery genre, by comparison, was discreetly vague and ladylike, composed mainly of recipes, and largely untouched by Calvinist household cleansing propaganda.[43]

The ascetic discipline was underlined by an austere dress code and a perfectly clean and neat appearance, described by Bacon as 'a civil cleanliness ever esteemed to proceed from a due reverence to God, to society, and to ourselves'. Erasmus had put his faith in early training in his influential humanist edu-cational handbook *On Civility in Children* (1532); and the Czech Protestant Comenius' *School of Infancy* (1633) likewise instruct-ed parents to teach temperance, cleanliness, and decorum from the very beginning of life:

> Immediately, in the first year, the foundations of cleanliness may be laid, by nursing the infant in as cleanly and neat a way as possible, which the bearers ought to know how to do, if they are not destitute of sense. In the second, third, and following years it is proper to

teach children to take their food decorously, not to soil their fingers with fat, and not, by scattering their food, to stain themselves... Similar cleanliness and neatness may be exacted in their dress; not to sweep the ground with their clothes, and not designedly to stain and soil them; which is usual in children by reason of their want of providence; and yet parents, through a remarkable supineness, connive at such things.[44]

The low-cut medieval gown disappeared very early in some European Protestant areas; in some northern German towns it was ordered that no female citizen could go around with a neckline any lower than the width of one finger below the collarbone. Plainer and purer Protestant sectarians had real moral objections to colour and pattern: 'Washing our garments to keep them sweet is cleanly, but it is the opposite to real cleanliness to hide dirt in them... Real cleanliness becometh a holy people; but hiding that which is not clean by colouring our garments seems contrary to the sweetness of sincerity.' Black and white became the dress code of Reformed asceticism; but where buttoning up was required, fine linen compensated. Sober black cloth had long been favoured by the clerically minded Catholic Spanish court; and the wealthy Dutch Protestant bourgeoisie who favoured the clerical style have since become famous through their portraiture—all rustling black silk, dark velvet, and covered-up modesty, strikingly set off by magnificent lace and linen cuffs, collars, and caps.[45]

There were no regular lustral baths to perform in Protestantism, but the act of washing was self-consciously symbolic, metaphysical, and erudite. Baptism was a key theme. Edward Topsell admonished the faithful to 'the outward cleansing and washing away of the filth of our bodies, being the saviour of sinne raigning in us'.[46] The zealous puritan Philip Stubbes urged washing because 'as the filthinesse and pollution of my bodie is washed and made clean by the element of water; so is my bodie and soule purified and washed from the spots and blemishes of sin,

by the precious blood of Jesus Christ . . . This washing putteth
me in rememberance of my baptism.' The metaphysical Protestant poet George Herbert wrote that on Sunday especially:

> Affect in all things about thee cleanliness,
> Let thy minde's sweetness have his operation
> Upon thy body, clothes and habitation . . .
> That all may gladly boarde thee, as a flowre . . . [47]

At a somewhat less exalted social level, the surgeon William
Bullein seems to have found it necessary to defend and promote
washing (but only with cold water) and put an unusually full and
earnest section on cleanly grooming into the morning regimen
of his small handbook *The Government of Health* (1558), aimed at
the student or the busy man of affairs about town:

Plaine people in the countrie, as carters, threshers, ditchers, colliers,
and plowmen, use seldom times to wash their hands, as appeareth
by their filthynes, and verie few times combe their heads, as is seen
by floxes, nittes, grease, feathers, straw, and such like, which hang-
eth in their haires. Whether is washing or combing things to
decorate or garnish the body, or else to bring health to the same?

Thou seest that the deere, horse, or cow, will use friction or
rubbing themselves against trees both for their ease and health.
Birdes and hawkes, after their bathing will prune and rowse themselves upon their branches and perches, and all for health. What
should man do, which is reasonable but to keep himself cleane, and
often to wash the handes, which is a thyng most comfortable . . . If
it be done often, the hands be also the instruments to the mouth
and the eies, with many other thinges commonly to serve the
bodie . . . Kembing of the head is good in the mornings, and doth
comfort memories, it is evil at night and openeth the pores. The
cutting of toes, haire, and the paring of nailes, cleane keeping of
eares, and teeth, be not only things comely and honest, but
also holesome rules of Physicke for the superfluous things of the
excrements.[48]

The English Puritans were no ragged dusty ascetic hermits, nor were they sleek priests. They often kept their beards, in imitation of the Jewish prophets; but they despised ornamental (long) hair-styles and were ostentatiously short-haired (or round-headed): 'Off with those deformed locks, those badges of pride and vanity which you have been so warned of...hate not to be reformed [and] become your Barber, as he has been to some amongst us...'.[49] In Comenius' catechism, baths were approved to 'wash off sluttishnesse and filth... [and] cleanse and scour away all dustinesse, sweat and foulness', but any other artificial cosmetics—curled hair, wigs, or perfume—were entirely banished. In the Calvinist world, sexual uncleanness was far more important than mere bodily cleanliness, and English anti-cosmetic tirades were worthy of the Church Fathers themselves, and were highly biblical. 'Plain Man' Arthur Dent was no doubt one of many puritan masters of their households who tended to quote Isaiah:

> And what say you of our artificial women, which will be better than God made them? They like not his handiwork, they will rend it, and have other complexions, other faces, other hair, other bones, other breasts, and other bellies than God made them... But they will humbled by the Lord... instead of sweet savours there shall be a stink, and instead of a girdle, a rent, and instead of dyeing the hair, baldness...[50]

Other English puritans were even more foul-mouthed about cosmetic waters and unctions 'wherewith they besmear their faces', musk perfume 'stinkyng before the face of God', linen starch for ruffs—'the Devil's liquor'—and earrings 'for which they are not ashamed to make holes in their ears'.[51]

It might seem as if Puritans had abandoned the sensuous body altogether by treating it largely as an asexual object in which all lusts and vanities could be controlled; but this was not entirely so. Many had a surprisingly primitive passion for the God of nature, and his natural works.[52] The European

Protestant sects who did not accept the spiritual and theological authority of Lutheran Calvinism (notably the Anabaptists, Baptists, Diggers, Seekers, Ranters, Quakers, Pietists, Adamites, the Family of Love, and many others) were idealists who refused to accept the doctrine that the Christian soul was predestined to be sinful at birth: they valued individual experience, questioned the Scriptures as they saw fit, disagreed with infant baptism, and tended to be more millenarian or utopian, believing in the 'simple plainheartedness or innocency' of the human soul before the Fall of Adam and Eve, and in the redemptive virtues of Love and communal brotherhood. The radical democrat leader of the English Diggers' sect, Winstanley, insisted that the supposedly heavenly Age of the Spirit existed, now, in all people:

> We may see Adam every day before our eyes walking up and down the street . . . This innocency or plain-heartedness in man was not an estate 6,000 years ago only, but every branch of mankind passes through it. . . . Oh ye hearsay preachers, deceive not the people any longer by telling them that this glory shall not be known and seen till the body is laid in the dust. I tell you, this great mystery has begun to appear, and it must be seen by the material eyes of this flesh . . . [53]

It was a fight over the soul and the body with some unexpected consequences for the later history of hygiene—the development of Christian naturism (if we can call it that). If he or she wanted, a pure-spirited Adam or Eve could even go naked, testifying their innocence, 'and live above sin and shame'. According to the historian Christopher Hill, there were many recorded occasions 'on which very respectable Quakers "went naked for a sign", with only a loin-cloth about their middles for decency. . . . In 1652 a lady stripped naked during a church service [in the chapel at Whitehall], crying "Welcome the resurrection!" . . . such occurrences were less rare at Ranter and Quaker weddings.'[54]

As Hill discovered, many English sectarians systematically proclaimed the right of natural man to live naturally, and to worship the God of nature; and nothing shows this more than the passionate debates over the hygiene and morality of pure food, cool air, and cold water. Confirming a general moral–thermal shift that seems to have begun in the later sixteenth century, English sectarians joined in the general Protestant attack on medieval (Catholic) Galenism, and loudly repudiated the old so-called 'Hot Regimen' in favour of a new and ascetic 'Cold Regimen'.

Pure Foods

Diet had long been linked to catharsis and purgation, and easily became a locus for puritanism. The seventeenth century was the time when many (if not most) of the Western world's 'Rich Restoratives' were introduced via the flourishing international trade routes. These new food drugs were cane sugar, tea, coffee, chocolate, and tobacco, and the new drinks made from the chemist's recent discovery of pure 'neat' alcohol—brandy, gin, fortified wines such as port or sherry, and herbal and fruit liqueurs such as aquavit and cherry brandy. All these items went down extremely well with the public, but were regarded by ascetics as excessively corrupting foods that produced over-heated brains and venal 'Hot, fantastick passions of love'. One seventeenth-century English physiologist's internalized moral hatred of the supine, sickly, effeminate, and above all Foreign 'Hot Regimen from Hot Climates' had very clear targets:

> Brandy, spirits, strong wines, smoking Tobacco, Hot Baths, wearing flannel and many clothes, keeping in the House, warming of beds, sitting by great fires, drinking continually of Tea and Coffee, want of due exercise of body, by too much study or passion of the mind, by marrying too young, or by too much Venery

(which injures Eyes, Digestion, Perspiration, and breeds Winds and
Crudities): and for all the effeminacy, Niceness, and weakness of
spirits that is produced in the Hysterical and Hypochondriacal . . . [55]

Uncompromising temperance and vegetarianism became the
badge of English radicalism in the seventeenth century. Pure
food or 'vegetable' beliefs either came through individual revelation or (increasingly as time wore on) through intellectual
persuasion and reference to the natural 'common sense' of 'our
forefathers'—'yea the most of them fed upon graine, corne,
roots, pulse, hearbes, weedes and such other baggage, and yet
lived longer than wee, were healthfuller than wee'. The ascetic
works of classical Pythagoreanism and Indian Vedic vegetarianism were beginning to be rediscovered and admired. The Famil-
ists and Adamites had vegetarian followers, mirroring the sects
and believers in Cromwell's Model Army who thought meat-
eating unlawful, and cold-water drinkers who abstained from
alcohol.[56] The famous radical Protestant hermit Roger Crab,
after a near-death experience while soldiering during the Civil
War, conducted the experiment of living alone on 'a smalle
Roode of ground . . . at Ickham near Uxbridge . . . in obedience
to the command of Christ', wearing sackcloth and eating
nothing but garden produce:

if naturall Adam had kept to his single naturall fruits of God's
appearance, namely fruits and herbs, we had not been corrupted.
Thus we see that by eating and drinking we are swallowed up in
corruption . . . [and] the flesh-destroying Spirits and Angels draweth
near us . . .

By praying, fasting, and suffering the pangs given to him by his
'Old Man' (his body), Crab became something of a celebrity
healer, preaching against meat and alcohol:

if my patients were any of them wounded or feaverish, I sayd,
eating flesh or drinking strong beer would inflame the blood,

venom their wounds, and encrease their disease, so there is no
proof like experience: so the eating of flesh is an absolute enemy
to pure nature; pure nature being the workmanship of a pure God,
and corrupt nature under the custody of the devil.[57]

Fasting was a particular sign of grace. There were many Protestant women who also felt the call of personal prophecy, and
embarked on a severe ascetic regime of virginal celibacy, isolation,
and, above all, fasting. Anne Wentworth embraced virginity
and public preaching; Martha Taylor carried out a 'Prodigious
Abstinence occasioned by twelve months fasting' and was
exhibited publicly in her home; the prophet Sarah Wight
starved herself as a penance, lost her sight and hearing, went
into a catatonic state, and spoke 'extempore in soliliquies'.[58]
Oxford and Cambridge universities were monastic and celibate
institutions steeped in the traditions of fasting and the philosophical or 'Mean Diet'. Protestant Cambridge was the centre of
a core group of ascetic Protestant natural philosophers later
known as the Neoplatonists, who strenuously opposed the
'clockwork' mechanism of Descartes, and argued for the material existence of a transcendent spirit world (including angels):
'The Platonists doe chiefly take notice of Three kindes of Ve-
hicles, Aetherial, Aerial, and Terrestrial, in every one whereof
there may be several degrees of purity and impurity...'. Platon-
ism and Pythagoreanism were closely aligned in Cambridge;
one leading member of the Neoplatonists, Henry More, was
known to be a strict vegetarian who considered it his bodily
duty to 'endeavour after the Highest Purity'.[59]

In the later seventeenth century, however, the main living
prophet of English vegetarianism was the self-taught shepherd,
hatter, and popular author Thomas Tryon (1634–1703), who
wrote dozens of books on Cleanness and Innocency for all
occasions:

> There is no other way to obtain the great mystery and Knowledge
> of God, his Law, and our Selves, but by Self-Denial, Cleanness,
> Temperance, and Sobriety; in Words, Imployments, Meats and
> Drinks; all which... [keep] our bodies in Health, and our minds
> in serenity; rendering us unpolluted Temples, for the Holy Spirit of
> God to communicate with.[60]

Condemning all hot 'Gluttenous and intoxicating Liquors [and]
fumes as those of Tobacco, Opium, and the like Poysons', he
followed Crab and preached an Adamite, hermetic, country life,
living on vegetables, grains, pulses, and cold water: 'he that lives
as he ought needs but a few things, and those easie to be
procured, a small cottage, a little Garden, a Spade, Corn, and
Water, white garments, a little wood, a straw-bed, will support
Nature to the highest degree'.[61] His Pythagorean philosophy led
him to abhor the violence and pollution of towns, with their
noise, smoke, and nauseous trades (including butchery), and to
become a pacifist. In *Pythagoras his Mystick Philosophy Reviv'd*
(1691), Tryon explained that this primarily meant living without killing anything:

> Let none of your food be attended with the groans of the innocent
> Creatures... endeavour and with equal constancy and earnestness
> to pursue after purity... to eschew things derived from violence;
> and therefore be considerate in the eating of Flesh or Fish, or any
> thing not procured but by the death of some of our fellow crea-
> tures; rather let them content themselves with the Delicacy of the
> Vegetables, which are full as nourishing, much more wholesome,
> and indisputably innocent...[62]

He once produced a plan for a Society of Clean and Innocent
Livers based on 'Rules of Cleanness, Self-Denial, and Separation'
and a Sublime merciful diet, but it was never put into practice;
though famous, and even fashionable (the poet Aphra Behn was
an admirer), he undoubtedly suffered some social derision on
account of his vegetarianism—not least because his wife,

though sober in other things, refused to give up meat.[63] But Tryon was certainly a proponent of Cold Regimen, and alert to the experimental work of the Moderns. His campaign against hot drinks, hot feather beds, and hot-coddling children and swaddling babies—'lapping of them up in several Double Clothes and Swathes, so tight, that a Man may write on them'—was firmly in tune with the medical teaching of his fellow Londoner Thomas Sydenham.

Cool Air

With the work of Galileo and the Italian anatomists, William Harvey's discovery of the blood circulation in 1628, René Descartes's philosophical work on mechanical physics in the 1640s, the work of the chemists, and the appearance of the practical microscope, seventeenth-century European science was more austerely rational, practical, and certainly more 'mechanical' than the speculative Paracelsianism of the sixteenth century. During the Civil War in England (1642–60) much serious and lengthy experimental work had gone into the Baconian project of capturing the power of nature, through agricultural reform, engineering, and statistical demography; but although Commonwealth debate had ranged widely over a number of idealistic, administrative plans for the health of the people, no parliamentary action was taken. It was a scientifically inclined prince, Charles II, who established a neo-Baconian research institute, the Royal Society, in 1662. One of the key experimental sites of seventeenth-century European science was the observation and testing of the qualities of the 'Element of Air'. Ordinary, simple, clean cool Air—the breath of heaven—is where English ascetic physiology finally made its mark.

The Greek model of good odours and bad miasmas was, in the seventeenth century, held to be true beyond doubt, a cornerstone of science, but one whose essential arcana and mechanisms had yet to be found. Sanctorius had proved that the body breathed out a miasma of perspiration; the chemists had discovered gases but had not yet discovered oxygen, and were in the processing of discovering that plants breathed too. In addition to pure science, there were pressing medical and social reasons for investigating air, namely the controversial medieval plague policy of 'aerial quarantine'—barricading the air into the house by closing the door on it, purifying it with good odours, and sealing it away from the contagions raging outside (or inside). Yet was it not also seen that air was worst when it was shut up and confined? Seventeenth-century writers on plague were highly concerned about the movement of wholesome air: 'oftentimes it is seene, that sick folks doe recover their former health onely by a change of air'.[64]

Thomas Sydenham (1624–89), the so-called Father of English Medicine, was a fever doctor and follower of Hippocrates who spent years measuring the epidemics of London and carefully observing his patients. Like the Methodists, he thought that the patient should not be trampled on by 'Physic', and that a doctor's aim should be to 'Assist Nature' through therapeutic nihilism: 'truly I sometimes thought, that we can scarcely proceed too slowly in driving away diseases, and that we should proceed slowly, more being often to be left to Nature, than is now generally imagined'.[65] By ignoring the medical rules and trusting to natural instinct Sydenham successfully dispensed with the conventional fever regimen, and obtained a huge reputation. The mistake of earlier physicians, he said, had been to have 'prescribed the hottest remedies and method for those Diseases, which required above others the coldest remedies and Regimen, [as] is evident enough both in the smallpox (which is one of the hottest diseases in Nature) and in the cure of Fevers'. The fever should not be stoked up with great fires, sealed rooms, hot drinks, thick odours, and loads of blankets: for 'how can we certainly tell that we may not kill the Man, while we endeavour to dispose the Humours to Sweat by a Hot Regimen, and hot cordials . . . it is clear to me, that the Fever alone has heat enough itself; not needs it any greater heat from abroad, by a Hot Regimen'. The patient only needed cool beds, plenty of cool drinks, cool air, and no bloodletting: 'the sick must keep up adays, at least some hours, or at least lie outside the Bed. . . forbidding the use of Broth of any kind, permitting in the meanwhile the accustomed exercise, and free Air, without so much as once using any Evacuations'.[66]

Sydenham's methods meant that the sickroom, or bedroom, became a very different place to the traditional sealed and heated chamber. We can imagine that many 'modern' house-holders threw open their windows with relief to let the fumes escape, especially in the summer. They may even have started aerating their old feather beds, for the cogent reasons given by Thomas Tryon in his domestic manual *A Treatise of Cleanness in Meats and Drinks, of the Preparation of Food, the Excellency of Good Airs, and the Benefits of Clean Sweet Beds. Also of the Generation of Bugs, and their Cure* (1682):

> Now Beds for the most part stand in Corners of Chambers, and being ponderous close substances, the refreshing Influences of the Air have no power to penetrate or destroy the gross humidity that all such Places contract . . . Not that everyone's Bed does smell indifferent well to himself; but when he lies in a strange Bed, let a Man but put his Nose into the Bed when he is thoroughly hot, and hardly any Common Vault is like it . . . You are to set your other sorts of Beds as near as you can to the most Airie Places of your Rooms, exposing them to the Air the most part of the day, with your Chamber-Windows open, that the Air may freely pass, which is a most excellent Element, that does sweeten all things and prevent Putre-faction. In the Night also you ought not to have your Window-Curtains drawn, nor your Curtains that are about your Beds; for it hinders the sweet refreshing Influences of the Air . . . [67]

Cold Water

According to one early eighteenth-century cold bather, John Hancocke, it was Sydenham and Richard Mead together 'who, so far as I know, broke the Ice, as to the cool Regimen'.[68] Cold Water joined naturally with cool beds, cool vegetables, and cool air, and rounded off the total commitment to 'cold' hygiene. Hancocke's own mentor was Sir John Floyer, the highly influential author of *An Enquiry into the Right Use and Abuse of Hot, Cold, and Temperate Baths in England* (1697) who had made it his mission to exhort 'The Present Age' to 'leave off the imprudent use of Hot Baths, and to regain their ancient natural vigour, strength, and hardiness by a frequent Use of Cold Bathing'. A stern mechanist and Sanctorian, he demonstrated how Cold Baths beneficially 'stopped the pores', compressed 'the juices and the internal rarefy'd Vapours', and gave a pleasurable afterglow—'a great warmth all over'—with the body becoming 'much more nimble, and [the] Joints more pliant'. The stimulating Cold Bath was excellent for the jaded appetite, and physical weakness, whereas hot baths made 'the body weaker, the Spirits exhausted'.[69]

The indications are that hardy cold bathing was already on the increase as Floyer wrote, partly owing to the increased European interest in river-swimming. In England, William Pearcy's *The Compleat Swimmer, or, The Arte of Swimming* appeared in 1658; and Melchisedech Thevenot's *The Art of Swimming...Done out of French*, in 1699. The Cambridge natural philosophers were keen swimmers in the 1680s. The rectangular stone-lined sunken pool in the Fellows' garden at Christ's College (adorned with busts of John Milton and the famous Platonist Master, Ralph Cudworth) was the first swimming pool in Cambridge; there was a swimming pool of similar date at Emmanuel College. As well as using the river 'backs', the students frequented a stone bath built at the Moor Barns cold spring a mile from the town.[70] In his next book,

The History of Cold Bathing: Both Ancient and Modern (1706), Floyer
gave the classical antecedents—'I publish no new doctrine, but
only design to revive the Ancient practice of Physick in using
Cold Baths'—and reported that the swimming pool building
craze was well under way:

> There are a great many Cold Baths lately erected in England, and
> next to Mr Baynard's, is that at Bathessen. 'Tis in the grounds of Dr
> Parton, and by him built ... The Honourable Charles Stanley Esq,
> brother to the present Earl of Derby, has made a Noble Cold Bath in
> Gripping Wood, near Ormskirk in Lancashire. I am told he had
> made it a very compleat Bath, with all the usual conveniences.[71]

The cooling doctrine in English physiology spread steadily
through the wider public from its first beginnings in the fever
literature. When Richard Mead published his *Short Discourse
concerning Pestilential Contagion* in 1720, advising a reversal of
the policy of confining people (and their air) during the plague,
it rushed through five editions in one year, bought by a grateful
public.[72] Tryon's bed campaign was also successful. During the
eighteenth century the free-standing bed, with a straw or horse-
hair mattress, a padded quilt, and without curtains, began to
come into general use. But the Stoic regime of physical 'hardiness' from cold bathing and cold air would not have progressed
quite so far in the next two centuries, had it not been for the
philosophy of John Locke.

John Locke's Cold Regimen

In *Some Thoughts concerning Education* (1693) John Locke commented: 'Everyone is now full of the miracles done by cold Baths
on decayed and weak constitutions, for the recovery of health
and strength; and therefore they cannot be impracticable or intolerable for the improving and hardening the bodies of those
who are in better circumstances.'[73] It was Locke (1632–1704)

who gave final weight and gravitas to the Cold Regimen, and prepared the ground for its general dispersal. His *Essay concerning Human Understanding* (1690) was a treatise on the philosophy and psychology of ideas which led not only to a new European physiology of sensation, but to the first stirrings of European ethnography. Locke's early career as a tutor and teacher was summarized in his next book, *Some Thoughts concerning Education*, which gave the English gentry advice on how to bring up their children in a bracing but humane Roman style. Although the physiological details have often been treated as harmless eccentricities, they were integral to the Lockean project of physically training the senses, in the classic traditions of gymnosophy. Like Erasmus, Locke believed in the concept of the *tabula rasa*—the clean, innocent, empty page of the child's mind. In Locke's view, the mind was gradually filled with whatever moral ideas society chose to impart; but whatever was first impressed on the human mind stayed for ever; and therefore careful training of the primary and secondary senses was essential. In classical gymnastics strength of mind went with strength of body: Locke liked to quote Juvenal's aphorism 'a healthy mind in a healthy body' (*mens sana in corpore sano*), calling it 'a short but full description of the most desirable state we are capable of in this life. He who has these two has little more to wish; and he that wants either of them will be but little better for anything else.'[74]

Many of Locke's ideas would have already been familiar to the humanist-trained, reform-minded, patriotic, late seventeenth-century English reader. His educational programme was designed to turn their sons into Stoic young warriors with 'strong constitutions, able to endure hardships and fatigue'—unlike 'most children [whose] constitutions are either spoiled, or at least harmed, by cockering and tenderness'. The boys should mostly play in the open air, 'and as little as may be by the fire . . . thus the body may be brought to bear almost anything'.[75] The whole plan was set out in a few easily observable rules: 'Plenty of open air, exercise and sleep, plain diet, no wine or strong drink, very little or no physick, not too warm or straight clothing, especially the head and feet kept cold, and the feet often used to cold water, and exposed to wet.'[76] The girls, too, were included in this regime: 'The nearer they come to the hardship of their brothers in their education, the greater advantage they will receive from it.' He was particularly disapproving of girls' strait-lacing and stays, stopping the circulation and compressing the stomach: 'That way of making slender wastes, and fine shapes, serves but the more effectually to spoil them.'[77]

The change in English children's fashion towards looser cotton clothing, for boys and for girls, dates from this period. Boy's clothing should be thin and light, with no cap, and open shoes—'with holes in his shoes so that they leak'—in other words, sandals. The stockings should be changed and the feet washed every day in cold water (a custom that may have led to the invention of boys' ankle socks): 'I fear, I shall have the mistress and maids too, against me . . . It is recommendable for its cleanliness; but that which I aim at in it, is health.' Locke approvingly quoted Seneca on cold baths in midwinter, on the cold-bathing of infants by the Germans, Irish, and Scots 'of old', and thought learning to swim was essential: 'It is that saves many a man's life, and the Romans thought it so necessary that they ranked it with letters . . . the advantages to health, by often bathing, in cold water during the heat of the summer, are so many, that I think nothing need be said to encourage it.'[78] Locke's Roman hardiness, his Greek athleticism, and his Protestant naturalism clearly appealed to large numbers of the English upper classes; it was a fitness regime that many English public schoolboys endured until quite recently, including daily morning plunges into cold water (even the sea), deep winter only excluded.[79]

There was an obvious transformation in the idea of cleanness in England in the seventeenth century. The association of coolness, cleanness, and innocence appears to have emerged directly from Protestant sectarianism, blended into a formal, neoclassical framework that had reincorporated the Greek regimen of the non-naturals. The more extreme health or hygiene beliefs (whether it was the Sanctorian Sober Diet, the Mean Diet, the Vegetable Diet, or the Cold Bath) were undoubtedly held only by a rather small constituency of ascetic self-experimenters, people of independent thought and means, or invalids who needed to mend their health. But the sheer numbers of references to the actual words 'Cleanliness' or 'Cleanness' had grown extraordinarily and were much more portentous than before, certainly when highlighted (as they so often were) with a capital letter. In the following century Cleanliness was to become far more Rational. Religious mysticism gave way to a strong presumption in favour of its usefulness in disease prevention as many further scientific 'proofs' of the utility of hygiene were presented, confirming the truth of Mead's dictum: 'as Nastiness is a great source of Infection, so Cleanliness is the greatest preservative: which is the true reason, why the Poor are most obnoxious to Disasters of this kind'. The general public in eighteenth-century England were to be targeted yet again by health educationalists, for the general good of an extremely affluent new commonwealth.

chapter 8
civil cleanliness

'That the inhabitants of this kingdom have of late years changed their way of living in a very remarkable manner, and greatly increased in luxury, is a truth of which every person, who has lived any time in it, must be sensible,' wrote the economist Adam Dickson in 1773.[1] By then the age of 'heroic' sectarian Protestantism had long passed; Quaker Friends no longer interrupted sermons or went naked in the street while they were busy making their fortunes. Borrowing a phrase from John Bunyan, the old Dissenters were crossing 'the plaine of Ease', at the edge of which lay 'a little hill called Lucre, and in that hill a silver mine', beyond which stood 'Doubting Castle'. The new United Kingdom's population rose steeply from c.10.5 million in 1750 to 15.5 million in 1801. There were only four new bodies of English local civic Improvement Commissioners set up between 1700 and 1749; over the next fifty years, by 1800, there were 567.[2]

The hygienic changes during the first fifty years of the eighteenth century were still mainly personal and economic ones—most of them occurring in people's minds and inside private homes. The result was a new market for health care. The thriving eighteenth-century health and leisure industries were blatantly connected to the fast-accelerating 'wheel of fashion'—a new vortex of consumerism that had emerged from unprecedented European mercantile expansion and surplus wealth.[3] But life was still harsh, brutal, and short if you were born at the bottom of the heap; and there was only the germ of an idea, around 1750, that these immemorial conditions could be 'improved'. In the second half of the century, in England, France, and Germany especially, there was renewed interest in the utility of public hygiene, coupled with the first tentative moves towards hygienic public health policies, based on statistics and natural science. Just to keep these wider social developments in perspective, however, the leap of the imagination required to make a connection between the old idea of private hygiene and new idea of public hygiene is reflected in this footnote from the amateur health bibliophile and reformer Sir John Sinclair, uncertainly attempting to redefine personal hygiene as a social science in 1802:

> Good health and longevity depends much upon personal cleanliness, and a variety of habits and customs, or minute attentions that it is impossible here to discuss. It were much to be wished, that some author would undertake the trouble of collecting the results of general experience upon that subject, and would point out to those habits, which, when taken singly, appear very trifling, yet when combined, there is every reason to believe, that much additional health and comfort would arise from their observance.[4]

Only five years later, however, he was confidently advocating the new European philosophy of 'medical police', namely,

> 1. Police of Climate. 2. Police of Physical Education. 3. Police of Diet. Police of Public Amusements. 4. Police of Habits and Customs. Police of Public Institutions. 7. Police for the Health of Soldiers and Sailors. 8. Police to Prevent Contagious Disorders. And, 10. Police of Medicine and the means of promoting its improvement.[5]

The Age of Elegance

The overriding image of eighteenth-century Europe is one of supreme elegance: the perfect 'Quality' lifestyle of the aristocracy, gentry, and educated middle classes, for whom personal cleanliness and orderliness were now very visible marks of being 'genteel'. The large personal fortunes made in eighteenth-century Europe were discreetly covered by the cloak of fashionable French *politesse*. In France a new style of 'liberal' or 'open' manners had slowly replaced the more rigid formal manners of the seventeenth century, and smoothed the way for wealthy upper-rank aspirants: the social formalities were to be entered into easily and naturally, in leisurely informal gatherings. In England liberal French manners sat easily with liberal English politics, and spread out from London into the provinces via the bustling English presses. Anxious queries about correct social manners peppered the pages of the *Spectator* magazine, where old-style courtiers were mocked as old-fashioned, since 'our Manners sit more loose upon us'; and in the 1714 issue the editor, Joseph Addison, tackled the subject of Cleanliness. He quoted the classics and called cleanliness a Half-Virtue, lying somewhere halfway between duty to God and duty to society:

> It is evident that Cleanliness, if it cannot be called one of the Virtues, must ever rank very near them: from age to age it has ever been admitted that 'Cleanliness is next to Godliness'; it is the mark of politeness; it produced love; and it bears analogy to purity of mind; Aristotle calls it one of the Half-Virtues. No-one, unadorned with this virtue, can go into company without giving manifest offence; and the easier or higher anyone's fortune, this duty rises proportionately. The more any country is civilised, the more they consult this part of politeness.[6]

The early eighteenth-century founder of Methodism, John Wesley, in turn quoted Addison, in a sermon on dress: cleanliness was, firstly, 'the mark of Politeness', secondly, the

'Foster-mother of Love', thirdly, indicated 'Purity of Mind', and fourthly, was a 'preserver of Health'. He was known to be personally fastidious, and was insistent on cleanliness among his followers: 'Be cleanly. In this let the Methodists take pattern from the Quakers. Avoid all nastiness, dirt, slovenliness, both in your person, clothes, house, and all about you. Do not stink above ground. This is a bad front of laziness; use all diligence to be clean . . . '.[7] In Addison's and Wesley's definitions, cleanliness was still very much cast in its traditional courtly mode, predominantly a social virtue, a sign of good breeding, and a sine qua non of beauty and elegance. Clean linen, clean hands, and precision grooming marked the gentleman, as well as good manners; this Ovidian model is recalled in one of Lord Chesterfield's famous letters to his son, in 1750:

My Dear Friend. You will possibly think that this letter turns upon strange, little, trifling objects; and you will think right, if you think of them separately; but if you take them aggregately you will be convinced that as parts, which conspire to form the whole, called the exterior of the man of fashion, they are of importance. I shall not now dwell upon those personal graces, that liberal air, and that engaging address, which I have so often recommended to you, but descend still lower, to your dress, cleanliness, and care of your person . . . Take care to have your stockings well gartered up, and your shoes well buckled; for nothing gives a more slovenly air to a man than ill-dressed legs. In your person you must be accurately clean; and your teeth, hands, and nails should be superlatively so. . . . The lowest peasant speaks, moves, dresses, eats, and drinks, as much as a man of the first fashion, but does them all quite differently; so that by doing and saying most things in a manner opposite to that of the vulgar, you have a great chance of doing and saying them right. There are gradations in awkwardness and vulgarism, as there are in everything else.[8]

But how could you tell what these subtle 'gradations in awkwardness' were? Eighteenth-century English fiction was full of nuanced and didactic examples of good manners, which were certainly used as an aid to self-education. Meanwhile, the slow seepage of 'polished' manners down the social scale opened up an even greater gulf between the literate 'polite' and those without these new manners, the illiterate vulgar.

The Private Parts

'The cleanliness of the rest of your person, which, by the way, will conduce greatly to your health, I refer from time to time to the bagnio,' remarked Chesterfield casually, but not urgently.[9] He might have known better than to send his son to France with that advice—or perhaps he assumed that French aristocratic males merely looked on while their womenfolk bathed and sluiced. In France the aristocratic *tendre* for cosmetic cleanliness that had developed during the seventeenth century had reached a new peak of perfection by the eighteenth century. It had virtually become a symbol of their class. The cultic aspects of the boudoir came from the French royal ritual of the *levée*, the morning toilette conducted in the royal bedroom suite with an audience of kin, intimate friends, and favoured counsellors, an old custom of monarchs that had been perfected by Louis XIV, and which spread throughout the French nobility—a new and highly favoured grooming pleasure zone, full of objets d'art.[10] Toilet sets were increasingly given as wedding gifts, individual items came as love gifts, and visitors were meant to be impressed by the immense profusion of silver, gold, and glassware on the toilet table:

> And now, unveiled, the Toilet stands displayed,
> Each Silver Vase in Mystic Order laid.
> First, rob'd in White, the Nymph intent adores
> With Head uncovered, the Cosmetic Powrs . . .
> This Casket India's glowing Gems unlock,

All Arabia breathes from yonder Box.
The Tortoise here and Elephant unite,
Transformed to Combs the speckled and the white.
Here Files of Pins extend their shining Rows,
Puffs, Powders, Patches, Bibies, Billet Doux...[11]

Well-made French cosmetics and perfumes were all highly desirable; they were imported (even smuggled), and then flaunted, by aristocracies all over Europe.

Perfumes, powders, and paints now arrived in easy-to-use luxury packaging; intrinsically they remained largely unchanged, but their application had become a high art form. Needless to say, strong perfume accompanied every possible item of the toilette, including scented mouth pastilles, toilet waters, and moisturizing creams. Clutching their white, red, and yellow greasepaints—their *pomades à la baton*—women designed the precise colouring of their faces—their *maquillage*—like artists in front of a canvas. Body depilation, eyebrow-plucking, eye black, rouge lip salves, and innumerable shades of rouge powder for the cheeks were de rigueur; and the new fashion for powdering the hair with scented powders and greasing it to form sculptural piles over inserted padding started early in the century. The infamous 'high' hairstyle, however, was only fashionable for a short-lived decade during the 1770s; women soon reverted to the more comfortable and easily maintained 'low' styles that had been normal between 1715 and 1770.

Underneath the façade things were not always so glamorous—we know enough about the fleas, lice, smeared paintwork, and powerful body odours to be sure of that. Some at least of the heavy painting can be attributed to the ravages of smallpox, then an endemic childhood disease, or to syphilitic disfigurement. There were certainly hygiene problems connected with wear and storage of clothes and wigs; although when well kept, with cropped hair underneath, wigs would have reduced nits and lice considerably. Although the parasite load was obviously still relatively high, multiplying with every increase in population and only held in check by constant manual grooming, it was now beginning to be deterred by regular domestic bathing. Among the female French aristocracy the bath had become an indispensable part of the toilette, and was constructed from the choicest materials: marble, bronze, painted and lacquered metal, or even crystal glass. Very select visitors were received in the luxurious surroundings of the *cabinet de bain*, which, as the ever-growing genre of titillating French bath paintings show, was an arena of unabashed sexual display. The profusion of new bathing furniture and toilet articles, however, indicated a more serious grooming intent. French cabinet-makers designed new and convenient washstands, holding a large jug and basin, with little drawers, mirrors, and other contrivances underneath, which were then copied by local manufacturers; they became an indispensable item for shaving and grooming in male quarters. The newly invented French bidet, a chairlike washstand for sluicing the private parts, was used by men and women alike; it was often taken on travels and military campaigns, and became a mark of supreme cleanliness among the French upper ranks.[12]

The other supremely private part was the mouth. Paris was the centre of advanced dentistry in the mid-eighteenth century, with patients arriving from all over Europe to get their teeth mended and their dental hygiene improved. A new vogue for *le sourire* (the smile) began to affect French manners; in 1787 the artist Elizabeth Louise Vigée Le Brun broke with formal tradition and painted the first romantic open smile, with gleaming white teeth, in European art history.[13] Rotting teeth and bad breath were an extremely common and painful problem, made worse by rising imports of sugar, and sticky fruits and sweetmeats, which the older methods of soft leaves, sticks, or cloths could scarcely deal with; and a lot of damage was done by using coarse or badly ground powders, ashes, and whiteners (chalk, salt, soda), which wore the enamel or irritated the gums. Chesterfield (and many others) badly damaged his teeth through the over-energetic use of 'sticks, irons, etc., which totally destroyed them, so that I have not now above six or seven left'. If a whole family suffered from poor teeth, the dentist's bills could be a minor financial disaster. Towards the end of the century standards of dental hygiene were improving among the upper classes, even outside France. English gentry-folk would have been aware of the surgeon John Hunter's handbook on the teeth *The Natural History of the Human Teeth: Explaining their Structure, Use, Formation, Growth, and Diseases*, after 1771; and new soft toothbrushes and purer pastes arrived slowly, in the last third of the century—William Cowper in rural retreat had to send for his new toothbrushes from London, commenting 'people do not brush their teeth at Olney'.[14]

The bidet may have been a step too far for many foreign consumers. Advanced cosmetic lore was still clearly absent in Protestant England, where heavy or excessive painting (including lip- or eye-painting) was generally frowned on, and more exotic cosmetic techniques (nail paint, depilation) were virtually unknown among the virtuous. All the exposed parts were expected to be kept as clean as possible, and there were plenty of washes, lotions, and whiteners available in the old receipt books that did just that; but the more intimate demands of the body were apparently often simply ignored, in chaste Christian fashion. On the regular female menstruation, 'the curse', and its personal hygiene problems and difficulties, there was (it seems) a general silence, according to the liberal physician William Buchan:

> there are no women in the world so inattentive to this discharge
> as the English; and they suffer accordingly, as a very great number
> of them are obstructed, and many prove barren in consequence...
> False modesty, inattention, and ignorance of what is beneficial or

hurtful at this time, are the sources of many diseases and misfortunes in life, which a few sensible lessons from an experienced matron might have prevented.

The normal method of dealing with menstrual flow was to cut out and sew a pad of rag, which was then pinned onto the underpetticoat and washed daily, a method which persisted well into the early twentieth century.[15]

But even in these small matters, things were improving. An imported Indian technology—lighter cotton cloth—was beginning to make 'shifting' far easier in Europe, at the same time as increasing the amount of underwear required to be frequently laundered. Cheaper cotton in the second half of the century was a godsend for the middling classes. Raw cotton imports to Britain soared as mass production took off: printed cotton, using engraved copper plates, arrived in the 1750s, and mechanized roller-printing started another boom in the 1780s, paving the way for mechanized spinning forty years later.[16] It was also during the 1780s, that the infamous *chemise à la reine*—a white muslin undergarment shockingly turned into a peasant-style outer garment—served as the precursor of all the lighter, softer, sprigged muslin fashions to come. Perhaps not uncoincidentally, cotton 'drawers' or underbreeches (pantaloons) for women first appeared at the end of the century—a usage previously confined to men.[17] During the seventeenth century the quantity of laundering per household had doubled, and had gradually developed into two forms: the Great Wash for larger items, and the Small or 'slop' Wash for small items of body linen, usually done by the month or the season. By the mid-eighteenth century town households would be regularly doing at least one of these washes once a week.[18]

In Britain the lessons of the plague had been learnt; and a passion for science had translated into a passion for 'improved' domestic architecture. Domestic engineering was reassessed hygienically in the Greek manner (the Palladian Greek style went down particularly well in the brand-new houses built by affluent eighteenth-century colonists in North America) resulting not only in many thousands of Greek frontal pediments but in the redesigning of gardens (for outdoor exercise); of larger windows and rooms (for light and air); of kitchen stoves and smaller fireplaces (for cleaner and more controllable heat); and of plumbing and laundries (for washing and sanitation). 'Convenience' was the word most often used to describe these new domestic changes: when something was convenient, it meant it was neater, cleaner, and easier to use or maintain. The large rise in the servant population reflected the quantities of new goods to clean and look after: acres of polished flooring, marquetry, ormolu, marble, glass, mirror, silver, porcelain, chandeliers, books, tableware, and musical instruments.[19] So much *ellu* everywhere: gold-leaf glinted throughout these domestic temples. And as each modern convenience or objet d'art arrived, it became a minor luxury that could shortly without too much difficulty be copied, redesigned, and installed to fit the demands of the rather smaller houses and tighter pockets of the increasing numbers of moderately prosperous gentlefolk—a market that Josiah Wedgwood and hundreds of other small domestic manufacturers quickly discovered and supplied. By 1861 in Britain, one in three women between the ages of 15 and 24 was a household servant.[20]

For most of the English (and colonial American) upper classes the bidet was probably regarded with stupefaction (they were still not thought *convenable* in Anglo-Saxon homes until the second half of the twentieth century). But the influence of rationalism and natural philosophy was nonetheless making itself felt. Even in early eighteenth-century England puritanical attacks on the Art of Beauty were beginning to seem old-fashioned, irrational, and irrelevant, and the dogmatic Christian doctrine on cosmetics was fading fast.[21] By the mid-century

quite a lot of English prejudice about warm bathing was starting
to be laid to rest as new 'foreign' habits and practices of balneology took hold. Queen Caroline had brought her German
bathing habits with her from Ansbach when she came to the
throne in 1727, and immediately ordered a full set of tubs for
the whole royal family so that they could bathe regularly: foot-
baths, small or half-baths, body baths, and even double tubs—
the 'very large body bath'. But there was still a long way to go in
converting the English gentry, and the warm bath was still a
novelty in 1741:

> I have suffered great disappointment about the warm bath, which
> I was advised to try, for the bathing tubs are so out of order we have
> not been able to make them hold water, but I hope this week they
> will serve the purpose . . . I pray Ivole for my bathing dress, tell her
> I must go in in chemise and jupon,

wrote the gentry traveller Elizabeth Montague, obviously taking
her warm bath very modestly in loose clothing, sitting on a
stool inside the normal draped and filled bath, with her handmaiden sluicing her with more hot water (how bathing-dresses
and caps helped or hindered these arrangements is a moot
point).[22] At the beginning of the century many English gentry
country houses had successfully begun to tackle the problems of
water engineering and plumbing, and by the 1730s many of
them could, in theory, have had running water on all floors and
as many baths and water closets as required; but apparently
most owners did not fully avail themselves of this technology
until the 1780s. Clearly the older methods, and more limited
water sources, still sufficed; at least until a far more efficient type
of ball-valve water closet latrine was invented by Joseph Bramah
in 1778, which was definitely a spur to reform: by 1797 Bramah
claimed to have made 6,000 closets. Flushed water closets, being
an English invention, were joyfully called *les lieux à l'anglaise* in
France (roughly translatable as the 'English shit place'); but the

built-in plumbing they required was not considered a necessity in France until the later nineteenth century.[23]

Further interesting balneological experiences occurred when West met East in British colonial India. British travellers and residents in early eighteenth-century India were at first over-whelmed by its culture; they lived in their houses in the Indian manner, wore Indian muslins, copied the umbrellas, and were fascinated by Indian vegetarianism, medicine, botany, and phil-osophy. It was an open window that was to close quite quickly at the end of the century as the British Raj got under way. European colonialists had rapidly discovered that perfect bodily cleanliness was expected of them in accordance with the caste system, and was essential to the authority of their rule. Among other things they were fascinated by the deft and rapid daily Indian strip wash, the expert Indian *champu*, or 'shampoo' mas-sage, and the ease of the Indian shower-bath, all of which became widely adopted in Indian colonial circles—habits which they then later brought back home.[24] Elsewhere, diplo-matic wives discovered the hot-vapour Turkish baths of Con-stantinople or northern Africa when they were invited into aristocratic female harems (like Lady Mary Wortley Montagu) and wrote about them in their correspondence.

Attitudes towards personal hygiene had thus changed dramat-ically during the course of the century, under French influence. Luxurious boudoir bathing was at its height in France under Napoleon in the 1790s, by which time baths (or showers) had become essential items in most aristocratic dressing rooms. The period 1792–1815 was the era of the famous Directoire or empire line, where the confining ribbon emphasized the breasts, and the lines of the naked body were shown sensuously beneath light muslin. Being ineffably hygienic and classical, the mode came complete with Grecian drapes and light Grecian sandals—open sandals on bare feet with which nailpolish was worn, and shorter, cleaner, haircuts—the Grecian tomboy look, or the

Grecian diadem-and-topknot. For men, the heavy brocaded
cloth, wigs, hair powder, and facepaint of the aristocracy were
abandoned, replaced by the plain, sober, but well-tailored
English morning suit (originally a sporting riding suit), immaculate linen, no powder, and windswept, romantic hairstyles.[25]
The fashion for hair powder thus slowly disappeared (the British
Army abandoned hair powder after hygienists pointed out that it
tended to turn to paste in the rain).[26] In the 1790s, even in
London, 'revolutionary' standards of French hygiene were
deemed fashionable: 'This simple and delightful affair of bathing the private parts and the fundament every morning, summer
and winter—is of more importance to the bodily health, youth-
ful beauty and sweet desirableness of men and WOMEN, than
anything I can possibly mention or inculcate.'[27] But up until
the end of the century it seems quite likely that the water that
mostly touched British (and Anglo-American) bodies 'all over at
once', during most of the eighteenth century, was probably cold;
and that the personal hygiene that they knew most about was
the one that came from books.

Hygiene and Hardiness
Travellers to eighteenth-century England constantly pointed
out—with a certain wonderment—how excessively fond of
strenuous physical exercise the English were. The romantic
English parkscape that developed in the first half of the century
had long informal paths that rambled around the estate towards
newly built plunge pools, cricket pitches, stables, and carriage
rides, fishing lakes, archery butts, boatsheds, and carefully
placed picnic pavilions. The aristocracy spent their time royally feasting and sporting and then recovering from it: 'The
Pretty Duchess of Devonshire . . . has hysteric fits in the morning
and dances in the evening; she bathes, rides, and dances for ten

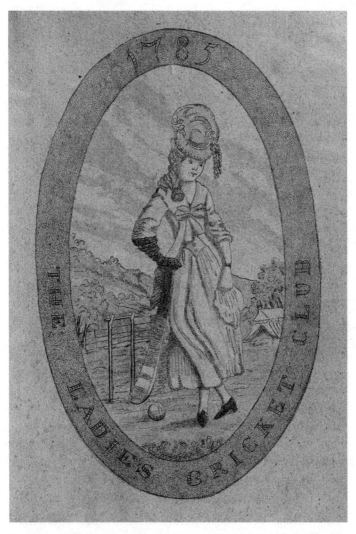

14 An unknown Ladies Cricket Club, 1785, showing the hygienic revival
of women's sports in later eighteenth-century England. Note the short
skirts and sensible shoes.

days, and lies in bed the next ten.'[28] What foreigners were seeing, in part, were the older forms of pleasure reinforced and given cachet by Locke's hygienic regimen.

The events of the seventeenth century had left the British upper classes well primed in science. Isaac Newton and John Locke had enshrined the status of science in Britain—Newton had had a state funeral, which profoundly impressed Voltaire. Between 1700 and 1770 the medical advice book market expanded intermittently but steadily, especially for works that took apart one or other of the non-naturals in detail—a style first explored in Richard Burton's *The Anatomy of Melancholy* (1621–38).[29] Readers were evidently sufficiently well versed in regimen to appreciate the growing debates on the Air, Diet, Exercise, Sleep, Evacuations, and Passions of the Mind, a trend picked up by the physician–author John Arbuthnot, who wrote two influential digests for general readers, *An Essay concerning the Nature of Aliments* (1731), and *An Essay concerning the Effects of Air on Human Bodies* (1733). An early best-seller was George Cheyne's *Essay on Health and Long Life* (1724), a semi-vegetarian Cornaroian text that explored diet, exercise, and weight loss using a quantity-controlled 'low' diet of milk, white meat, vegetables, and fruit. He told patients to monitor their weight using a Sanctorian chair, and to 'make exercise a part of their religion'.[30]

Francis Fuller's *Medicina Gymnastica* (1705; six editions by 1750) set the tone when he announced the arrival of modern Rational mechanical doctrines and denounced old humoral methods—'our too partial Consideration of the Body of Man, by attributing too much to the Fluids, and too little to the Solids'. The Cartesian–Newtonian Rational physiology emerging from the new northern Protestant universities recently opened in Leiden, Edinburgh, and elsewhere now saw the solid body in mechanical terms of pumps, ducts, and vessels, mass and flow, contraction and relaxation, entrances and exits. The pores of the skin, for example, were now likened to little valves, opening and closing on the surface; or smoky chimneys exhaling the hot vaporous excrements.[31] Muscular vigour was essential: a vigorous circulation carried off the poisons quicker and 'braced' the solids to perform their proper actions. Although Galenic bleeding and dieting was still a prop which many physicians (and patients) were loath to abandon, anything 'bracing' was considered excellent for stimulating the evacuations of the insensible perspiration—given off in a healthy, sweaty 'glow'. Fuller was greatly in favour of cold bathing for this purpose, 'a severe Method of Cure taken up lately among us . . . yet we see now the tenderest of the Fair Sex dares commit herself to that terrible element'. According to the bibliographer Charles Mullet, British bathing book lists reflect the influence of John Floyer from the 1720s, followed by a mid-century burst of scientific activity, after which 'the tide of balneological literature flows ever higher'.[32]

In the most widely read and quoted health poem of the century, John Armstrong's *The Art of Preserving Health* (1744), Hygieia was a stern and chilly goddess, and hardiness was her second name:

'Tis not for those, whom gelid skys embrace . . . to cultivate a skin
Too soft; or to teach the recremental fume
Too fast to croud through such precarious ways . . .
Study then your sky, form to its manners your obsequious frame,
And learn to suffer what you cannot shun.

Hardiness in a cold climate appeared to make perfect sense. Eighteenth-century Britain was the golden age of commercial freelance medicine (university-trained or otherwise), unrestrained by legislation or strict codes of professional ethics; and faced with a bewildering array of medical operators many people preferred to put their trust in the new hardy preventive regimen.[33] Personal regimen had now become a constant topic of conversation, like the weather, when there was little else to say; some eighteenth-century diaries and journals often recorded little else but their owner's non-natural health regime. It was often accompanied by the culture of invalidism, or the habit of constant 'complaining' about infirmities (probably the best-known regimen bore in literature is Jane Austen's valetudinarian Mr Woodhouse, with his very accommodating surgeon, Perry).[34] Though the sources have yet to be thoroughly combed for devotees of the Lockean or Spartan lifestyle, it can emerge offhandedly in letters. Thus we find out that the indefatigable Horace Walpole was indeed indefatigable, and had trained himself to be so, since the 1730s. Writing in 1777 at the age of 60 to a friend who was obviously urging him to take things easy, he replied:

> I know my own constitution exactly, and have formed my way of life accordingly. No weather, nothing gives me cold; because, for these nine and thirty years, I have hardened myself so, by braving all weathers and taking no precautions against cold, that the extremest and most sudden changes do not affect me in that respect. Yet damp, without giving me cold, affects my nerves; and, the moment I feel it, I go to town...I am preached to about taking no care against catching cold, and am told that I shall one day or other be caught—possibly: but I must die of something; why should not what has done to sixty, be right? My regimen and practice have been formed on experience and success...everything cold, inwardly and outwardly, suits me. Cold water and air are my specifics, and I shall die when I am not master of myself to employ them...

And to another friend, still at it at the age of 65:

> A hat you know I never wear, my breast I never button, nor wear great-coats, &c. I have often the gout in my face (as last week) and eyes, and instantly dip my head into a pail of cold water, which always cures it, and does not send it anywhere else. All this I dare do, because I have so for these forty years, weak as I look...

And once, from the heart:

> Christ ! Can I ever stoop to the regimen of old age ? . . . to sit in one's
> room, clothed warmly, expecting visits from folks I don't wish to
> see.[35]

He died, alas, an incapacitated valetudinarian who had to be
carried from room to room—but no doubt on his own terms.

Cold water was now being copiously applied as a universal cure-
all. In his famous work *Primitive Physic* (1747), which is known to
have reached a very wide sectarian audience, especially among
the rural puritan colonies of North America, John Wesley believed
in drinking cold water for almost anything and prescribed the
cold bath continuously, for example, 'Cancer. Use the Cold Bath.
This has cured many. This cured Miss Bates of Leicestershire of a
Cancer in her breasts, a Consumption, a Sciatica, and Rheumatism, which she had had near 20 years. She bathed daily for a
month, and drank only Water.' The book praised Cheyne and 'the
great and good Dr Sydenham' but also promoted radical Protestant health beliefs, railing against the doctors with their abstruse
science ('abundance of Technical Terms, utterly unintelligible to
Plain Men'), their evil compound medicines ('scarce possible for
Common people to know'), and their wicked slander of wise
'Empiricks' and the simple folk remedies formerly used in an
Arcadian state of grace and health.[36] In Wesley cold water was
being lauded as a folk remedy; and its contemporary revival may
well have resurrected certain deep-seated water beliefs. By the
mid-century in Britain the cold bathing of children and infants
had apparently reached the fetish stage in the well-staffed nurser-
ies of the rich at least, where, according to one critic, cold water
had attained a semi-mystic value, and become almost a rite:

> I have known some [nurses] who would not dry a child's skin after
> bathing it, lest it should destroy the effect of the water. Others will
> even put clothes dipt in the water upon the child, and either put it to

bed, or suffer it to go about in that condition. Some believe, that the whole virtue of the water depends upon it being dedicated to a particular saint; while others place their confidence in a certain number of dips, as three, seven, nine, or the like; and the world could not persuade them, if these do not succeed, to try it a little longer... We ought not, however, entirely to set aside the cold bath, because the nurses make a wrong use of it. Every child, when in health, should at least have its extremities daily washed in cold water. This is a partial use of the cold bath, and is better than none. In winter this may suffice; but, in the warm season, if a child be relaxed, or seem to have the tendency of rickets or scrofula, its whole body ought to be frequently immersed in cold water.[37]

See that body glow. Being rubbed raw after a freezing morning bath, every day, year after year—possibly even for life—was the lot of many British infants and adults, from the eighteenth century onwards.

The other main barometer of eighteenth-century British cold-water balneology is the existence of the baths themselves. The equipment for cold-water therapy was either very simple—like Walpole's bucket—or very elaborate. Stone-built cold plunge baths were either put in small bathing pavilions near the house (as at Kenwood House in Hampstead), or built as small rectangular swimming pools in sylvan settings overlooking the countryside, with or without charming shell-encrusted grottoes and waterfalls.[38] Commercial outdoor facilities were quickly provided for the carriage trade: the river baths run by an apothecary, John King from Bungay in Suffolk, were advertised to the 'Physicians and Gentry in our neighbourhood' with all the necessary conveniences: changing and eating pavilions, carriage access, bridges, gardens, plantations, boats, and bathing platforms. He had already added 'a warm Bath, together with a Bagnio or Hummumms...accommodation rarely to be met with unless in the Metropolis or very popular places'. Surely a day out with a difference in 1737. Over on the other side of the country, the Salop

Infirmary near Shrewsbury, in Shropshire, began opening its baths to the paying public from 1748; as had the mid-eighteenth-century Liverpool Infirmary, with its suite of cold baths on the ground floor, both paid for by public subscriptions. The Salop baths were opened at 1s. per person (later reduced to 6d. for adults and 3d. for children) with an extra 6d. for a hot bath: middle-class prices. The inclusion of hot baths must have seemed wonderfully practical, as well as delightfully exotic and novel, explaining the mid-century success of Bartolomeo Dominicetti's suites of urban commercial Turkish baths for the gentry in Chelsea and Knightsbridge, and 'particularly at York, Manchester, Newcastle upon Tyne, Bristol, and et cetera'.[39]

The fact that the various balneological routines were described so carefully suggests that full-body immersion did not necessarily come naturally, and was a technique that had to be learnt by the general public (or so the doctors certainly thought). The cold 'dip' was just as exhaustively described for the upper and middle classes in the eighteenth century, as shower-baths and the strip wash were in popular working-class advice books in the nineteenth century. Cold bathing, of course, was tremulously associated with the frightful 'shock of the cold'. In 1771 the Delaware resident Elizabeth Drinker screwed up her courage to take the cold plunge—and hated it: 'S. Merriot Snr., Molly Hall, Anna Humber, and Self went this Afternoon into the Bath, I found the shock much greater than I expected.... took a ride this morning to the Bath, had not courage to go in ... went into the Bath; with fear and trembling, but felt cleaver after it.' She soon gave up her attempts at cold bathing, and did not try again for twenty-eight years. She was not alone: in 1796 young Henry Tucker in Williamsburg wrote, 'Mama has taken a bath and enjoyed it very much though at first she was quite frightened.'[40] But more and more it was the lure of the sea, and the seaside, that gave cold bathing that extra zest. The main reason why fearful people forced themselves to be braced and battered by cold water was that it had become a social event, as firmly attached to communal pleasures and merrymaking as the hot stoves had ever been.

Sea Bathing and Fresh Air

Unlike the mineral-water spa, sea-bathing resorts were not confined to certain geographical areas, and the history of British resort development is above all one of steady geographical spread. People were already cold-dipping in the sea in Lancashire and Wales at the beginning of the eighteenth century, in what seems to have been an entirely local custom. While walking the Welsh coastline in the 1790s, the poet, swimmer, and philosopher Samuel Taylor Coleridge came upon an unusual scene which he greatly admired for its innocence:

> At Holywell I bathed in the famous St Winifred's Well—it is an excellent cold bath. At Rudland is a fine ruined castle. Abergeley is a large village on the sea coast. Walking on the sea sands, I was surprized to see a number of fine women bathing promiscuously with men and boys—perfectly naked! Doubtless, the citadels of their chastity are so impregnably strong, that they need not the ornamental outworks of modesty. But seriously speaking, where sexual distinctions are least observed, men and women live together in the greatest purity. Concealments set the imagination a'working, and, as it were, *canthardizes* our desires.[41]

By the 1730s Scarborough and Margate on the east coasts were developing recognizable sea-bathing seasons, while Brighton on the south coast took the fashionable lead after Dr Richard Russell eulogized it in 1752, and became the hub of a coastal growth that spread lengthways east and west.[42] In the second half of the century the seaside became closely associated with the new European Romanticism, making it even more appealing and 'sublime'. In the 1790s a second wave of seaside resorts and inland 'watering places' was developed for a mass urban clientele, each successive village inexorably swallowed up in turn, as gentry health-seekers sought ever quieter or more exclusive scenery. Partly in response to British travellers' demands, in the early nineteenth century seaside resorts began to spread steadily along the northern coasts of France and Germany, and rapidly extended to fashionable health resort developments on the southern Mediterranean French coast, the French and German Alps, the Italian coastline, and the Italian Lakes. But the most popular beaches of all were near the larger cities. In America the early inland spas and river baths were dramatically eclipsed by sea-bathing resorts springing up on the east coast: in 1794 the crowds coming out from New York to sea bathe, drink tea, and admire the views in the coastal resort at Long Island were so great 'as to keep four large ferry boats, holding twenty persons each, in constant employ'. There were similar crowds on the coast near Liverpool during a hot August in 1791:

> For a week past, upon the most moderate calculation, here has not been less than five thousand persons out of the country, for the express purpose of bathing in the sea. If to these we add five thousand of the inhabitants . . . ten thousand persons have daily been immersed in the briny element; and that on an extent of shore not much exceeding half a mile.[43]

Nothing stimulated the economy like health resorts. George Carey's famous resort guidebook *The Balnea: or, An Impartial Description of All the Popular Watering Places in England* (1801) was a lively (and sarcastic) progress report on the genteel state of each of these thriving new settlements. Jane Austen's last, half-finished novel about a mythical coastal resort, Sanditon, written during the renewed resort boom in Britain after the Napoleonic Wars in 1816–17, would undoubtedly have been a satiric masterpiece on the subject of coastal resorts and health-faddery in general. In what is left of it, it still is. Austen's tongue-in-cheek descriptions gently but unerringly undermine all the pretensions of late eighteenth-century British balneological tourism:

'But Sanditon itself—everybody has heard of Sanditon. The favourite—for a young and rising bathing place—certainly the favourite spot of all that are to be found along the coast of Sussex...'...
Mr Parker's character and history were soon unfolded...he was perceived to be an enthusiast, a complete enthusiast. Sanditon, the success of Sanditon as a small fashionable bathing place, was the object for which he seemed to live. A very few years ago it had been a quiet village of no pretension...circumstances having suggested to himself and the other principal landowner the probability of its becoming a profitable speculation, they had engaged in it, and planned and built, and praised and puffed, and raised it to something of young renown; and Mr Parker could now think of very little besides....'Civilization, civilization indeed!' cried Mr Parker, delighted. 'Look, my dear Mary, look at William Heeley's windows. Blue shoes, and nankin boots! Who would have expected such a sight at a shoemaker's in old Sanditon! This is new within a month. There was no blue shoe when we passed this way a month ago. Glorious indeed! Well, I think I have done something in my day. Now for our hill, our health-breathing hill'...

Trafalgar House, on the most elevated spot on the down, was a light elegant building, standing in a small lawn with a very young plantation around it, about a hundred yards from the brow of a steep but not very lofty cliff...Charlotte, having received possession of her apartment, found amusement enough in standing in her ample Venetian window and looking over the miscellaneous foreground of unfinished buildings, waving linen and tops of houses, to the sea, dancing and sparkling in sunshine and freshness.[44]

Academic Physiologies

In the second half of the century two particular scientific developments had greatly strengthened the impact of hygiene, and given the European—and American—public a whole new set of medical words to play with. Firstly, physiology took a turn towards the social sciences, towards seeing the human body en masse, observing the effects of personal hygiene from a distance. Secondly, a new phase of physiology opened up through the mid-century discovery of the nervous system, which ultimately led to the softening of the 'heroic' form of cold hygienic regimen. The first development opened up the public mind; the other appealed to more private sensibilities.

In the new 'Westernized' world that was now so closely interconnected by science on both sides of the Atlantic, health advice book publications rose steeply from c.1770 to 1800. Most of them were now written by university-trained medical professionals.[45] During the first half of the century, hundreds of university graduate theses had begun to focus on the Hippocratic relationship between human disease and the physical environment, including the social environment. While some were attempting to systematize the classification of diseases through theory, others were empirically searching for disease *causus* elsewhere. Study of the air had led to study of the climate and 'emanations' from foul waters and places, without dislodging earlier theories of direct contagion through touch, bites, or poisons.[46] Epidemic quarantine had long been imposed for leprosy and plague, but the full political apparatus of quarantine in Europe is generally held to have emerged with the mercantile plague regulations of the early modern Italian city-states; and for similar commercial reasons, increasingly elaborate pan-European quarantine regulations were gradually adopted during the seventeenth and eighteenth centuries.[47] But the hardest-hitting proofs of environmental impact in the eighteenth century, and which ultimately led to the revision of European quarantine legislation in the nineteenth century, came from the neoclassical revival of military hygiene—the old Roman classical category of 'ships, camps, and armies'.

The key experiments were those of the Scottish physician Dr John Pringle (1707–82), physician-general of the British Army from 1742 to 1758, who used his position to study the effects of mass crowding on disease and fevers and, especially, the means of 'antisepsis' (as elsewhere, Dr James Lind was experimenting with 'antiscorbutic' fruit—limes—to stem appalling naval losses due to scurvy). Pringle's influential *Observations on the Diseases of the Army* (1752) described how he had applied Sydenham's cooling regime to his soldiers, and found that it worked, including bathing them in the sea. Mortality fell, and rates of casual infection fell. He also found that a systematic regime of cleanliness was of utmost importance in preserving the gains. His subsequent chemical and mechanical analysis of putrefaction, infection, and contagious particles was also persuasive: 'It was never imagined, until Dr Pringle shewed it, that the Antiseptic Power is so extensive.'[48] Specific antiseptic matter could be found, according to Pringle, in mineral salts and in the fluids of most vegetables, which could be used in the form of good antiseptic odours or fumes (sulphur), or astringent washes (vinegar). More generally, coolness on its own could retard and prevent putrescence: cold water and cold air both had antiseptic properties, but the air was most antiseptic because it also dried. The diseases that responded to hygiene best were the 'low' enteric diseases, and diseases of the skin, all of which were prevalent in overcrowded conditions. The remedies were the ancient ones: personal cleanliness and clean clothes, exercise and fresh air, and constant vigilance to eradicate all sources of dirt.

The next generation carried on testing, and took Pringle's 'gospel of cleanliness' into all sorts of places. Captain James Cook used full hygienic principles on board his zealously scrubbed ship, with its equally scoured crew (taking Lind's fruit with him as an extra onboard experiment) in his first voyage round the globe in 1770, returning triumphantly with only one man lost and all the rest in good health. Other naval officers followed suit, and late eighteenth-century British naval hygiene became a thorough exercise in the health management of men and resources—carrying antiscorbutic oranges, lemons and limes, and fresh vegetables; enforcing drill, swimming, and athletics; cleaning linen and inspecting quarters, and detecting early signs of fevers, all of which revolutionized morale on board ship. By the end of the century the army officers were demanding full-scale hygienic reforms too. The civilian hospital movement was also spurred on by naval hygiene; mainly by Pringle's reformed naval hospitals, but also by the success of Dr John Haygarth's antiseptic regime at his fever hospital at Chester in the 1770s—especially his investigations into actively infectious 'zones' around the patient (which he concluded was roughly one yard).[49] In the 1780s the long campaign to hygienically reform the British and European prison systems began, started by the philanthropist John Howard and the Quaker reformer Elizabeth Fry.

The 'animal' nervous system was first clearly described by Albrecht von Haller in 1752, and turned into the central physiological problem of the eighteenth century. By the second half of the century it was widely assumed that 'nervous' energy was one of the key agencies through which the human animal interpreted the environment, via the nerves connected to the senses: it was what made humans 'sensible'—or 'sensate', as we would now call it. Moral feeling ran high over potential implications. A whole new nervous pathology was required, and with it a new sensate interpretation of personal hygiene and regimen. As always, excess was blamed. Overwrought nerves, or nervous 'sensibilities', were now the cause of a new range of 'diseases of civilization'—nervous havoc caused by over-sensuous, luxurious, and 'artificial' modes of urban life (later called 'asthenia').[50] In 1780s London, quack 'sensualist' doctors adroitly took money off sensitive well-off 'New Age' readers whose health interests included the occult, herbalism, primitive diet, balneology, pneumatics, magnetism, and electricity. The medical showman James Graham, 'the Hygienist', treated the sexual disorders of the aristocracy on, and in, his famous electric 'galvanized' bed (surrounded by flashing lights) in his Electrical Temple of Health and Hymen in London's fashionable West End. He also guaranteed total cure for nervous prostration from a hectic, overheated social life with other elemental purifications, such as vegetarian foods, water bathing, sun and air bathing—and his unique therapy of earth bathing (being buried up to the neck in earth to absorb its goodness).[51] Deep below this urban health faddery, however, lay the many different 'proofs' and debates that had originally encouraged Jean-Jacques Rousseau to dream of a new relationship with nature.

Child Health

Rousseau's famous *Émile, ou, L'Éducation* (1762), a health book in the form of a novel, can be credited with the invention of the *vis medica naturae* at the heart of the Romantic movement. His determination to restore natural medicine sprang, he said, from his own unhappy and confined childhood; and John Locke gave him the physiological framework of nervous and innate sensation that he built on. His concise opinion of nature and nurture was contained in the opening paragraph: 'The inner growth of our organs and faculties is the education of nature; the use we make of this growth is the education of men; what we gain by our experience of our surroundings is the education of things.'[52] Emile and Sophy, his girl partner and 'helpmeet', were to be given back all their natural sensations, in full. They were breastfed, never swaddled, lived hardily mainly outdoors, and were allowed to run, jump, shout, laugh, and question freely and instinctively, learning through play—Rousseau's axiom was that 'children learn nothing from books that experience cannot teach them'. Even regimen was another of those rigid conventions that bound men hand and foot in society; over-careful habits were artificial, and 'the only habit the child should be allowed to contract is that of having no habits'. Rousseauian experiments throughout Europe later inspired the Pestalozzian school of educational philosophy, for which *Émile* was considered to be 'the children's charter'.

Rousseau was certainly a wake-up call to newly conscience-stricken mothers in the eighteenth century. The role of the 'Devoted Mother' was strengthened: she was a new partner in the education of the child. Old nurses who fussed and fretted and knew nothing of higher scientific, moral, or educational motives were out. Rational mothers, fathers, tutors, and doctors were in:

We write to Reason: Hence ye doating train
Of Midwives and of Nurses ignorant!... Thine is the nursery's
charge; Important trust !...
To this then bend thy care, O parent Mind;
Array thy Child in Health. Wouldst thou thy children blest?
The sacred voice of Nature calls thee; Where she points the way,
Tread confident... [53]

Large numbers of mothers apparently followed Rousseau's programme to the letter, taking to breastfeeding and vegetarianism along with everything else.[54] The French Romantic poet Lamartine, for example, was a vegetarian, having been brought up by a Rousseauian vegetarian mother:

[I had] a philosophical education corrected and softened down by motherly feelings. Physically, this education flowed in a great measure from Pythagoras and *Émile*. Consequently the greatest simplicity in dress and the most rigorous frugality in food formed its basis... Mother was convinced that killing animals to feed on their flesh was wrong and barbarous, and implanted hard-heartedness.[55]

Like Émile, she took him to a slaughterhouse at an early age, in order to disgust him (which it did). A whole new generation of Rousseauian-educated children became young men and women in late eighteenth-century Europe, deeply inspired by personal freedom, political liberty, democracy, poetry, science, and a love of 'sublime' nature. In England vegetarianism reappeared on the revolutionary agenda at the end of the century, as 'a necessary step in the moral perfection of humanity', part of a utopian New Age in which animal rights were to be fully equal with human democratic rights.[56] John Oswald's Jacobin-inspired text *The Cry of Nature; or, An Appeal to Mercy and Justice, on Behalf of the Persecuted Animals* (1791) stimulated a new group of English vegetarian radicals such as Thomas Young (*An Essay on Humanity to Animals*, 1798), Joseph Ritson (*Essay on Abstinence from Animal Foods as a Moral Duty*, 1802), John Frank Newton (*The Return to Nature, or, A Defence of the Vegetable Regimen*, 1811), and, not least, the hardy and unconventional nature poets enrapturing the London *ton* at the turn of the century: notably Coleridge (1772–1834), Lord George Byron (1788–1824), and Percy Bysshe Shelley (1792–1822). Shelley was the author of the influential vegetarian essay *Vindication of a Natural Diet* (1813), the atheistic poem *Queen Mab*, and the pacifist poem *The Revolt of Islam* (which influenced George Bernard Shaw and Mahatma Ghandi), all of which made him a famously romantic vegetarian, especially after his early death.[57]

William Buchan

Thanks to the influence of John Locke, children's health and medicine (paediatrics) had become a strong clinical speciality in Britain. William Cadogan's famous *Essay upon Nursing, and the Management of Children*, which urged natural breastfeeding and was against unnatural swaddling, was published in 1748, some fourteen years before Rousseau; while William Buchan's

Domestic Medicine (1769), written by an enlightened and sensitive Edinburgh children's doctor, became the best-selling British practical health manual of the second half of the century. *Domestic Medicine* was translated into many European languages, republished successfully in America, and lasted well into the nineteenth century. If anyone had doubted the importance of a good regimen, or found it difficult to understand medicine, or to talk about their health problems, after 1769 they had their private help and ever-present consultant in Buchan. Buchan and all the other professional authors who wrote in the great surge of health publications in the last thirty years of the century (including, in France, Simon Tissot's *Avis au peuple sur la santé*, 1761) were already determined that the hygiene-and-cleanliness message hitherto given to those under parental or state care should reach far into the middling classes, and become a general social habit.

Buchan thought instinctively in public health terms, and in a strongly journalistic style. The first page of *Domestic Medicine* had a heart-stopper in the second paragraph: 'It appears from the annual registers of the dead, that almost one half of the children born in Great Britain die under twelve years of age. To many, indeed, this may appear to be a natural evil; but on due examination it will be found to be one of our own creating.' Buchan combined Rousseauian hygienic sensibilities with brisk, pragmatic common sense, and was yet another Celsus. His elegantly written instructions and discussions on the hygienic *vis medicatrix naturae* showed him to be a moderate regimenist, a cautious prescriber, and a reluctant bloodletter. Liberal advice on personal cleanliness, good diet, proper sleep patterns, and plenty of exercise sent children out to romp in fresh air away from their books, and kept girls out of tight-fitting stays—'that wretched custom which prevailed some years ago of squeezing every girl into as small a size in the middle as possible'. Menstruation was approached hygienically and practically, banishing secrecy, urging cleanliness, good diet, and exercise; he even talked openly about the menopause, calling it a difficult and dangerous period of life: 'Hence it comes to pass, that so many women either fall into chronic disorders, or die about this time'; continuing, a little more reassuringly, 'Such of them as survive it, however, often become more healthy and hardy than they were before, and enjoy strength and vigour to a very great age.'[58]

Three special chapters on 'Intemperance', 'Cleanliness', and 'Infection' enlarged on three themes dear to Edinburgh medicine: Buchan reverently visited and interviewed the ageing Sir John Pringle, and enshrined his theories throughout *Domestic Medicine*. Human slovenliness and ignorance were the main culprits behind disease: 'the peasants in most countries seem to hold cleanliness in a sort of contempt ... everybody may be clean, even in rags, or in the meanest abode'. Of streets and towns: 'We are sorry to say, that the importance of cleanliness does not seem to be sufficiently understood by the magistrates of most great towns in Britain; though health, pleasure, and delicacy, all conspire to recommend it.' In true patrician style, the all-important question of urban water supply that was to feature so largely in the nineteenth century was politely mentioned, while the idle poor were crushingly accused:

Most great towns in Britain are so situated as to be easily supplied with water; and those persons who will not make a proper use of it after it is brought to their hand, certainly deserve to be severely punished ... It is not sufficient that I be clean myself, while the want of it in my neighbour affects my health as well as his. If dirty people cannot be removed as a common nuisance, they ought at least to be avoided as infectious. All who regard their health should keep a distance even from their habitations.

But the Buchanite poor were to have good done unto them, whether they liked it or not. Buchan regarded nursing as a Christian mission:

> There cannot be a more noble, or more god-like action, than to minister to the wants of our fellow creatures in distress . . . to instil into their minds some just ideas of the importance of proper food, fresh air, cleanliness, and other pieces of regimen necessary in diseases, would be a work of great merit, and productive of many happy consequences.

This was a direct appeal from the pious Nonconformist Buchan to the many thousands of godly women and men with time on their hands and zeal in their hearts, and certainly helped to educate and support the generation of social reformers who became active towards the end of the century. Buchan ended his chapter on cleanliness with a rousing (and very much quoted) appeal to enlightened civility and common sense:

> Cleanliness is certainly agreeable to our nature . . . It sooner attracts our regard than finery itself, and often gains esteem where that fails. It is an ornament to the highest as well as the lowest in station, and cannot be dispensed with in either. Few virtues are of more importance than general cleanliness. It ought to be carefully cultivated everywhere; but in populous cities it should be almost revered.[59]

Revolutionary Hygiene and *Naturphilosophie*

After 1789 the French Revolution gave hygiene a new political status. Revolutionary French hygienists enthusiastically followed the plan of rational medicine set by the *philosophes*, and used hygiene and preventive medicine as a stick with which to beat the forces of conservatism. Revolutionary hygiene progressed from being a lengthy article in the *Encyclopédie méthodique* in the 1780s to becoming officially adopted as one of the rights of the healthy citizen, and one of the duties of the state, by the National Convention's Committee on Salubrity in 1793. Behind the scenes public hygiene had been a long time maturing. Plague deaths (and commercial life insurance tables) had stimulated the first studies of 'political arithmetic' in seventeenth-century England, and a similar trend towards population quantification emerged in the pious economic 'cameralism', or benevolent despotism, of the early eighteenth-century Protestant German states, who began to devise pious political policies (medical police) to encourage 'vigorous growth . . . virtuous conduct . . . praiseworthy education . . . [and] abundance of necessary, useful and superfluous means of life' for their populations.

In 1732 Peter Sussmilch produced the first demographic study using population statistics; in 1738 Friedrich Hoffman published *Medicus Politicus* ('The State Doctor'); in 1749 first Sweden and then Finland completed the first European censuses, which formed the basis of their early and comprehensive national health systems, and the rest of Europe followed during the course of the century. At the time of the French Revolution, Johann-Peter Frank was halfway through his six-volume *System einer vollständigen medizinischen Polizei* ('A System of Complete Medical Police', 1779–1821), which was to form the basis of a newly established public health university course for trainee Habsburg imperial administrators. In it he discussed the hygienic necessity for the public regulation of marriage, pregnancy, and lying-in services, personal hygiene, clothing, nutrition, food control, drainage, pure water supplies, street cleaning, venereal disease, prostitution, orphans, housing, and the sanitary regulations of hospitals. Frank became the hero of the *partie d'hygiène* in France, based at the new Department of Hygiene at the Royal Academy of Medicine, which put French hygiene on a solidly professional footing after the Napoleonic Wars.[60]

But at the heart of European hygiene in the revolutionary period *c.*1790–1820 was a 'transcendent' or 'vitalist' *Naturphilosophie* that galvanized the natural sciences and inspired the Romantic concept of 'sublime nature'. German *Naturphilosophie*—nature philosophy—laid the foundations of nineteenth-century eugenics and naturopathy, and (incidentally) finally legitimized the warm bath. Vitalism was the old seventeenth-century scientific philosophy that argued for the material existence of the divine or supernatural, against the prevailing Cartesian, or mechanistic, scientific paradigm; and in the eighteenth century it had become deeply engaged with the contemporary discoveries of 'universal forces' in physics (such as chemistry, pneumatics, electricity, and magnetism). Vitalism was reinvigorated by the philosopher Immanuel Kant (1724–1804), a fervent admirer of Rousseau, in his seminal work, the *Critique of Pure Reason* (1781). Kant seemed to provide a rational solution to the problem of material–immaterial existence by defining 'pure reason' (or pure science) as a priori: pure reason was not contingent, it existed of itself, and was 'absolute' in itself, like pure mathematics or logic, and humans used natural rationalism and intuition to comprehend a priori truths about the invisible forces of the universe (which Kant saw as consisting of eternal motions of attraction and repulsion). Many of Kant's followers (including the philosopher Hegel and the great physical geographer Alexander von Humboldt, who wrote a massive five-volume work on the integrated ecology of the cosmos) therefore dedicated their lives to the rational progress of a priori knowledge in the modern era; or (like the poet Samuel Taylor Coleridge, or the painter Joseph Turner) found inspiration in 'sublime' visions of nature.

The most speculative form of pure *Naturphilosophie*, however, was developed by Friedrich Schelling in his *System of Transcendental Idealism* (1800), which involved devising a complete theoretical model of the synthetic macrobiological universe, infused with the 'pure spirit of nature', governed by harmonious principles of logic and universal polarities ('antinomies')—often demonstrated by followers in the form of complex tables, diagrams, and flow charts.[61] Transcendental *Naturphilosophie* saw the whole world as an endless cycle of matter, or, as one health book author put it,

> we find [Nature] moves in a circle; that the smallest particle, though invisible to our eyes, is usefully employed by her restless activity; and that death itself, or the destruction of forms and figures, is no more than a careful decomposition, and a designed regeneration of individual parts, in order to produce new substances, in a manner no less skilful than surprising... all Nature is united by indissoluble ties, [hence] we justly conclude, that man himself is not an insulated being, but that he is a necessary link in the great chain which connects the universe.[62]

Subsequently airbrushed out of materialist history, 'pure reason' *Naturphilosophie* became an almost forgotten scientific episode until the more complex questions it raised concerning holistic, balanced, or 'organized' systems quietly re-emerged in early twentieth-century biology.[63] But its vitalist health practices and nature philosophies lived on; for the spiritual and philosophical holism that so disgusted the nineteenth-century professional materialists had a much greater and more long-lasting appeal for lay men and women.

Vitalist Health Care

The medical bible of the end-of-century European *Naturphilosophie* vitalists was the health book by Goethe's friend Christian Wilhelm Hufeland (1762–1836), called *Makrobiotik, oder, Die Kunst, das menschliche Leben zu Verlängern* (1794), translated into English as *The Art of Prolonging Life* in 1797 (thus taking the strange foreign word *Makrobiotik* out of the title).[64] *Makrobiotik* was a handbook on how to control the 'rapid or slow vital consumption' of the life force, and how to regulate the 'vital operations' and 'vital organization' of the body. It held out the hope not only of personally prolonging life, but of being able to perfect it universally, in the future, through physical culture: 'by culture alone, [man] becomes even physically perfect...physical and moral health are as nearly related as body and soul. They flow from the same sources; become blended together; and when united, the result is, HUMAN NATURE ENNOBLED AND RAISED TO PERFECTION.'[65] There was a new emphasis, in vitalist health care, on what we might call the regimen of future genetics—the guiding and regulation of the conditions of birth as well as life. Hufeland's basic 'Means of Prolonging Life', for example, started with: 'Good physical descent'. The British vitalist author A. F. M. Willich spelt out these 'Means' more clearly:

A certain bodily and mental disposition to longevity. A sort of hereditary disposition. A perfect birth of child, and proper conduct in the mother. A gradual culture of the physical and mental faculties. A constant habit of brooking and resisting the various impressions of external agency. A steady and equal progress of life. A sound state of digestion. Equanimity of mind—avoiding violent exertions.

In the highly symmetrical style of vitalist physiology, the exact opposite regimen, of course, spelt doom:

Bad descent, debilitating education, impure air, bad nourishment, sedentary mode of life, immoderate or deficient sleep, immoderate activity, care of skin neglected, passions and excessive sensibility, venereal dissipation, pain, unnecessary and superfluous use of medicines, poisons, infectious poisons...

The vitalists were constantly lamenting the loss of 'national debility—the debility of the age' in which man was 'no longer the son of nature' and 'nothing remains except affected sensations'. The poor had 'immoral habits and relaxed principles', while the upper classes were cultivated but supine. 'I hope I may be forgiven', said Willich, 'when I assert that the present age appears to labour under a certain mental and corporeal imbecility.'[66]

The vitalists were great enthusiasts for all types of bath, cold, warm, and hot—especially the new vapour baths and shower-baths. The science of dermatology was riding high at the turn of the century, as a newly revived subspecialism of physiology focused on the still-virulent skin diseases of the poor. Through vitalist dermatology the warm bath at last reappeared in public, medically reinstated in full.[67] The skin, readers were now told, was one of the most important organs of the body: 'the greatest medium for purifying our bodies'—'the seat of feeling, the most general of all our senses, or that which in an essential manner connects us with surrounding nature'. Willich even pointed out the natural connection between human and animal grooming.[68] He gave the warm bath an unqualified seal of approval, in the now standard chapter 'Cleanliness in General':

Cleanliness... claims our attention in every place which we occupy, and wherein we breathe... Let the body, and particularly the joints, be frequently washed with pure water... The face, neck and hands... the ears... the whole head... the mouth... the nose... the tongue... the feet... the beard and nails... it would be of great service, if the use of baths were more general and frequent, and this beneficial practice not confined to particular places or seasons, as a mere matter of fashion. Considered as a species of domestic remedy, as one which forms the basis of cleanliness, bathing, in its different forms, may be pronounced one of the most extensive and beneficial restorers of health... The warm, that is the tepid, or luke-warm state, being about the temperature of blood, between 96 and 93 of Fahrenheit, has usually been considered as apt to weaken and relax the body; but this is certainly an ill-founded notion... On the contrary, the lukewarm or tepid bath from 85 to 96 is always safe; and so far from relaxing the tone of the solids it may be justly considered as one of the most powerful and universal restoratives with which we are acquainted.

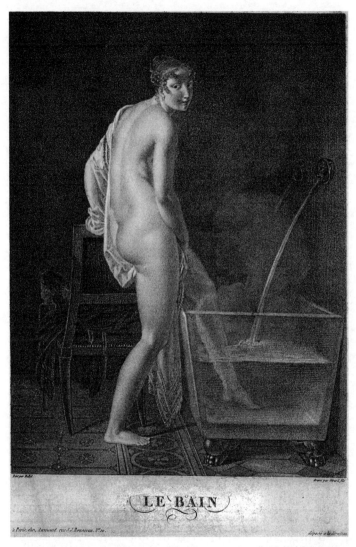

LE BAIN

15 An early nineteenth-century neoclassical nude with a classical hair-style and a crystal bath—but the lion-head taps are attached to a modern hot-and-cold plumbing system.

Children should be washed in warm water daily, adults once a week, 'and it will be of considerable service to add to it three or four ounces of soap'. Precisely accurate temperatures were essential in maintaining exactly the right mean body temperature, along a supposed sliding scale of nervous or 'sthenic' irritability (hence the new diagnosis of 'asthenia'). The 'vital signs' of the human body were also thought to react to air temperature, barometric pressure, and air quality, which led some vitalists to start experimenting with the improvement of domestic ventilation, and even with outdoor air baths: 'By exposing the naked body for a short time to an agreeable cool or even cold air, we perceive effects somewhat similar to those produced by the cold bath . . . [It is] a species of bath that certainly deserves a fair trial.'[69]

With such high standards, the general public's personal hygiene was inevitably assessed and found wanting: 'among the greater part of men, the pores of the skin are half-closed and unfit for use'. Virtually all commentators were now agreed that the general levels of personal cleanliness among the 'mass of the people' were unacceptably low; and together with the clinical dermatologists, vitalist doctors reopened the debate on public baths.[70] In an unmistakable reference to German traditions of stoving, both Willich and Hufeland called for re-establishment of public warm baths, 'that poor people might enjoy this benefit, and thereby be rendered strong and sound, as was the case some centuries ago'. But in the absence of public hot baths, most people had to tackle these problems on their own; and even the middle-class Drinker family in America found increased bathing and washing an educational challenge, as they took up each successive craze. Henry and the children swam in outdoor public locations in the 1770s and 1780s; and in 1798 they bought a new 'shower box' for the back yard (eliciting Elizabeth's comment: 'I bore it better than I expected, not having been wett all over at once, for 28 years past'). Then came the 'portable bath' in 1803, which could be used with warm water, indoors. This was an instant success: 'It is very good I believe for young and old,' announced Elizabeth, and from then on the family used it constantly.[71] It would seem that the respectable reappearance of the domestic warm bath was greeted with great relief by the middling classes, especially those who were neither young nor fit, and was the obvious solution to all their personal cleanliness problems. All that remained in the nineteenth century was to extend these benefits to the lower classes.

From c.1500 onwards public health education had transmuted and transmitted successive waves of thought and eloquence—humanism, puritanism, neoclassicism, romanticism—catching many people in its wake. The eighteenth-century Enlightenment, however, had produced a public health education movement and a gospel of cleanliness and hygiene that still only really affected the middling and aristocratic groups in society. Radical hygienists knew that the next stage was to reach the poor 'in every one of our considerable towns'. In *Hygëia: or, Essays Moral and Medical* (1802) the democrat and experimenter Dr Thomas Beddoes stated:

> It should now be possible to provide each individual with a set of ideas, exhibiting how the precise relation in which his system, and the several organs of which it is compounded, stand to external agents...and that these set of ideas be so placed in his head, that he may refer to them with as little difficulty as to the watch he wears in his pocket.[72]

A little optimistic perhaps. Possibly the simplest and original *Regimen Sanitatis Salerni* had provided just that, once upon a time. Instead a nascent public health and hygiene movement evolved into a general 'sanitarian' movement during the course of the next century, working pragmatically towards the goal of a complete medical police or 'welfare state', while most of the population were still absorbing the personal hygiene lessons of the previous century.

chapter 9
health crusaders

The legislative story of British public health reform has often been told; but the moral mission to cleanse and save the nation emerged from a whole penumbra of health reformers stretching far beyond the public façade of Sanitarianism. They included the many millions of silent consumers whose private health care arrangements were already making their contribution to the new health industries—and to demographic statistics. In nineteenth-century Europe the average population growth rate was roughly 60–70 per cent; but in Britain the growth rate was nearer a staggering 140 per cent (from c.15.5 million in 1801 to 41.4 million by 1901). Town dwellers were 20 per cent of the UK population in 1801, 54 per cent in 1851, 80 per cent by 1901.[1] In 1800 European public health philosophy was enlightened but barely off the drawing board; but the immediate problem facing Britain as its population grew so rapidly was the looming question of long-term health investment, above and beyond the norm. Who was going to pay for the necessary bricks and mortar, and water supplies? Ever since 1688, political pragmatism had ruled in British affairs. Legislation was tentative at first; but in the end the utilitarian (or mercantilist) economic arguments were decisive. No public investment—no sanitation, no cleansing, no civilizing process, no trade.

Whig Politics and Mutual Aid

The Whigs represented the liberal elite of the eighteenth-century aristocracy and mercantile classes, who were very well placed to witness destitution on their own lands. They took an early lead. The red-leather, gold-tooled volumes of the Society for Bettering the Condition and Improving the Comforts of the Poor (SBCICP, 1790) were reports from scores of small local charities devoted to welfare relief, job creation experiments, and educational schemes operated by benevolent landowners. The first three pieces of health legislation in which early reformers were involved at the beginning of the century—the first national Census (1801), the Health and Morals of Apprentices Act (1802), and the National Vaccine Establishment (1808)—neatly represent the three main engines behind future policy-making: statistics, applied science, and pure science. But education was the mantra of early nineteenth-century reformers. The long-running Society for the Reformation of Manners had been superseded by a wave of mid-to late eighteenth-century morality, and education had become the preserve of religious evangelical women reformers (notably Hannah More) via the enormously popular late eighteenth-century Sunday School movement, which laid great stress on clean dress, clean skin, good manners, and moral obedience. The rapid development of religious tract societies gave a further excuse for large numbers of charitable middle- and upper-class women to go among the poor and 'witness' their unclean homes and habits.[2] At this stage the health debate was firmly circumscribed by voluntarism, or charitable philanthropy; the principle of voluntarism was built into most of the nineteenth-century British legislation that enabled—but did not absolutely require—specific environmental improvements (such as baths, parks, and public toilets), leaving their actual provision to public philanthropists, or voluntary associations of ratepayers.[3]

But Whig views on individual rights of laissez-faire and the sanctity of private property still ruled in the early nineteenth century, and the SBCICP looked backwards for its models. It had begun a long and inconclusive debate on the provision of 'houses of recovery' reminiscent of the times of the plague, that would quarantine and clean infected or dirty people and their houses; and when Dr Christopher Stanger, a European émigré, published *Remarks on the Necessity and Means of Suppressing Contagious fever*, on the desirability of establishing permanent local health committees and a more comprehensive medical po-lice, he was politely ignored. His progressive measures not only included regular inspection of the local housing, streets, cellars, and the supervision of nuisances, burials, and all public buildings; but also extended to eliminating Window Tax, providing open-air recreation, and teaching habits of personal cleanliness—specific-ally, the use of fresh air, frictions, washing, and warm bathing. The idea of houses of recovery was dismissed as useless:

> Without such domestic regulations, enforced by a vigorous police, for promoting cleanliness and ventilation in the dwellings of the poor, Contagious Fever, tho' greatly diminished, cannot be effec-tually suppressed by the removal of the sick, and purification of their cloaths, furniture, and apartments.

He went on to suggest a plan for public baths and wash-houses:

> Cleanliness might also be greatly promoted by supplying water in abundance in the districts of the poor, and by erecting baths, which they might use without trouble and expense ... workhouses ... more especially ought to contain baths for the benefit of their inhabitants, and of all the indigent parishioners. They might also contain machines and employ paupers, capable of working, in cleansing many articles of dress and furniture belonging to the poor, gratuitously, or at a trifling expense ... Where the total sum of private philanthropy is insufficient, parliament will, unques-tionably, assist in completing the benevolent plan.[4]

All of Stanger's suggestions were carried out by later generations of reformers.

'The poor', however, were not content to wait for charity to trickle fitfully into their communities; and some of them were starting to take matters into their own hands. In a revolutionary spirit the young merchant Robert Owen (1771–1858) had built a much-visited and talked-about utopian factory community at New Lanark; and in *A New View of Society* (1813) had described the cottages, and all the sanitary conveniences and built-in recreational pursuits, that would serve as the future model for humane and health-conscious 'Villages of Co-operation'. Thirty years later he found himself the hero of a new generation of working-class cooperative trading experimenters, and thereafter wrote, lectured, toured, and preached for a rational New World of socialism brought about by the 'construction of a great social and moral machine, calculated to produce wealth, knowledge, and happiness, with unprecedented precision and rapidity'.[5] After 1830 Owenite gatherings in small villages and large towns were often the places where working-class reformers first saw the light, as part of a personal philosophical journey.

Physical Puritanism

The sectarian religious revival of the nineteenth century was a ferment that had worked its way through every aspect of working-class life, reopening many old wounds. One of them was the old Protestant democratic argument with the medical faculty over the rights to medical knowledge and self-medication, and rights of control over one's own body—particularly the puritanical control over the body as the path to self-enlightenment. The multidimensional, universalist, and markedly utopian aims of pure-spirited health reform were typified by the masthead of *The People* (1848), a small magazine dedicated to 'Phrenology, Teetotalism, Theological Reform, Dietetics . . . and all that contributes to the free and full development of the whole human being and of the whole human family'.[6] In 1852 a journalist, Samuel Brown, coined the phrase 'Physical Puritanism':

A new sort of puritanism has arisen in our times, and its influence is as extensive as its origin is various. In some of its features it is as ancient as history, in others as modern as yesterday, and in all not inexpressive of certain of the wants and aspirations of society. It is the puritanism of the body; but the common purpose of all its manifestations is the healing, cleansing, and restoration of the animal man.[7]

The most active physical puritans (according to Brown) were the vegetarians, hydropaths, mesmerists, phrenologists, teetotallers, homoeopaths, and popular physiologists. But the dense mass of medical 'irregulars' that accumulated over the course of the century also included the old herbalists (medical botanists), bone-setters (chiropractors and osteopaths), occulists and aurists, the spiritualists, anti-vaccinationists, anti-vivisectionists, animal rights activists, Christian Socialists, Christian Scientists, and many other minor health-conscious sects and morally inspired associations.

One historian has described nineteenth-century plebeian science as 'the problematic of imponderables'—an open-ended science combining a sense of holistic wonder with a Baconian sense of limitless natural possibilities.[8] Essentially they shared the same self-taught, eighteenth-century Aristotelian–Baconian–mechanistic physiology, underpinned by puritanism, and overlaid with transcendental vitalism. Their staunch empiricism encouraged craft cooperation and made space for the older manual arts; which was why bone-setting, for example, could be aligned with mesmerism; or why the animal magnetists, with their touching, 'hands-on' methods of healing, seem to have been associated with a revival of manual frictions—especially spinal frictions—which led to the late-century revival of massage therapy.[9] It is very difficult—probably impossible—to say how many fellow-travellers there actually were in the active health reform movements, though the medical botanists and the Temperance Leagues were already claiming tens of thousands of followers in the 1820s and 1830s; while the great outpouring of British health magazines in the first half of the century shows clearly how the physical puritans grew in public confidence and momentum, reaching a peak of enthusiasm in the 1840s and 1850s.[10]

Inner Cleanliness

The transcendental vegetarians and the medical herbalists were the true political heirs of seventeenth-century medical dissent. Both believed in inner cleanliness in the ancient sense of ingesting 'clean' foods and drinking pure drinks (and had no trouble in adding outer cleansing to their list of reforms). Vegetarianism was cocooned within Dissent—almost any ascetic sectarian was a potential convert. Methodism, for example, did not make vegetarianism a religious issue, but tacitly supported it; it was also subliminal in Quakerism, and in many of the Anabaptist-derived and other European sects in America. It had also found a powerful new prophet in the works of the eighteenth-century evangelical spiritualist Emanuel Swedenborg (1688–1772), whose millenarian vision of a New Church of faith, love, and vegetable innocence leading to a New Jerusalem was laid down in his spirit-inspired *Arcana Coelestia* (1747–58). Swedenborgianism was transplanted to the London Church of New Jerusalem in the 1780s (possibly attended by the artists William Blake and Joseph Turner), and then to northern England, where it became the basis of a cooperative vegetarian movement, the Bible Christians. The Bible Christians crossed the Atlantic in 1817 with a congregation from Yorkshire whose leader, William Metcalfe, founded the American Vegetarian Society in 1850.

Joseph Brotherton, former pastor to the Salford Chapel of Bible Christians, chaired the inaugural meeting of the English Vegetarian Society in 1847.[11]

Samuel Hahnemann's homoeopathy, when it arrived, with its tinctures and essences, was a very refined version of the vegetable healing mission. In Britain homoeopathy's main feature was the early and dramatic conversion of large numbers of aristocrats and royalty, patrons of its fashionable hospitals. But it, too, could find a foothold within the broad church of democratic herbalism.[12] Nineteenth-century herbal democrats not only believed in treatment with herbs, they violently opposed 'unnatural' mineral medicines, emphasized hygiene, and actively distrusted all doctors. The old international Protestant networks had become immensely active during this time of high migration, and nineteenth-century cooperative Protestantism was a powerful force in the revival of Anglo-American physical puritanism. During the 1820s the American self-taught healer Samuel Thomson founded groups of Thomsonian 'medical botanists' in both America and northern Britain, dedicated to the use of pure vegetable medicines, indigenous natural herbal remedies, and the use of God's own water, fresh air, and exercise—a popularized version of Wesley's *Primitive Physic*.[13] The next Thomsonian American evangelist, Dr Isaiah Coffin, who settled in Leeds in the 1840s, added temperance and anti-alcohol teetotalism to the cause, and set up a network of botanic agents and medical 'friendly societies' which trained a new generation of empiric, working-class 'medical botanists' with their own herbal casework, drawings, collections, clubs, conferences, and publications. Eventually the herbalists became part of a moderated 'eclectic' medical reform movement (which carefully argued the right to choose 'any remedial agent irrespective of origin or class of medical practitioner') and fought hard to be registered under the Medical Act of 1858 (they failed).[14]

The emotional and spiritual appeal of vegetarian purity was kept alive in England by the utopian socialists. The famous Ham Common 'Concordium' communal retreat in London, founded by James Pierrepont Greaves ('Apostle Greaves'), was a vegetarian showcase and a reformers' meeting-place in the 1840s. Greaves believed in the transcendental Creative Power of the universe, and thought of himself as a scientific socialist in the manner of the contemporary French socialist Charles Fourier, whose socialist theories of the progressive stages of civilization occupied the same intellectual space as the old Protestant Adamites: mankind was progressing from Edenism, Savagery, Patriarchy, and Barbarism, to Civilization, Cooperation, and Association. The Concordium, of course, was the model for harmonious cooperation, and was designed to create 'the true practical socialist' in 'buildings cheerful, light, and spacious', with 'harmonic industrial occupations', 'intellectual and scientific pursuits', and a strict vegetarian and cold-bath regime, uncut beards, open sandals, and 'pervious and flowing Cotton garments undyed'. Greaves's Pythagorean emphasis on purity also involved celibacy: married couples were not allowed within the inner circle at the Concordium, only Platonic 'Unions of affectionate and intelligently adapted natures'; or, more perfectly, 'Unions of Spirits of selected pairs in sympathetical harmony with LOVE'.[15]

The few issues of the *New Age and Concordium Gazette* (1843–4) were full of American abstracts and news. In nineteenth-century America, health reform 'rang with the rhetoric of democracy'. Ralph Waldo Emerson was the prophet of the Transcendentalists of New England, while the hygienists Sylvester Graham and William Alcott famously travelled up and down the east coast of America during the 1830s and 1840s promoting temperance leagues, temperance hotels, vegetarian dining rooms, and vegetarian products. But the argument remained a spiritual one on both sides of the Atlantic. Bronson

81

Conditions unsuitable for Developing Noble, Moral, Healthy Natures.

Conditions suitable for Developing the three orders of Progressive Humanity.

	AIR.	WATER.	FOOD.	CLOTHING.	HABITATION.	EMPLOYMENT.	EDUCATION.	RELIGION.	MARRIAGE.
(1) For all natures.	Low, marshy, and damp localities; ill-ventilated apartments; atmosphere corrupted by coal dust, smoke, tobacco, and all vitiating ingredients.	Warm, foul, and stagnant.	Fermented and cooked Fruits, Vegetables, and Roots; Flesh of all kinds; Fermented Liquors.	Woollen fabrics, Stays and tight Dresses of every description; animal Skins; superfluous ornaments.	Towns & cities, dirty, dense, and dark; luxurious mansions and dilapidated cottages.	Competitive trades and all oppressive labor for unjust and selfish acquisition.	Repressive, compressive, punishing, and coercive disciplines.	Physical and intellectual misrepresentations & deadening ceremonies.	Formed on worldly and interested motives & for self gratification, without reference to Divine end.
(2) For the Life or monad natures.	Pure, sweet, bracing atmosphere.	Cold from a spring; abundantly and daily applied to the whole body.	Vegetables, Fruits, and Farinaceous food; fresh Water.	Cotton or Lempen dress undyed.	Buildings cheerful, light, and spacious, adapted to Educative and Industrial purposes.	Harmonic, Industrial occupations.	Conditions for developing the Life organism with respect to moral & intellectual progress.	Devotion towards God and kindness towards man.	Unions of affection and adaptation.
For the Life and Light natures.	Softened effulgence; etherealized conditions.	Cold shower bath every day, with occasional plunge bath in the open air.	Solarized Vegetables, Fruits, and Nuts: fresh Water.	Pervious and flowing Cotton garments undyed.	Buildings cheerful, light, and spacious, adapted for Scientific studies.	Intellectual, Scientific, and Industrial pursuits.	Conditions for developing the Life and Light organism with respect to moral and Divine progress.	Intelligent devotion and brotherly kindness.	Unions of affectionate & intelligently adapted natures.
For the Life, Light, and Love or triad natures.	Celestialized elements.	Cold shower bath every day, with frequent ablutions in various ways.	Ripe saccharine Fruits and Nuts: fresh Water.	Pure undyed Linen robes.	Buildings cheerful, light, and spacious, adapted to Genetic natures.	Exercise of Love sympathy and intelligent faculties.	Conditions for developing the Life, Light, and Love organism with respect to Spirit.	Universal passivity and active obedience to the Spirit.	Unions of Spirit selected pairs in sympathetic harmony with LOVE.

VOL. II.   M

16 Early socialist hygiene c.1840—the theory of 'Conditional Law' laid out for James Pierrepoint Greaves's utopian vegetarian commune.

Alcott's honorary address to a Ham Common Concordium gala in 1842 spoke for them all: 'Our trust is in purity not vengeance. Together with pure beings will come pure habits. A better body shall be built up from the orchard and the garden . . . flesh and blood we will reject as the accursed thing. A pure mind has no faith in them.'[16]

Drugs and Cholera

Radical physical puritans may have been a tiny minority, but public scepticism in Britain about 'regular' therapeutics was reinforced by the four epidemics of cholera (1831–2, 1848–9, 1853–4, and 1866–7). The first epidemic in particular caused great public anxiety, and was met by considerable legislative confusion over the activities of the (temporary) local boards of health; John Snow's definitive reports on water transmission were published in 1849–55.[17] Cholera also highlighted the deficiencies of nineteenth-century Galenic therapeutics— especially the new wave of 'heroic' bloodletting promoted by the French vitalist physiologist F. J. V. Broussais (1772–1838). What was particularly worrying was that the favourite drugs were useless, and bloodletting patently did not work—the blood in cholera victims was far too thick and tarry. The experience of trying to bleed in cholera, it was noticed, had 'shattered the faith of many believers'.[18] Many young doctors nevertheless still relied firmly on drugs and the scalpel. The commercial market for drugs had grown enormously. Drugs were now available over the counter ready for self-dosing—powerful medicines 'which, under a great variety of seducing forms and titles, are constantly employed'. Laudanum (opium), calomel (mercury), antimony (arsenic), and the bark (aspirin) were the main stocks-in-trade, but new chemical laboratories in the 1820s and 1830s were just starting to produce the new chemical alkaloids—the active therapeutic agents in natural drugs such as quinine, codeine, caffeine, and cocaine.[19]

Many university-trained doctors, on both sides of the Atlantic, thought the profession was on the wrong track, and floundering. Like the disillusioned Dr William Dale, they saw popular and professional quackery flourishing everywhere throughout the 'Upas Tree' of medicine, bringing down the rotting apples of 'Confusion', 'Disappointment', and 'Ruin'.[20] Thomas Wakely's London magazine *The Lancet* was founded in 1823 to stimulate professional reform on all fronts. For progressive doctors, reducing the use of drugs and reinstating hygiene as a branch of regular medicine seemed to be the only way out of this professional impasse; but this also required retraining the medical profession itself (as Thomas Beddoes had noted thirty years earlier). Hygiene was not yet on either the British or the American medical curriculum. The health author Andrew Combe complained that 'foreign universities' had chairs of hygiene, but 'there is scarcely a medical school in the country in which any special provision is made for teaching it'. (Edwin Chadwick had to go to Paris in the 1820s in order to take a course on medical police.) In Britain, Combe lamented, 'both the teacher and student fix upon [cure] as their chief object; and are consequently apt to overlook...the laws of health. [The medical man] works it out for himself; but in general attains it later than he ought to do, and seldom so completely as he would have done had it been made a part of his elementary education.' Another doctor remarked bitterly that when it came to prescribing hygiene, most doctors seemed to 'despise the subject, or think that it forms no necessary part of his professional lore'. If someone asked them about prevention, they 'immediately put the person down as a hypochondriac' and refused to have anything to do with 'the twaddling maxims of old women... But who else is so better qualified?...If hygiene is now despicable in the eyes of the Physician, he has himself to blame for her state; for he left her in bad company, where she has been seduced and corrupted.'[21]

Popular Physiology

Health reformers from both sides of the professional fence moved instinctively into the new cheaper magazine market to reach a new mass audience of urbanites apparently desperate for all forms of self-help information. The term 'popular physiology' described a type of middle-of-the-road health philosophy that required no severe ascetic practices, had no membership requirements, and excluded no one. 'Popular physiology' was the new title, but the modern works fitted seamlessly into the old genre of health handbooks. The burst of middle-class 3d. to 1s. monthly health magazines shows how successful these large, slim, well-decorated publications were; when bound at the end of their run, with additional illustrations, they also made a handsome health encyclopedia.[22] Magazines such as *The Family Oracle of Health; Economy, Medicine, and Good Living; Adapted to All Ranks of Society, from the Palace to the Cottage* (1824–6) give a strong impression of popular health concerns. The *Oracle* was a jolly little publication, full of wise-cracking jokes which carefully trod the professional middle way, its main aim being to moderate drug-taking and promote self-help and personal hygiene in its broadest sense. It was packed with small, easy-to-read essays, and was calendrical—always starting with 'Problems of the Month':

> *Diseases of August*; Hydrophobia or water-fear; Philosophy of Bathing, No. 2; Poultry buying; Pimples; Art of Medical Training, No. 1; Training adapted to Ladies; Beauty training; Ruined constitutions; Indigestion; Diseases of the unmarried state (green sickness); Cock a leeky soup; Mrs Pringle—quack; Philosophy of the Hour, No. 4; Hereditary dunces and Borough Jobbery.

Diseases of September; Fever; Sauces; Indigestion; Effects of Drugging on Beauty; Coughs and consumptions; Typhus fever; Weak moving; Venison and grain; Art of Medical Training No. 2; Choosing spectacles; School diseases from school vices; Evils of boarding schools exposed ... Examination of food, exercise, etc. in 11 fashionable schools; Economical elder wine; The Philosophy of Hearing ... [23]

One major innovation in popular physiology was the teaching of 'popular anatomy'. Dr Andrew Combe's best-seller *The Principles of Physiology Applied to the Preservation of Health, and the Improvement of Physical and Mental Education* (1833) went into five editions in three years (with American, German, and French editions). It combined a moderate vitalist regimen with simple anatomy (describing in detail the structures and functions of the skin, muscles, bones, lungs, and nervous system). By the late 1840s, readers of domestic medicine could marvel at the microscopic anatomy of the skin, and thrill to the functions of the insensible perspiration:

> ... I counted the perspiratory pores in the palm of the hand, and found 3528 in a square inch. Now each of these pores being an aperture of a little tube about a quarter of an inch long, it follows that ... there exists a length of tube equal to 882 inches, or 73 and a half feet. Surely such an amount of drainage as 73 feet every square inch of skin ... is something wonderful, and the thought naturally intrudes itself—what if this drainage were obstructed? The number of square inches of surface in a man of ordinary height and bulk is 2,500; the number of pores therefore is 300,000 and the number of inches of perspiratory tube 1,750,000, that is 145,833 feet, or 48,600 yards, or nearly 28 miles ... from this explanation the necessity and value of cleanliness to health must be self-evident. [24]

In Combe exercise was now firmly linked to mental training— 'the physiology of mind as well as body'; Combe's brother was George Combe, whose *Constitution of Man* (1828) imported the controversial and astonishingly popular mental 'phrenology' of Franz Joseph Gall and J. C. Spurzheim, which linked the brain's organic structure to its mental powers (diagnosed through bumps on the skull).[25] The principles of hygiene had long been used to treat the unbalanced passions of the insane, the hysteric, or the depressed; it was only another short step to apply the principle of *mens sana in corpore sano* to stressed-out urban civilians.

From the 1830s onwards, middle-class families faced a barrage of indoctrination on the subject of sober, temperate personal hygiene—now often called the 'economic' life; fewer drugs and less food (the 'economic' diet); leanness instead of corpulency; training instead of relaxation; mental and physical fitness. As always, obesity problems were closely connected with rising standards of living, and the message was the same: 'If exercise conduces to throw off all superfluities in the system, temperance in diet prevents their accumulation and renders it less necessary; if exercise cleans the vessels, temperance neither satiates nor overstrains them.' People were exhorted to plan regular daily patterns of physical exercise. Swimming, walking, and other sports were already well established; but the great craze in the 1820s and 1830s was gymnastics (or 'callisthenics' as it was more frequently called), which was imported into Britain and America from Per Henrik Ling's Gymnastiska Centralinstitut in Stockholm; followed later by Friedrich Ludwig Jahn's 'Turnplatz' ('Turning') equipment, with wooden beams, bars, and horses (the type of gymnastics that we now see in the Olympics) which in Germany were often situated outside in natural forest settings. Military-style outdoor gymnastic 'drill', which was simply brisk walking in disciplined formations, became highly popular with schoolteachers; and all gymnastic exercise routines were thought to be particularly suitable for children and women, producing a mild strength, suppleness, and graceful lines, rather than visible muscles. To start with women's callisthenics and 'turning' were the hobby of the

health enthusiast; but gymnastics provided the future foundation for sports in girls' schools.[26]

In Britain, the popular physiologists saw exercise not only as
a personal hygienic discipline but as a public hygiene require-
ment, which they busily and actively promoted via the so-called
'Rational Recreation' movement. Village sports and entertainments were dying as their populations shrank, and in the towns
there was nothing to replace them, reformers argued, but the
public alehouse. Rational Recreationists encouraged the building of pleasure parks, sports fields, baths, libraries, museums,
and meeting halls. Local, national, and international sports
leagues were developed between 1820 and 1890; and every
single British county had a football league by the 1880s. Much
of this popular success was to do with the acculturation of
school sports. School hygiene had already been raised by popular physiologists at the beginning of the century, and organized
school sports were originally conceived as rational recreation
for boys. Thomas Arnold, headmaster at Rugby in the 1840s,
recognized that the discipline would be useful against the unfet-
tered 'vandalism' of the boys (who were traditionally allowed to
roam free in the afternoons) and allowed his masters to develop
it. Rugby produced a new generation of notably athletic British
public schools, with a strong ethos of 'muscular Christianity'
that was also later exported into the American sporting college
system. In 1855 Dr Oliver Wendell Holmes compared the rosy,
muscular, well-fed, and large British visitors that he saw with
puny, pale-faced, American youths: 'They fill their coats vigorously, they walk more briskly... they are warm, jolly, and athletic.'[27] However, popular physiology, rational recreation, and
sanitary reform were all very much part of the same hygienic
project. From the 1840s onwards the broad popular front of
sanitary reform turned its attention to two remedies for filth
that were long overdue: the provision of clean water, and
cleansing public baths.

Sanitation and Water

Health reform in Britain came to a head in the distressed years of the 1840s—a time of economic growth, population increase, and the return of cholera. The numbers of peripheral supporters of health reform crusades increased dramatically as a great battle for public health legislation began. During the 1840s drains, baths, and water were constant headline news: the 'conquest of water' was the first lesson for the newly founded sanitarian lobby. The early 1840s were dominated by Edwin Chadwick's famous 1842 *Report on the Sanitary Condition of the Labouring Classes*, which forced the public to recognize that there truly was an urban crisis. The overcrowded poor, living in hutlike conditions unchanged over the centuries, were grossly deprived of sufficient sources of fresh water, while the rich were polluting the old public watercourses with their overflowing waste. Thanks to the mass production of water-flushed latrines, by the 1840s 'some 250 tons of faecal matter daily found their way into the Thames'; twenty years later that fecal matter could be measured in many thousands of tons.[28] As doctor after doctor in the Report described their local slums, and their rivers of sewage, people saw filth with new eyes: they suddenly noticed it everywhere, in the air, water, in the streets, on clothes and skin, in food.

From the time that the Health of Towns Commission sat between 1843 and 1846, and for years after the sanitary reformers' Health of Towns Association was formed in 1844, a physiological picture of poverty emerged which not only deepened public concern but confirmed conditions that charity visitors had seen (and physiological reformers had suspected) for years. It was noted that deprivation had stunted growth as well as scything through the weakest bodies during epidemic attacks—the poor were some 5 inches shorter on average. Far more than the rest of the population, they suffered from multiple disabilities. Many had bent limbs from suffering rickets in a malnourished childhood, and workshop diseases and deformities were normal. Women and girls in particular were thin and small through malnourishment, with small pelvises that made childbirth more difficult and low birth weight inevitable. Because of close proximity to infected persons, open rubbish heaps, common use of all utensils, and above all lack of water, all the old skin diseases were still rife among the poor, who 'quietly suffer the penalties annexed to the want of cleanliness, as disagreeable smells, perpetual irritation with chaps and fissures on the skin, boils, and eruptions of painful, inflamed pustules, the Itch and Prurigo, the Lepra, the dry Tetter, the running Tetter, the Dandriff, and Scald-head'. Physiology had long ago embraced vitalist doctrines of race-theory, heredity, and the diseases of civilization, and reformers could virtuously point to an easily recognizable physical type: the asthenic, the debilitated, the aetiolated poor:

> the national habit of body is depreciated. Our people are etiolated; every tenth man is a pauper; every seventy-fourth is a drunkard; three generations of pauperism is producing the Negro type, without its redeeming black or brown, in some parts of Ireland; and no whole family is free from the strumulous or emasculating or morbific taint . . . It is clear that the national circumstances and manner of life are to blame for this dreadful result . . . [29]

Disease, minimal amounts of dry grooming, and unwashed rags and underlinen meant that the bodies of the poorest smelled intensely, with strong animal odours, compared to the washed or scented population. The very poorest were sometimes described by fearful people as 'savages', 'brutes', or 'animals'—traditional terms describing those beyond the boundaries of society, the untouchables, the impure. Now they also became known as the 'great unwashed'.

There had been much discussion about public baths among the mercantile utilitarians in the 1830s; and, following the model of New Lanark, various philanthropic manufacturers had set up workforce baths. Applying the new technology of steam to public baths had become an exciting project for health progressives: 'What if this same engine, whilst it clothes the British labourer with garments as rich and as fine as those worn by the Kings of Tyre and Sidon, should likewise give him what was the next Eastern luxury and refinement—the warm bath!' There was also an unsuccessful attempt by Rational Recreational hygienists to legislate for baths in the newly reformed Parliament in 1835, with a bill to promote 'Public Walks, Playgrounds, Baths, and places of healthy recreation and Amusement', with another bill for 'Institutions for the diffusion of literary and scientific information, including Libraries and Museums, with commodious Halls and Places of Public Meeting'. But the two bills were quietly dropped in 1837; hygienic idealism bowed before empiricism, and the statisticians were given their way.[30] Chadwick's Report five years later provided a clearer and more universal focus, with 'cleanliness' identified as the central agent of the civilizing process.

The year 1842 was key for British health reform. It was the starting block not only for Chadwick but also for the public baths movement, both simultaneously moving in different directions. In 1842 Liverpool Corporation opened a municipal laundry or wash-house (with baths attached), which was so successful that they soon opened another one six times the size. Not to be outdone, in 1844 the City of London started a royally patronized Association for Promoting Cleanliness among the People, which quickly built a similarly successful wash-house in a slum called Glass-House Yard, followed by another in Goulston Square. The public baths reformers quickly set up a broad front, led by the reforming wing of the Anglican Church, with powerful speakers in Archdeacon Samuel Wilberforce and the bishop of London, Dr Charles Blomfield—cleanliness was so clearly a 'moral purity' issue. By 1845 the so-called Clean Party was well into its stride, and had set up the Association for the Establishment of Public Baths and Washhouses, which closely supervised the national legislation of 1846–7. The Act simply empowered any parish or borough to build public baths (including vapour baths) if the ratepayers voted in favour, with maximum charges (6*d.*) and a tiered pricing system (1*d.* cold bath, 2*d.* warm bath, children half price) to ensure that they remained poor baths. There were muted objections from commercial baths operators, and some puritanical diehards objected that the baths would be 'gossip shops' and 'sinks of corruption'; but the vote was passed decisively. From then on the Act was left to fend for itself and often had a rough ride at local meetings, as in the London parish of St George's in the East where the Dirty Party met in the pub, while the Clean Party met in the church. But in the end these poor baths proved more difficult to build and operate than foreseen; they lost money in the winter, were overcrowded in the summer, shunned during epidemics, were high-maintenance and dependent on an efficient water company, and rarely made a profit. They were only a real success after a second Act prompted a new wave of building in the 1870s.[31]

It is difficult to get past the liberal reformer's top-down view of the baths-and-cleanliness movement. The equally dedicated Dirty Party was usually composed of anyone who objected to raising the rates (shopkeepers and small businessmen); or who feared increased overheads (manufacturers); or who believed that the expense would send jobs elsewhere (including Chartists and many others); or those who simply thought that dirt was a necessary sacrifice on the altar of prosperity, the price that had to be paid—'where there was muck there was brass'. With hindsight it is remarkable how much got done at all before the civic-minded 1870s, in the face of widespread political indifference and open hostility.[32] It was probably the new Labour vote after the 1832 electoral reforms that tipped the balance towards action. The Baths for the Working Classes movement in Edinburgh, for instance, was started with a petition signed by '2400 working men', many of whom turned up to the inaugural meeting, and seemingly had no objection whatsoever to a shining moral vision of cleanliness. When the surgeon James Simpson referred to temperance, he was received by 'loud and long-continued cheers', while his 'view of... well-built houses, sewers, water in abundance, pure air and light... [and] of better things for the working man's dwelling, produced a strong sensation in the audience'. The chairman, Lord Dunfermline, thought that cleanliness was not only necessary for the

comfort, health, and respectability of the people, [but] I look upon it as a necessary preliminary to alliances between the working classes, and those whose province it is to inculcate religious and moral conviction on the people.—(Loud Cheers)...I have no doubt [that] we are about to carry the day—that henceforth we shall have established far more method, far more order, far more cleanliness in the domestic economy of the people.[33]

The religious feeling does seem to shine through: sobriety, temperance, cleanness, thrift, and respectability were sober old Calvinist virtues. It did not necessarily mean that all the labouring classes shared the same 'soap-ori-fic' cross-class political viewpoint. As one working-class poet warned in a burst of Jacobin satire on the general lack of moral cleanliness in high places, baths and wash-houses were 'but a small instalment due, sir':

... But sure the chap's no silly 'un,
Who to cleanliness a railroad planned
A washhouse for the million.
Chorus: Ri tooral, looral, looral, loo
Ri tooral, looral, lido
Sure purity outside and in,
Should be a people's pride oh.
But stay—'tis not the vulgar herd
Alone who lack a scrubbing,

We've great ones too who want a bath
And pretty hard dry-rubbing...
...To scour such knaves, as I have heard—
At all observe, no snarl-I-ment—
A thumping bath is being built
In the New Houses of Parliament.
Ri tooral, looral, etc....
So let us praise the general scheme,
As a small instalment due, sirs,
From wealth and rank to poverty—
And hope still more they'll do, sirs.
Chorus: And then we'll own, in bath and park,
That to serve your poor neighbour
A duty is—and bless the man,
Who helps the sons of Labour.
Ri tooral, looral, etc.[34]

From the 1840s onwards public speakers referred to 'cleanliness' constantly: it became a litany that few members of the public, literate or otherwise, could have avoided, or failed to have learnt. Cleanliness would make everyone happier. It would create a more disciplined workforce and save them from the demon drink. Mental and physical dispositions were linked in a strong moral polarity:

A clean, fresh, and well-ordered house [has] a direct tendency to make the members of a family sober, peaceful, and considerate of the feelings and happiness of each other...whereas a filthy, squalid, unwholesome dwelling...tends directly to make every dweller in such a hovel regardless of the feelings and happiness of each other, selfish and sensual. And the connection is obvious between the constant indulgences of appetites and passions of this class, and the formation of habits of idleness, dishonesty, debauchery, and violence.

Cleanliness kept the civilized man safely at home. The 'rosy' view of the beautiful clean home with its beautifully clean contents became the source of a rich 'trope' or type of cleanliness prose in novels and fiction, as well as campaigning journalism, directed at young women and young wives especially:

> Who . . . has contemplated the wide difference in the aspect of everything, where the presiding spirit, the wife, is a votary of Cleanliness, and the state of things where she is not. How ill-favoured the handsomest furniture looks, covered with dust and stains—the most beautiful carpet, by crumbs and shred. On the contrary, the polished oak table, the well-rubbed floor, on which the light of heaven shines through a clear glass; the white hearth, and shining fire-irons; the bright fire, which blushes not for the ashes that lay scattered before it, but smiles because only its own clear face can be seen, render the poorest cabin an earthly paradise . . . [35]

This was a neglected and disorderly home—not a poor one. Good housekeeping was rewarded by shining oak tables and glowing Turkey carpets; an overt appeal to the consumer, that eager self-improver, and one which was used constantly by utilitarian reformers promoting 'the engine of Trade'.

Environmental Hygiene

Environmental public hygiene policies were pursued in Britain in the second half of the century with grim determination, long after the baths fuss had died down. European and American cities were also starting to feel the impact of urban growth; but in Britain certain clear priorities had already emerged. The early 1850s were particularly busy years, and the national press became a major force in environmental crusading. As is well known, *The Times* made Florence Nightingale into a heroine when she used scrubbing brushes and cleanliness to reduce death rates at Scutari Hospital in the Crimean War of 1854. *The Lancet* underwrote the work of Dr Arthur Hill Hassall, who had provided the famous microscopic slides of Thames water for Chadwick in 1849–50, and who between 1851 and 1855 became *The Lancet*'s one-man Analytic Sanitary Commission, analysing over fifty different types of common food, naming and shaming nearly 3,000 commercial traders, and discovering 'an amount of adulteration which certainly no person was prepared for'. Hassall virtually invented the office of the public analyst, and paved the way for the three food and drug Adulteration Acts of 1860, 1875, and 1899. In 1852 Joseph Bazalgette was appointed Surveyor to the Metropolitan Sewers, and was soon to present his master plan for sewering the whole of London, a plan which came into its own after the Great Stink of the Thames in 1858; it was completed in 1859–75, and all of its affairs were very closely monitored by the press.[36]

Chadwick's successor Sir John Simon rallied the profession to hygiene, employed chemical laboratories, demanded and got trained medical officers of health, successfully created the discipline of state medicine, and put in such sterling work attempting to remove various national 'Nuisances' that his large raft of legislation had to be consolidated into the 1875 Public Health Act, which finally made local boards of health mandatory. Most importantly, reformers took advantage of the widening tax base of a prosperous economy, to tempt local councils into taking on low-cost loans for public works; the Public Works (Manufacturing Districts) Act of 1863 has been pinpointed as the turning point in British civic reform. The whole task of cleansing towns was thus turned over to local government civic reformers and municipal socialists, who pushed through wide-ranging slum clearance, housing schemes, water and gas schemes, drainage and cesspit renewal schemes, with the accompanying hygienic cultural programme of public libraries, museums, parks, and baths. Private philanthropy supported these schemes and (on a lesser scale) the provision of park bandstands, public latrines, drinking fountains, and horse troughs. This was the Romanesque or monumental phase of sanitary history, when grandiose architects, designers, and their clients spent large sums of money developing the

Victorian city as we know it.[37] The bigger the projects, the more Roman-like were the stone tablets put up to record the munificence of the local worthies—local politicians who had rediscovered an old truth, that public health schemes brought prestige, local employment, and increased powers of patronage. Even sewage outfalls or water towers could be objects of local pride (municipal rubbish dumps, however, were not).

In 1847 Dr Ignaz Semmelweis had discovered a simple antiseptic routine using cleanliness and carbolic acid; but it was only when the surgeon Joseph Lister perfected antisepsis procedures in the 1860s, wearing white gowns and drenching everything in carbolic spray (thereby making routine operations far safer and more difficult medical conditions 'operable'), that the public really sat up and took notice of the new 'cellular' microbiological sciences opening up under the guidance of Rudolf Virchow, Louis Pasteur, and Claude Bernard. Most of these advanced medical discoveries did not as yet help a great many people until the end of the century. Preventive medicine in the laboratory was barely conceivable compared to preventive hygiene in the city, and at home. Keeping well and avoiding infection seemed the only alternative to paying large medical bills or dying young. Health faddery, for those who could afford it, retained its appeal. Domestic sanitation became big business. By the 1850s many bourgeois health consumption patterns had already been framed, and were simply set to rise.

La Luxe Anglaise

'Comfort' had now been added to 'convenience'. The English house was well on the way to becoming the fully furnished, massively ornamental, thickly carpeted, heavily curtained, well-serviced, and ingeniously plumbed home which typified *la luxe anglaise* to Europeans, and which was displayed to international view at London's Great Exhibition in the Crystal Palace in 1851.

French authors put it all down (logically) to the nasty cold climate 'chez les peuples du Nord', and particularly praised the control of temperature and ventilation.[38] 'Comfort' was considered to be the happy medium between luxury and poverty. Many London houses had underground drainage and piped water as a standard convenience after the 1850s. No self-respecting Victorian could have done without his or her domestic bathing arrangements.

Sanitary habits were already changing in the 1820s and 1830s, although older, unplumbed habits died hard: 'jerries' and close stools (night tables) in late eighteenth-century marquetry designs still delighted nineteenth-century consumers. But whatever most people had managed in the way of grooming before, they were now expected to try just that little bit harder, as J. S. Forsyth put it (in 1829): 'Cleanliness of person, and in all concerned with it, is a principal duty of man...It is better to wash twenty times a day than to allow a dirty spot to remain on the skin...'.[39] The bath had finally 'come to rest' in the purpose-built bathroom—but only if space was available; strip washing in the bedroom was still the cheapest and most convenient option. Significantly, it was in the 1830s that the simple bedroom washstand started to become the much more imposing washstand table, with a wooden or tiled back and drawers underneath, holding a larger bowl, a larger jug, a soap dish, a sponge dish, tooth glass, and towel rail. Other households found that they could put a portable metal shower-bath in the corner of a bedroom, following the advice of magazines who assured their readers that 'baths on a large and expensive scale' were 'by no means necessary'. Wooden portable baths, with wheels, a drain-hole, and brass fittings (and from the 1850s gas heating attached underneath), were perfect for moderately well-off clients, and had a long and honourable existence throughout the century. The cheaper painted tin baths seen in so many nineteenth-century illustrations were mass-produced from the mid-century in many different shapes and sizes: the full-length lounge bath, the shallow sponge bath, the foot- or slipper bath—and the highly popular, oval, sit-down hip or 'Sitz' bath, with a high back and small elbow rests also serving as soap dishes: 'Many older persons will remember a hip bath set out in a cosy bedroom, on a waterproof bath-sheet, with the brass or copper cans gleaming in the light of a good fire, and a thick towel warming on the sideboard.'[40]

In wealthy upper-class families in the second half of the century, the baths were monumental, and the exotic bathrooms were large—big enough for crinolines, or even for callisthenics. Thomas Crapper made his fortune after 1866 by redesigning and supplying top-of-the-range plumbed-in products, including the now fashionable cast-iron bath–shower combination, with elaborate shower screens and metal sprays; and cast-iron pedestal washbasins, hugely ornate, with mirrors and hot and cold mixer taps. Porcelain slowly replaced metal in the fixtures and fittings and opened a new window for designers—luxuriant colours and patterns in the latter half of the century giving way to clinical white at the end of the century. John Shanks and Thomas Twyford became household names by designing porcelain valve closets, which finally trapped all smells, for their pedestal flush toilets in the 1870s. The problems of supplying hot water were partially eased by the introduction of gas geysers, from the same late-century supply that also brought new, 'clean', artificial gas lighting and heating. For the enthusiastic home DIYer (and, like George Grossmith's fictional Mr Pooter, there were many of these) the era of the large domestic water boiler had just begun, and there would be many more household 'bangs' and disasters before it was more or less perfected.[41]

The toilette that accompanied the bath was now a rite of modest purity and perfection. Victorian painters and novelists put great aesthetic emphasis on the translucent 'bloom' of the female skin—simple 'natural' beauty from soap and water, with

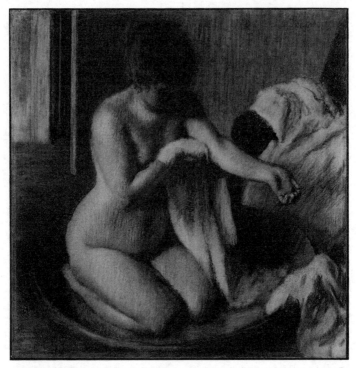

17 Edgar Dégas's *Woman in a Tub* (*c*.1883), one of his many intimate depictions of women grooming in the bedroom. The strip wash in a shallow basin was still the simplest and cheapest method of washing for those without any plumbing.

shining, well-brushed hair. Eighteenth-century cosmetic fashions were long gone. Lip paint was forbidden; eye paint should be invisible; heavy rouge was frowned on; lightly scented cold cream and a touch of powder were allowable. But only for married women: modest and virtuous girls should never 'paint' (though young women started to rebel at the end of the century). Instead of paint, toilet soap production rose steadily after soap duties were halved in 1834; and took off dramatically when Gladstone's free trade policy abolished the old Soap Tax in

1852. Perfume was increasingly contained not in the bottle but in the soap. Light floral scents were preferred, and several new herbal and mineral soap odours (including peppermint, coal tar, and the antiseptically pungent Old Brown Windsor Soap) were on show in the Great Exhibition.[42] Tablets of scented soap (especially new transparent soaps) became objects of desire in the Victorian middle-class home, and to lower-middle-class aspirants: country village girls still cherished their own bars of scented soap in the 1920s.

The 1830s had seen the start of a new trend in male hairstyles: the expertly barbered moustache, longer hair, and the beginning of the Victorian cult of the beard. Like the recently reintroduced corsets and 20-inch waists for women, with enormous hooped crinolines laden with frills, flounces, and trimmings, beards and moustaches were not at all hygienic, but they were overt grooming displays. After so many centuries of being clean-shaven, what did the reappearance of beards signify? Primitive virility? (Or puritan indifference?) It does seem to be true that the more material goods later nineteenth-century Victorians possessed, the more perfectly groomed they were, the more they yearned to get back to nature. In their personal habits, and in their rich inner life, many of them were staunch Greek primitives, with the added spice of romantic vitalism. Those who could afford it returned to their primitive roots at the hydros.

The Hydro

The spa and seaside craze had continued unabated in the 1820s–1830s, and by 1850 the British coastline was lined with scores of small, genteel resorts, all reachable by rail; while the inland spas rapidly expanded with elegant infilling and residential development. The major seaside resorts had doubled in size; by the 1880s they had doubled or trebled again; really cheap

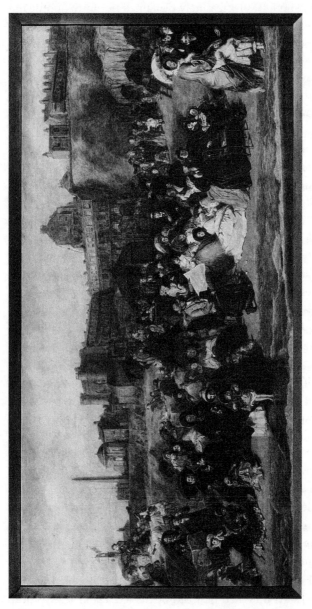

18 Ramsgate Sands, 1854, in its early heyday as a seaside resort reachable by railway and steamboat from London. Sea breezes and a view of the sea were obviously hygienic enough—only one child is going for a paddle, and none of the adults have altered their dress in any way.

working-class excursions came at the end of the century.[43]
European spas, lakes, and mountains were now also reachable
by rail, and Baden-Baden, Karlovy Vary (Carlsbad), Wiesbaden,
Mariánské Lázně (Marienbad), and Aix-les Bains became select
health retreats for the upper classes. But a hydro was not a spa;
it was the purists who despised the spas and spa life who first
went to the hydros.

In the early 1840s the first eulogies of Vincenz Priessnitz's 'wet-
wrap' cure in the mountains of Austria began to appear in the
European press. Priessnitz was an illiterate peasant farmer from
Gräfenberg who had devised a new version of 'heroic' cold bathing in the early 1820s, when he cured himself of the pain of four
broken ribs (after resetting them himself by manipulation) by
keeping cold, wet bandages constantly wrapped round his body
while they healed. He then started to heal others as paying guests
on his farm, using the same 'wet-wrap' methods along with a
fierce regime of outdoor walks, outdoor showers, and a simple
peasant diet. His success stung the local medical profession into a
barrage of legal attacks, but his fame was sealed after the local
aristocracy tried the cure, and immediately started sending their
own chronic sick. You had to be very ill, or desperate, to go to
Priessnitz. People were not expected to enjoy what they endured
(though most seem to have found it an extraordinary and fascinating experience), but the therapy of detoxification was impressive, and moreover seemed to work. Cold water was applied in
almost every way except bathing. Fierce jets of cold water, or cold
outdoor 'waterfall' showers, were favourite stimulants for the
circulatory system. Inside their daily cold-water-doused 'wraps'
the patients quietly steamed, stimulating the kidneys to evacuate
large quantities of fluids. The treatment was found particularly
effective for gout, syphilis, and all those suffering from mercury
poisoning—which was about half the clientele: 'Priessnitz
assured a friend of Sir Charles Scudamore that he had seen mer-
curial globules issue at the ends of the fingers after a long

continued course of the water-cure, years after the use of mercury had been abandoned.'[44] People developed muscles at Gräfenberg. It re-created peasant life with all its promise of longevity through a cure that was very like hard physical labour.

News of the water cure spread quickly and inspired many similar operators throughout Europe and America. The best sites were defunct springs or spas, on a hill or mountainside. In Ireland, Dr Richard Barter was an early convert to hydropathy (as it became known) and opened the first water cure hydro on the site of the holy well on St Anne's Hill, in 1842. He later developed an interest in the Irish sweat lodge tradition, and ended up leading a late-century popular Turkish vapour baths movement throughout Ireland, Scotland, and England; scattered remnants of this movement can still be found in British cities. England's first hydro on the site of an old spa in the Malvern Hills was opened in 1842–3 after a quick visit to Gräfenberg by two fashionable London doctors, James Wilson and James Manby Gully. The London literary and scientific set (Alfred Tennyson, Thomas Carlyle, Florence Nightingale, Samuel Wilberforce, Charles Darwin) became their loyal patients. Yet another proprietor, John Smedley, redeveloped an old spa at Matlock in Derbyshire in 1851. Smedley was a successful spinning magnate, the builder of a model factory community, a strict Methodist, and a hater of doctors, and an enthusiastic convert to hydropathy (though not to Priessnitz). Matlock was much patronized by puritanical northern industrialists like himself, and by the 1870s was the biggest hydro in Britain.[45] In America hydropathy was also an immediate success. During the 1850s twenty-seven hydros were built by springs, lakes, and mountains; later hydros, such as Round-Hill Water-Cure Retreat in Northampton, Massachusetts, were based on the larger German water cure resorts, where exercise took the form of sporting play rather than gruelling work.

Women in particular flocked to the hydros whenever they could, and appreciated its unconventional freedoms. The American suffragette trousers, or 'Bloomers', were originally a hydro-pathic style. The 'wet dress' worn over the steaming compresses beneath was in the Turkish or oriental style—a loose-fitting tunic or coat reaching below the knees, which was worn over loose trousers gathered at the ankles. 'Wearers usually cut their hair short for easy drying, and felt themselves emancipated from the bondage of trailing skirts, petticoats, corsets, and corkscrew curls.' This Turkish outfit was apparently introduced into fash-ionable American circles by a reformer's daughter, Elizabeth Smith, and was subsequently taken up by the feminist Amelia Bloomer, who dared to wear the trousers publicly in the street.[46] These and other late-century sports clothes were the beginning of a new phase in hygienic dress reform.

Late-Century Reform

On the whole, physical reformers in the last twenty or so years of the century could look back on a lot of specific achievements in the field of public hygiene, many of which had been (or were in the process of becoming) institutionalized. The key reform in Britain was obviously the capture of central and local government and the creation of an ethos of sanitary need. Municipal socialists and commercial developers were now starting to rebuild the towns through mass slum clear-ances, all new housing was fully plumbed and drained, and a whole cadre of doctors had moved into public health. A great deal of municipal and state effort was now also being put into adult physical fitness training, and in the new state and Church schools children were now being exercised and taught the basic rules of hygiene and popular physiology, collectively, for the first time. The Early Hours Movement released—and in part was designed to release—male and female clerks and shop assistants from their work in order to join in regular sporting activities and other rational recreations, attracting millions of people in their weekly 'time off'. The reformers had thus succeeded in creating an ethos of personal 'fitness'—what the philosopher William James called 'the religion of healthy-mindedness'.[47]

The sporting nineteenth century ended with the triumphant Olympic Games of 1896. These international games were held as the result of Baron Pierre de Coubertin's personal crusade to reinvigorate the French race through cricket and cold baths, and to put Greek sporting ideals on a world pedestal. There seems to be a distinct possibility that Coubertin's idea of the Olympics finally took shape in the summer of 1890, after an invitation from an English Rational Recreationalist, Dr W. P. Brookes, to visit the village of Much Wenlock in Shropshire and view their annual festival of 'Olympic Games', which he had started in 1849. Brookes had for years been trying to export the idea of an Olympic Games to be held at Athens, and in Coubertin he had finally found a fellow enthusiast.[48] It took Coubertin four years to assemble the first International Olympic Committee of 1894, which inaugurated and organized the first worldwide festival of sport. The First Olympiad was opened in Athens in 1896, on the site of the ancient festival, and went thereafter to Paris (1900), St Louis (1904), London (1908), and Stockholm (1912), with constant fixtures (excepting 1916 and 1940) to the present day.

But even while the sanitarian and physical hygiene reforms were steadily unrolling, the last twenty years of the century were filled with urgent social anxieties, uncertainties that had arisen directly from the onslaught of late nineteenth-century science. Not only had the Darwinian evolution debate raised unwelcome atheistic thoughts; but equally worryingly, the still-popular, if fading, Aristotelian–Galenic scientific paradigm was being fatally attacked and undermined by the rise of bacteriology and microbiological medicine from *c*.1880 onwards. Professional science had never been the monolith that radicals liked to think. If there was a problem interpreting the natural world, it had always been a communal one—and nothing was more communal than germ theory.[49] Germ theory unwittingly aroused the psychology of pollution fear in a new and acute form.

Germs

The old 'filth diseases' had been redefined by sanitarians during the course of the nineteenth century as 'zymotic' or 'pythogenic' diseases that were thought to generate spontaneously from human excrement and general filth, spread through miasma. Prince Albert's death from 'bowel fever' (typhoid), supposedly caught from the antique sewer system at Windsor Castle, frighteningly emphasized the importance of good sanitary provision in the home. Plumbing, sewerage, and cesspits were earnestly discussed in the press, and sales of water closet sewer traps soared. Another domestic fear, 'ptomaine poisoning', was raised after chemists had isolated the natural toxic substances produced by bacterial degradation in the intestinal tract, a piece of science which immediately took root in the public mind in the form of 'autointoxication'—a cesspit inside the body: 'one cannot live over a cesspit in good health. How much more difficult to remain well if we carry our cesspit about inside us—especially when, as so often happens, the cesspit is unpleasantly full?' Constipation (and the bowel and laxative market) was to remain a popular health obsession well into the next century.[50] But bacterial fermentation proved to be a fruitful lead towards germ theory, greatly helped by improved microscopes; but it was the effective practical and experimental work of Louis Pasteur, in particular, helped to popularize the new 'bacteriology' and led to much public debate in the 1880s about living 'vibrio', 'germs', and other microscopic zymotic particles. Germs were likened to tiny invisible seeds or amiculae that flourished, flew, and wriggled everywhere, thriving on unwholesome matter or weakened human constitutions.

Pasteur's work on germs was soon extended by Robert Koch's experimental finding of specific disease bacilli, with the result that specific disease micro-organisms were being discovered at the phenomenal rate of one a year between 1879 and 1900.[51]

Germs in fact fitted very easily into older popular notions of *contagium vivum*; but Koch's discovery of specificity—germs as separate species with a life of their own—was more threatening to the older miasmatist sanitarians. Sir Benjamin Ward Richardson, the author of *Hygeia: A City of Health* (1876), a mission statement for future macro-environmental hygienic town planning and architecture, was an old-fashioned sanitarian who placed all his faith in environmental cleansing, and considered germ-ridden laboratories immoral:

> Let us drain our country on a plan of such uniformity, that every particle of pollution shall pass from our houses as it is produced there; let us cleanse our outward garments, our bodies, our food, our drink, and keep them cleansed; let us cleanse our minds as well as our garments, and keep them clean; let us isolate the contagious sick as they become contagious. Then all elaborate experiments for the prevention of disease will appear, as they are, mysterious additions to evil which ought not to exist, and which of themselves might re-introduce death into a deathless paradise.[52]

The specificity of germs attacked both humoralism and hygiene by denying spontaneous generation—no balancing of hot, cold, wet, or dry was required to deactivate or activate a specific contagion; nor (so it seemed) the observation of the seasons, ordering of temperaments, diet or exercise—indeed the whole paraphernalia of Hippocratic environmental and personal hygiene. The amoral biological determinism that germ theory implied (like the extreme forms of contemporary evolutionism) appeared irreligious and inhumane. For people like the anti-vivisectionist John Ruskin (who resigned his art professorship because the university appointed a professor of anatomy) and

Florence Nightingale (then designing her 'pavilion' hospitals of light and air), microbiological science had no place in the city of Hygieia. The anti-scientific research lobby in Britain was so strong that the first British microbiological research laboratory in the 1890s was called the Lister Institute of Preventive Medicine: the word 'research' was specifically kept out of the name to avoid a backlash from anti-vivisection groups.[53] But by then the public's belief in the existence of 'germs' was strong and unstoppable, and mostly far more concerned with the microscopic world than the transcendental one.

Germs were now the invisible enemy, fought at every turn. Germ theory reinforced every single lesson of the old gospel of cleanliness, but the 'eternal vigilance' now required made house-cleansing a heavy burden of responsibility; its neglect was akin to murder. In the new procedures of 'domestic science' the basic old routines of the 'home hospital' were now to be applied to every room, but especially to kitchens, water closets, and bedrooms. There was an emphasis on the old axis of wet–dry purification. Strong light and continual fresh air dried up and 'cleaned' dark and dank cellars, rooms, and privies; antiseptic washes for floors and all surfaces mopped up lurking germs. Water sources must be pure, or if necessary purified, and all plumbing fixtures and fittings regularly inspected; for greater safety, plain white porcelain and tiling was now specified for super-cleanliness in and around the water closet, bathing, and food preparation areas. Laundry had to have ten minutes of boiling to kill germs (and vegetables only slightly less). Every kitchen saucepan and utensil had to be burnished and sterilized, every work surface cleaned off and disinfected daily, food cooled and covered with cloths to prevent germs from settling and breeding; new kitchen food refrigerators were found necessary in the hotter American climate. Since bacilli were also now known to live on in dry form, household dust was considered especially lethal. Thick curtains, wallpaper, heavy carpeting, ornate furniture, and knick-knacks were discouraged; and the use of damp cloths and mops were urged instead of sweeping and dusting—or even better, the new vacuum cleaner, for those who could afford it. Even dress length was affected, after domestic science reformers criticized long hems that brushed in the dirt and dust, bringing potential disease from the street directly into the home.

Complete isolation, or 'asepsis'—the bodily procedures that soon put germ-conscious surgical staff into gloves, masks, and gowns—was obviously not feasible for daily life; but nonetheless certain procedures closely resembled the ancient purity rules. Contact with any other person's body was dangerous. Kissing and hugging, even among members of the family, could be a risk, with strangers even more so; public handshaking was perilous (women were advised to wear gloves), and public coughing and spitting even worse (carrying a clean handkerchief was essential). Household food had to come from 'clean' retailers and shopworkers (hygienically produced 'branded' goods were safest) and preferably clean-wrapped in front of your eyes (transparent cellophane soon met this need). The whole suspect outer world—neatly summed up as 'flies, fingers, food'—obviously included the old insect pests such as fleas, the bedbug, nits, and body lice. Flies were a new fear that had been raised by agricultural science and the experience of fighting mosquitoes; they were now known to leave their invisible sticky footprints everywhere, randomly, and the life cycle of the fly was widely discussed in the press. The 'house-fly danger' campaign led to much covering of food and drink with beaded lace doilies, muslin over the baby's perambulator, fly screens, and campaigns against street refuse, manure heaps, and horse droppings. A new deluge of toxic sprays, gases, waters, and powders was directed at all these old and new insect enemies, including paraffin, arsenic, and lead compounds, as well as the traditional disinfectants (vinegar, soap, lime, derris dust).[54]

Levels of pollution fear among the general public must have been raised exceptionally high in those early days, even though an outpouring of domestic technical innovation was providing new solutions and familiarity gradually softened the new scientific routines. Bacteriology could increasingly identify and thus help prevent disease causation; but specific chemical therapeutics ('magic bullets') only arrived halfway through the next century, when the subsequent development of immun-ology—with its idea of the 'fighting body'—also reduced anx-iety and somewhat restored the human status quo. But scientific uncertainty left a good deal of room for divided opinion, perhaps even for a divided mind: you could be sanguine and optimistic one day, or for some reason fearful and pessimistic the next. Hygienic health reform fragmented and intensified, but the main body of sanitarians took the common-sense, broadly optimistic approach and threw themselves into prac-tical action. The civic hygiene and domestic science reformers in Britain and particularly North America operated through an avalanche of national and local committees, mass meetings, posters, tracts, books, magazines, newspapers, and advertising campaigns, and finally succeeded in changing domestic habits and manners and raising levels of domestic cleanliness to a degree undreamt of, in a remarkably short time (at least among urban populations—rural populations were not so accessible). A mass civic campaign against tuberculosis at the turn of the century hammered the message home.[55]

The pessimists were equally active, and just as desperate. There was still a large rump of physical puritan reformers campaigning hard against all the depravities of modern civilization, and the array of purity crusaders in Britain and America that arose during the last two decades of the century (and carried on well into the next century) was truly formidable. The ethics of personal hygiene and purity were stretched to the limit by (among others) birth control and eugenic 'social hygiene' enthusiasts, sexual purity campaigners against public prostitution and private 'onanism' (masturbation), the anti-science lobby of the anti-vaccination, anti-vivisection, and animal welfare movements, and the purest of the pure, the extreme vegetarians who refused any contact with animal matter (the vegans), or to inflict any pain on living things (the fruitarians). In Britain a joint alliance, the Humanitarian League, gave them a unified public platform in 1890.[56] But empiric healers such as herbalists, homoeopaths, osteopaths, spiritualists, and hydropaths were now truly locked out of modern science—satirized as dogmatic medical 'cults', under fire from medical licensing authorities, and completely outpaced by medical technology and new standards of rigorous scientific training in the medical colleges. Some awareness of the isolated position of the old medical democrats can be seen in the so-called Eclectic Movement at the end of the century, which united all their skills in a brand-new identity eventually called Naturopathy. Given the widespread popularity of the drug-free nature cure, one of the more emotional, or instinctive, public reactions to extreme materialism was evidently self-purification, and another bout of rugged, rural, primitivism.

Naturism

The two key empirics who reinvented the nature cure were Arnold Rikli, who opened his 'sanatorium' in the Swiss mountains at Veldes in the 1870s, and Adolf Just, author of the mystic *Return to Nature* (1896), who opened Jungborn in the Austrian Harz Mountains in the 1880s. Both took their cue from Priessnitzian hydropathy but took it a step further. They preferred patients to take their baths naked and exposed to the elements: Adolf Just even revived the eighteenth-century vitalist earth bath (being buried up to the neck). At Veldes patients lived in 'air huts' (three wooden walls with an open front) on the shore of a lake, and sunbathed on two large platforms, naked except for modesty aprons and protected with smoked sunglasses and straw hats. Veldes was so successful that Rikli had to open another, winter establishment where patients could outdo each other in their endurance of snow and cold air.[57] But the huge popular success of the nature cure came with the charitable, or free, regime devised by the celebrated Father Sebastian Kneipp (1821–97) at Wörishofen in the Austrian Alps in the 1890s.[58] The thoroughly vitalist and Priessnitzian Kneipp sent his patients and followers out for strenuous walks and swims in the mountains wearing minimal loose hygienic clothing, such as 'Father Kneipp Swimming Trousers' or the Reformed (porous) vests, shirts, and shorts invented by Dr Gustav Jaeger and promoted by Just, but preferably wearing nothing at all—he disapproved of clothes. Kneipp also invented the 'dew bath' (walking with bare feet over dewy wet grass, wet stones, or even fresh snow), and insisted on the 'vitality' of bare feet.[59] Heavily popularized in the press, the naked air bath movement spread rapidly throughout Germany via societies for natural methods of healing and living, which encouraged municipal councils to set up public air baths in grassland enclosures on the outskirts of the town, surrounded by very high board fences. Photographs show naked brass band rehearsals and newspaper-reading, as well as bowling, turning, and gymnastics. Amateur sunbathing at the end of the century required professional instructions as grave and careful as any eighteenth-century balneologist:

Sun baths should not be confounded with air baths, for they are essentially different types of baths. If the body is kept exposed in the open air to the action of the sun's rays, the bath becomes a sunlight bath. It is well known that the energy of light rays is beneficial to the human system . . . The position of the body should be frequently changed so as to expose it on all sides. The duration of the sun bath should not exceed 20 to 30 minutes, at the end of which usually free perspiration has set in. After the bath one should take a full water bath of 90 to 95 Fahr., and finish up with friction rubbing. . . . Modifications of the air bath, which require but brief mention, are . . . the 'genuine rain bath', i.e. walking in air-bath costume during a rainstorm, which is only intended for those with strong constitutions; the earth, sand, and moor baths; and finally the snow bath . . . One may either roll in the snow outside, or else gather a pail of it, bring it into the room and rub the body with the soft and warm snow.[60]

By 1900 the mountain-top air bath movement had become one of main convalescent techniques of turn-of-the-century main-stream medicine—the super-hygienic tuberculosis sanatorium, architecturally designed with the emphasis on the open-air life and sunlight baths, with the nature cure as a model.[61] But a Kneipp enthusiast, Benedict Lust, took naturism into the twentieth century by amalgamating the essential elements of the nature cure and changing its name, opening his American School of Naturopathy in New York in 1901, and founding the Naturopathic Society of America in 1902. In Lust's *Naturopath and Herald of Health* magazine, artificial modern drugs were unutterable poisons and the higher moral goal of naturopathy was 'ideal living' or complete wellness: 'Massive muscle, Surging Blood, Tingling Nerve, Zestful Digestion, Superb Sex, Beautiful Body, Sublime Thought, Pulsating Power'.[62] Kneippism was represented in Britain by the brief *Nature Cure Annual* of 1907–8, but had quickly spread along the grapevine among 'the more enlightened of the Bohemian class', including the beard-and-sandals vegetarian socialism of Bernard Shaw and members of the Fabian Society and their 'set'; or the artistic 'Pagan' students and their set, who swam and sunbathed naked on the Cambridge backs. Many were proud to call themselves 'neo-pagans' at the end of the century (though not many were as vehemently anti-Christian as the hardy hiker Friedrich Wilhelm Nietzsche, 1844–1900).[63] But the simple natural life—simplicity de luxe—also attracted such millionaire Nonconformists as the Reformed food manufacturer Dr Harvey Kellogg; or the Liverpool soap manufacturer Lord Leverhulme, who slept in a specially designed open-air bedroom containing little else but a simple iron bed and an enormous marble bath.[64]

Poverty and Doubt

Amidst all this frenzy of political, social, and economic activity and reform the very poorest were still completely powerless. Although by the end of the century Britain was, to the outward eye, a clean and washed nation, the inhabitants knew better. The immaculate Victorian home was a middle-class dream, with a big shortfall. As one cleric dourly noted in 1889:

> The rich man's family may grow up unbroken around the hearth...The children of the poor must die...What is it to the poor that it has been proved how cleanliness is the secret of health? They cannot have the latest sanitary appliances. They cannot take baths, or have a constant change of clothing...The poor, by bad air, by dirt, by accident, cannot live out half their days. The good news about health which science preaches to the rich is not preached to them.[65]

The political mood at the end of the century was sombre; and the rise of the racial purity crusaders, the eugenicists, reflected a profound crisis of confidence. Several peaks of the sanitary crusade had been and gone, and there was anxiety about what should follow. The sense of outstanding sins of omission towards the poor sustained the British evangelical slum settlement movement at the end of the century that produced grim reports such as those of William Booth and many others—a sort of national reckoning of the state of the poor. It was not that municipal sanitary reform had not worked (of that they were sure); but that the job was half done, and the central features of poverty had not disappeared despite the high expectations (experience of lifelong work in the charity sector convinced Sidney and Beatrice Webb that only full state intervention would succeed). These problems were tackled with further reforms in the next century. Meanwhile, the infrastructure that the nineteenth-century engineers and politicians built still sustains many of us, on a daily basis.

chapter 10
the body beautiful

In this last chapter we face, to some extent, a final reckoning—and we can barely do justice to it in the space that remains. The twentieth and twenty-first centuries are by far the best documented and probably the most grimly fascinating of all the centuries embraced by the history of personal cleansing. They are probably also the most interesting period for us as individuals, as well as recalling many of our parents' (and grandparents') own personal experiences. The sense of déjà vu is enormous. We can see older habits and customs persisting in domestic housing, cosmetic care, health education, therapeutics, and general self-care—but the scale is utterly different. It is global, again. The tried and tested hygienic 'middle-class' lifestyle of the Western industrial urban classes for the first time became feasible for a much larger proportion of the world population, beneficiaries of scientific medicine and a booming global economy. The economic equation between personal cleansing and domestic income is inescapable in these last centuries, as it was in every other era. But behaviourism also still plays a vital part in our responses. Purificatory ideologies also went global: anti-pollution ecology became an international crusade, pollution fears have brought major world food industries to their knees, and, tragically, purity rules have also inspired mass 'ethnic cleansing'.

The twentieth century itself was probably the most hygienic and cleansing-conscious era on record in all industrialized countries. It was punctuated by two world wars, both leading to periods of significant social transition. The whole period 1945–2006 has often been portrayed as one of extreme materialism and fully secularized personal hygiene—a new form of highly individualistic narcissism. But this may just be a trick of the light—many more people obviously embraced by economic consumerism, while the health objectives remained the same. The period 1900–39 was also individualistic and narcissistic, and saw a huge rise in health consumerism and the ideology of the fit and beautiful body. Personal hygiene had now reached the stage of a general consensus.

Eugenics and Preventive Medicine

Among advanced industrialized nations, public hygiene had gradually turned into an international crusade. Following a series of International Sanitary Conferences, the north–south Pan-American Sanitary Bureau was founded in 1902; and the first European Office International d'Hygiène Publique was founded in Rome in 1907, later becoming the League of Nations Health Organization Committee. Both bodies were replaced in 1948 by the World Health Organization. The nineteenth century had shown decisively that investing in public hygiene—not only in housing and drains but in personal hygiene as well—made sound economic sense. Andrew Carnegie, Johns Hopkins, Henry Wellcome, and John D. Rockefeller were only some of dozens of global industrialists in the first half of the twentieth century who threw unprecedented amounts of money at international (and national) public health scientific research programmes, for profitable as well as philanthropic ends. Revolutionary twentieth-century communist governments likewise put personal and public hygiene at the top of their agenda for building fit nations.[1] But the century had also opened with another optimistic liberal welfare initiative designed to 'do something for the people', as Lloyd George put it—state and private medical insurance, which took off like a rocket throughout Europe and the United States.

Medical insurance was a new form of commercial medicine— medical care at a discounted, cut-rate 'group' price; the idea came from the old working-class self-help burial clubs and cooperative saving schemes. By paying small regular amounts into a general fund, insurance brought the right to enjoy a far freer access to hospital medical services, and almost everywhere in Europe and the United States voluntary hospital admissions doubled, specialist treatment and convalescent clinics multiplied, and a large group of new middling classes— lower-middle-class office workers, managers, and skilled craftsmen—were brought into the professional medical orbit.[2] At the heart of this newly confident medical service industry were the laboratories, slowly but inexorably unlocking the chemistry of disease through effective vaccines, and the constant search for 'magic bullets' (the effective 'sulpha' drugs and antibiotics that finally arrived in the 1940s and 1950s).

The professional pride of the inter-war period is shown in the contents page of C. E. A. Winslow's student textbook of 1923: 'I. The Dark Ages of Public Health. II. The Great Sanitary Awakening. III. Pasteur and the Scientific bases of Prevention. IV. The Golden Age of Bacteriology. V. The New Public Health'. The New Public Health concentrated less on drains than on bacteria, and was inspired by the new discipline of scientific behaviourism, sociology, which drew on the experience of public health workers, measured observable trends, and refocused social policy towards the actual bodies and the life cycles of welfare recipients, inside their domestic surroundings, and within their local environment. Major preventive domestic health campaigns focused on hospital medical insurance cover, maternity and child health services, handwashing, venereal diseases, food hygiene, and milk supplies with much publicity from semi-public bodies such as the Health and Cleanliness Council (1928–46) in Britain, and the Cleanliness Institute (1926–) in the United States, run by the American soap industry.[3] But life was still a lottery for most people in the inter-war years. There was no welfare safety net, no magic bullets, and the economic 'boom–bust' cycle was very sharp—new industries boomed as old industries slumped. All the luxuries of modern housing and health insurance disappeared overnight if you were unemployed; and health insurance was generally too expensive to cover women and children.

During the early years of the century it became evident that certain pockets of relative deprivation were very marked indeed, with inner cities, older industrial cities, and agricultural districts suffering most; they were 'the submerged tenth' described by Charles Booth as still existing 'like a hidden sore, poor, dirty, and crude in its habits, an intolerable and degrading burden to decent people forced by poverty to neighbour with it'. At the beginning of the First World War, the very poorest in Britain were apparently not even fit enough to defend the state, which immediately rang alarm bells among the ruling classes. Pessimism about the state of the nation's health reached an all-time low in the famous 1904 Report of the Inter-Departmental Committee on Physical Deterioration, which led to the foundation of the Eugenics Education Society in 1907, followed by the highly influential *Eugenics Review* in 1909.[4]

Eugenicists in Europe and North America came from many existing schools of vitalist doctrines of racial genetics and biological holism, physiological reform, and physical puritanism, and understood each other well. They leant heavily on Herbert Spencer's well-known philosophy of Social Darwinism, or the survival of the fittest, which annexed Darwin's theory of human evolution and physiological modification, and created eugenics as a form of social hygiene. As the British eugenicist Havelock Ellis put it in 1912:

> all social hygiene, in its fullest sense, is but an increasingly complex and extended method of purification—the purification of the conditions of life ... the purification of our own minds ... the purification of our hearts ... and the purification of the race itself by enlightened eugenics, consciously aiding Nature in her manifest effort to embody new ideals of life.[5]

Eugenicists considered preventive medicine to be thwarting their aims by artificially prolonging the lives of the unfittest; they also wanted to eliminate prostitution, control alien immigration, sterilize 'mental degenerates' and segregate them in mental asylums; and they often raised the issue of racial physical degeneration through bad housing—which the sanitarians roundly rejected.[6] When the First World War was over many eugenicists in Europe and the United States joined the growing naturopathic 'physical culture' movement, such as the eugenics-inspired People's Health League, founded in 1917.[7]

The social surveys tacitly supported the sanitarians by showing that some of the worst hygienic conditions prevailed in rural areas where the housing infrastructure had remained untouched for centuries—earth floors, communal sleeping rooms accessed by stepladders, outdoor taps, outdoor toilets, barely any heating, and no baths. (In some parts of rural Ireland in the 1950s and 1960s there were no toilets at all—'under a bush as often as not, using a dockleaf'—and only on Sundays would children 'wash our face and neck, our hands up to our elbows, and our feet up to our knees ... relatives [said] how our congregation stank—of cow dung, I suppose'.) In most of these homes the only hot-water source was the kettle on the fire; but the very high population densities of the inner cities made personal hygiene equally difficult. In Shoreditch in London in 1938,

only 14 per cent of families had baths: 'Some had a footbath or
small tub, but as it was awkward to use...it was frequently
reserved for the children, whilst the parents went out to the
public baths or else never bathed.' In many tenements or small
apartments lack of space meant the coal really did go in the
bath:

> A bathroom in the house is not necessarily a great advantage as far
> as cleanliness goes—it strikes the more thrifty as a convenient coal-
> cellar...Baths are only found in about a dozen houses inhabited
> by working class families in this area. Out of these twelve, it is
> known that at least nine are used for storage purposes, and not
> as baths...The expense of heating the water...and lack of
> privacy...are great drawbacks.

Despite this, one East End mother of thirteen children with only
a cold tap in the yard still managed to run a house that was
spotless, with sheets starched 'white as snow'.[8] But many of the
children of these inter-war urban poor, when evacuated in 1940,
arrived in rags or, like several children from the slums of northern England, 'sewn into a piece of calico with a coat on top and
no other clothes at all'; and were often found to be dirty, ver-
minous, suffering from scabies, impetigo, and other skin diseases, incontinent day and night, 'ill-clad and ill-shod, [with]
never a change of underwear or any night clothes and had been
used to sleep on the floor'. A 1915 national survey of public
baths provision had come to a sober verdict: most public baths
were well used by only about a third of the population in their
surrounding areas, they had cost over £2 million to build, and
were consistently unprofitable: 'It is worthy of note [that] their
income is less than 50 per cent of their expenditure. Whether a
relatively high percentage under this heading is to be regarded
as a measure of success or failure will depend largely on whether
the baths are considered as a trading concern or as a department
of Public Health.'[9]

The Suburbs

If you were lucky, and had a job, you probably aspired to live in a spacious suburban settlement, infilling the big arterial roads lined or dotted with factories, bringing a stream of modern consumables into the cities. Most towns and cities in Britain (and elsewhere) acquired an outer ring of housing in this period, and outer-suburb growth was phenomenal; at its peak in London in the 1930s when mortgage restrictions were eased, detached or semi-detached houses were built at the rate of 1,500 houses a week. Their owners came from the older inner cities, young couples on their way up, out of the slums and rented lodgings. Suburbanites were dedicated above all others to personal hygienic health care. They came for the bathrooms with the hot water ('first thing, you went into the bathroom, and turned on the hot taps'), the indoor water closets ('we actually had a toilet on the first floor'), the clean electricity supply ('such an excitement—fantastic!'), the floor-length French windows, sun terraces, and balconies; the garden flowers, the nearby fields and fresh air; and the tennis, croquet, bowling, and golf clubs. The kitchens were small and convenient ('everything within easy reach—it was a special feature'), and their shops were built into the new 'parade' nearby.[10]

Very high standards of hygiene and presentation were expected in these pest-free, fully sanitized homes. The new servantless lady wife did most of the light domestic work, with some 'help' with the heavier chores, using an increasing range of 'labour-saving' cellophane-packed foods, cleaning agents, and mechanical equipment. The suburban husband's domestic role was simply to eat, relax, and look after the new garden.[11] His income paid for the modern electrical machines and sleekly designed streamline metal and bakelite gadgetry that rapidly appeared, promoted by photographic advertising that played heavily on the dangers of germs and dirt: the early electric radios, fires, fridges, water heaters, early washing machines, kettles, and irons; also the improved gas cookers, lights, and fires, the tiling, the parquet, and the latest easy-clean rubber linoleum. Hygienic plastic goods, such as Tupperware, came in during the second half of the century (along with wash spinners, dishwashers, and freezers). The only domestic dirt source often left largely unreformed (in Britain at least) in the inter-war years was the traditional open coal or wood fire in the comfortable modern 'lounge' or 'sitting room'; but for the rest of the house, modern electricity provided 'clean' heat and 'clean' lighting, and revolutionized domestic cooking, cleaning, and laundering.[12] The British electricity industry mounted a huge publicity campaign during the 1920s and 1930s, aimed squarely at the upper classes and middle-class suburbanites:

USE THE ELECTRIC METHOD to clean your house this Spring, and keep it healthy all year round...

With the help of Electricity you can do the housework without making more work and clean the Home without making yourself dirty.

Banish dust, dirt, and disease by using an ELECTRIC SUCTION CLEANER which lifts all the dirt direct into a sealed bag without a particle escaping.

ELECTRICITY is the cleanest, hardest working, most willing and cheapest servant under the sun. Always on duty, ready for instant service, day and night at the touch of a switch.

But electricity was expensive and more than a bit dangerous (1928 was 'a particularly bad year' for fatalities); even by 1931, less than 30 per cent of homes were wired, and less than one in a thousand was all-electric. Mass provision only got going after a boom in 1936, while in many industrial regions the working class remained loyal to coal and gas, and sceptical towards electricity, until the campaigns and Clean Air legislation of the 1950s and 1960s. One very obvious reason for this was that coal was a third of the price of gas or electricity, and that homes had to be laboriously and expensively adapted for a new 'clean fuel' supply.[13] It was similar to the introduction of domestic plumbing during the eighteenth century; all of these new domestic conveniences were acquired, as they had always been in the consumer surges of the past, on a sliding scale of income— which meant that most people at this stage could not yet afford them, and continued to clean up dust, grime, and soot in the old back-breaking ways: dustpans and brushes, soap and water (now with a dash of Jeyes' Fluid added). Large numbers of isolated rural cottages and farms in Britain, the United States, and elsewhere did not get piped water or electricity until well into the second half of the century, and continued to use wood, paraffin, or oil lamps, and local springs and wells.

Life in the suburbs followed an almost clockwork sanitary regime. Housework was ideally followed by an afternoon of genteel activities such as shopping (at nearby town department stores, which were also booming), or going to the local hairdressing and beauty 'salons' (sprung up to serve those without personal maids, and bristling with modern electrical beauty equipment) to get a fixed-wave 'perm' for the new shorter hairstyles. Electrical technology was a boon for the personal toilette; and better evening lighting clearly extended the hours of grooming preparation, and display, and possibly enforced higher standards as well. Essential preparations included an early evening heated bath in the new tiled and glittering bathroom with WC (featured heavily in estate promotional literature), next door to the well-lit bedroom, with its large-mirrored Art Deco dressing table and toilet sets, displaying quantities of face powder, 'scents', and deep-red lipstick and nail varnish. Heavy cosmetic painting came back with a vengeance from the 1920s, much influenced by the stage make-up used by the new film industry, and cleverly exploited by the Hollywood entrepreneur Max Factor. But the leaders of fashion in the

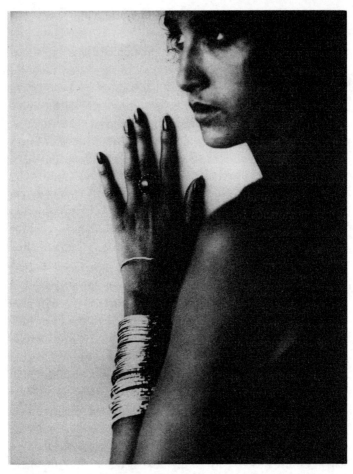

19 The fashion model Renée, photographed in 1938 in a sportive modernist style (ribbed cotton athletic vest, heavy exotic jewellery, and dark varnished nails) that is equally chic today.

1920s had already started to abandon the *ancien régime* of the milky-white complexion in favour of the natural all-over healthy body tan—first defiantly displayed by the fashion designer Coco Chanel after a long holiday on board a friend's yacht.[14] A respectable state of cosmetic undress was paraded in flamboyant female dressing gowns, with a new range of flimsy, sheath-like, underwear (favourite colour flesh pink). Convenient disposable sanitary goods had also been developed, such as paper tissues (originally for tuberculosis patients), paper toilet rolls, and commercially made sanitary pads, specifically designed for the busy and active 'New Woman'.[15] For women, hygienic dress reform had brought shorter hemlines and looser clothing without corsets; but sports hygiene had meanwhile exploded into sportswear. Sportswear fashions accentuated comfort and lightness: lighter (and artificial) fabrics, new stretch woollens, light colours, liberating trousers, bare arms, necks, and backs, legs bared in 'shorts', and feet bared in sandals and beach mules. It was entirely possible that the local dress shop could run up (or order) the latest line in Schiaparelli woollens, Jaeger tennis and walking outfits; or stock elasticated Jantzen or Hermès beach wear, with beach pyjamas, beach robes, American playsuits, sun and swim hats, and satin-ruched ('aqua-satin'), halter-neck, bare-back, bathing costumes.[16]

Suburban Children

If there were children in the suburban household, the afternoon and early evening feeding and grooming routines centred on them—until their father came home, when they were promptly sent to bed to have their good long healthy sleep. Many 'modern' mothers in the 1920s and 1930s carried on late nineteenth-century trends in child hygiene and followed the advice book author Dr Truby King's famously strict (and thoroughly vitalist) hygienic recommendations to the letter—a heavily disciplined training process which started directly after birth with time-regulated feeding and evacuations (potty training) and which in the hands of a conscientious or germ-obsessed mother could become a nightmare.[17] Powerful smells, plus elbow grease and kitchen cabinet staples, and possibly a few of the new aspirin tablets (acetyl salicylic powder was synthesized in 1896), were still the family's front-line defence against sickness. But nylon toothbrushes and hairbrushes, superior dental powders and pastes, cheaper soaps and heavily antiseptic-smelling, dandruff-clearing liquid hair shampoos (Sebbix, Vosene) were making basic grooming a little easier and more effective; and supported a vigorous campaign in schools and homes to combat the continuing problems of children's body odours, head lice, and bad teeth. Progressive dentists recommended (in books, magazines, but now also over the radio) a preventive oral hygiene regime of a wholesome diet, plus twice-daily brushing and a biannual check-up: 'the intelligent and steadfast practice of the means indicated in these rules would result in far fewer teeth being lost'. Championed by Army dentists during the Second World War, the oral or dental hygiene movement took off in post-war private dental practice, heavily influenced (in Britain and elsewhere) by high standards of cosmetic dentistry in the United States. Since being available at a subsidized price on the National Health Service in Britain as an auxiliary service for dentists, oral hygiene has greatly reduced the number of teeth being pulled and the number of fillings done, compared with pre-war days.[18]

When their children grew up and went to the local school, quite a lot of parents might have been lucky enough to find that the local council had already adapted to the modern style of educational architecture, with plenty of large, low windows, open verandas, grass lawns, sandpits, paddling pools, kitchens, showers, toys, and Montessori reading and numeracy aids. Madame Montessori's infant school movement started in 1912 (as a successor to Johann Heinrich Pestalozzi's and Friedrich

Froebel's 'kindergartens') was a modern educational milestone; it emphasized the need to catch and train the 'human animal' when young. It trained through educating the senses, Rousseau-style, and put children into a relaxed but intensive hygienic regime of feeding, sleeping, correct dress, play, and exercise, thrusting the infants and toddlers out into the sunlight and fresh air whenever possible, to get tanned and hardened—a belief that had only been strengthened by the tuberculosis sanatorium movement and naturism. Photographs show ranks of cots placed outside in gardens, and orderly groups of toddlers in white aprons blinking uncertainly into the sunlight behind the camera. By all accounts they often transformed the lives of those poorer children lucky enough to attend them, as well as slowly transforming primary school educational philosophy.[19]

Inter-war babies were bathed as ferociously in fresh air and sunlight as their eighteenth-century predecessors had been in cold water. Doctors, teachers, and parents were at one on the importance of the Lockean outdoor life for children. In the 1930s the journalist John Gale (himself a notably 'clean young Englishman' brought up barefoot and athletic in the early 1920s) and his wife were extraordinarily determined to do the right thing for their newborn child:

Because the flat was so small and had neither garden nor balcony, we decided to keep Joanna in a cage outside the window. It was an exaggerated parrot cage, made of what is known as elephant wire.... An expert, a man in a small brown hat, came to fix it up. He assembled it in a few easy movements, and screwed it onto the window-sill, adding a couple of metal supports for good measure...Certainly the cage was extraordinarily secure.... at last, holding our breath, we picked up the basket containing Joanna, then less than a month old, and thrust her into space. Simultaneously, a number of startled and elderly female faces appeared from behind lace curtains in the windows opposite. Although they became familiar with the sight of the caged baby, the faces never altogether lost their look of shocked surprise . . . Yet, whatever the psychological risks of the cage, Joanna did well enough. She was nicely sunburnt; she became apparently immune to frost, instantly pulling off any glove or woollen boot and dropping it at the feet of the milkman; she watched traffic; she was a fine imitator of dogs and rag and bone men and a passionate admirer of the Salvation Army . . . When there was snow or an east wind, Jill zipped her up in a sort of sack with armholes, made from a worn-out blanket; even in this she humped around quite actively, abusing people in the street below, and getting more opportunity for exercise than could be provided by the largest pram . . . [After a year old] she grew out of it altogether. But it gave her an admirable start.[20]

Swimming facilities had become the norm for many British city children—like Angela Rodaway's young sisters, who 'went about in the summer wearing nothing but a pair of swimming trunks. Many children did this. I could not help comparing it with the flannel petticoats in which I had been dressed.' To get a swim, suburbanite families could take a trip to the vast new local open-air lidos built by towns and boroughs from 1929 onwards, with their aerating fountains, lawns, Imperial-sized pools, and terraced cafés. Some towns, starting recreational parks from scratch, added public tennis courts, bowling greens, infant paddling pools, and play areas. In 1935 the massive Jubilee Lido, jutting out into the sea at Penzance, was opened; and Cheltenham Lido had 100,000 visitors in its first opening season—with 10,000 cars.[21] Outdoor lidos were a substitute for going to the seaside; but of course many people now went there for a week or so on holiday, as well. The inter-war years were a holiday boom time for car, caravan, coach, and rail trips to coastal resorts, beach huts, and holiday camps; two-thirds of all British holidays were taken by the seaside.[22] Cycling and hiking were especially popular among young workers; and the Youth Hostels Association (YHA), copied from the German

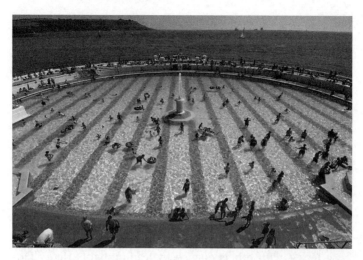

20 The Tinside Lido jutting out into the sea at Plymouth, built in 1935 at the height of the swimming boom, now fully restored and in use during a heatwave in 2006.

youth Wandervogel movement, was founded for hikers in 1930, with almost 300 hostels by 1940 providing over half a million overnight stops—the YHA found that its initials were popularly translated by young women as 'Your Husband Assured'. There was more than a fair chance that they would meet up with a handsome young socialist, or young professional, well away from inquisitive family eyes—just as upper-class girls were courting on the golf course, the swimming pools, car race tracks, or tennis courts.

Naturists and Nudity

The new suburban lifestyle was strongly supported by the ethos of 'modernism'. Modernism is usually associated with reforms in art, architecture, and design, but also incorporated a whole raft of politically Progressive hygienic beliefs centring on social democracy, individual freedom of conscience, sexual politics, and of course naturism.[23] Naturism won steady converts during the first half of the century. Many committed naturist individuals—and indeed whole families—drew on a rich and ancient mixture of health beliefs absorbed and formed over generations. The disappearance of the last clothing layer, revealing once again the primitive naked skin of the animal body— bare arms, legs, torso, feet, and uncovered loose hair—was to a large extent continually spurred on by naturism and naturopathy among the more adventurous, or wealthier, classes of western Europe and America.[24] Turn-of-the-century naturopathy flourished in luxurious, exclusive health resorts such as Lust's famous Yungborn retreat in America, opened in 1896 in New Jersey, with others opened by leading lights Henry Lindlahr and Bernarr Macfadden. Macfadden opened his first 'Health Home' in Britain in 1907, and one of his managers, Stanley Lief (editor of the long-running magazine *Health for All*, later called *Here's Health*), opened the still-existing 'health farm' at Champneys, Hertfordshire, in 1925. Naturopathy was set firmly in Protestant medical traditions, spurning the use of any artificial drugs (and vaccines), and was thus just as eclectic and empirical as its predecessors, drawing on all the old physical therapies and adding many other modern (or revived) techniques such as body massage, 'radiant heat' or 'artificial sunlight', yoga and breath control, the Alexander method of vocal exercises, and the Bates method of eye exercises—all of which became well known to the select few.

Because of the general exodus of patients to other health-seeking sites, many of the old British inland spas languished in the inter-war years, sustained only as convalescent centres for the elderly or war-wounded, although in Europe professional hydropathy was kept alive in the larger spas of Germany, France, Italy, and Hungary.[25] In 1993 cold-water hydrotherapy in Britain was somewhat naively relaunched as a brand new 'thermo-regulatory hydrotherapy training' for boosting the immune system. 'It is very interesting to read that this discovery has been made in England and I am extremely excited about the findings... similar findings were borne out at the turn of the century by our own scientists,' politely commented the director of the Kneipp Hydrotherapy Centre at Bad Wörishofen in Germany, opened by Kneipp in 1889 (now with two research departments and 160,000 members of over 600 Kneipp clubs worldwide, and growing).

Naturopathy remained securely fixed in its transcendentalism. In food reform circles Dr Max Bircher-Benner was a charismatic figure. In 1906 he had founded his Force de Vie Privat-Klinik outside Zurich, having been snubbed by Zurich Medical Society for giving a paper in which he quoted the second law of thermodynamics and described fruit and vegetables as 'living matter'—'living food'—with a Life Force of their own which was completely destroyed by cooking. His patients went on a 'Detoxication' nature cure consisting of exercise, elemental bathing, three days of raw fruit and vegetables, one day fasting, and two days of the Bircher-Benner diet. This was the famous Birchermuesli, made of porridge oats, milk (or yoghurt), honey, nuts, and raw fruits, which, in true empiric fashion, he had once shared and enjoyed with a peasant in the mountains (just as he had once eaten a raw apple which made him well). Bircher-Benner's regime inspired other naturopathic clinics in Europe and America, and the 'macrobiotic' diet, and 'vitamin' salads, emphasizing the principle of 'holistic' raw and unrefined foods, became an intriguing new addition to the vegetarian cuisine. During the 1920s nutritional science had gradually isolated the essential nutrient 'vitamins' (A, B, C, D, E) found in raw foods, and seemed at last able to establish a scientific basis for vegetarianism; ironically, by the 1930s synthetic vitamin supplements had become major profit-earners for the big pharmaceutical companies.[26]

For the true naturist, however, the real action had already gone elsewhere—to sun worship and the 'Joy of Light'.

> A healthy brown body beside the blue lake, in the green of the forest, on the mountain tops: nothing is more splendid ... All who have seen it, seen with their whole souls, know why human beings are not born with clothes on—they know that man is a creature of light ... Gaze into the clear joyous eyes of young people accustomed to the light, and you will behold a new radiant purity— something that no merely 'civilised' person can even guess at.[27]

Werner Zimmerman's glowing description of his Joy of Light colony on the shores of Lake Neuchâtel was one of the inspirations for the Swiss League of Light, founded a year later, in 1928. Its members believed in sunlight, cooperation, pacifism, free love, vegetarianism, the elimination of stimulant drugs— and the power of the naked body: 'A new humanity shall come out of nakedness; the nakedness that courageously stands up for the "new spirit" in the face of a corrupt world.' Naked sunbathing caught the public imagination like nothing had done since cold bathing. Nudity broke through the Christian taboos that had accumulated around the naked body in Europe, and its beauty and muscularity was now celebrated and exposed for the first time since the fall of Rome. With the rediscovery of pagan Greek ideals also came renewed demands for sexual freedom and sexual equality, and freedom from the burden of Christian sin, guilt, and shame. For women in particular, pure-minded healthy nakedness was an astounding bodily liberation, while feminist 'free love' theory (and birth control reform) was intended to release them from the old ascetic bonds of virginity and celibacy.

Because of its vitalist traditions and its nineteenth-century Natural Healing Movement, Germany was the leader in what now became known as the 'free body culture' (*Freikorperkultur*). The cult of nudity (*Nacktkultur*) was well advanced in Germany by the 1900s, and the first public mixed sunbathing area, the Free Light Park (Freilichtpark), which opened in Berlin in 1903, drew many thousands of bathers. The first-ever sunbathing club, the Friends of the Rising Light, was formed in 1906. A series of outdoor lodges around Berlin led to the forming of the Nude Airbathing Association of Berlin, where the first international Congress of Nudity and Education took place in 1921. The old German youth hiking movement, the Wandervogel, had been stripping off for years; and Major Hans Suren, chief of the German Army School for Physical Exercise between 1919 and 1924, raised a whole generation of soldier cadets who trained naked in all weathers. By the early 1930s there were an estimated 3 million nudists in Germany.[28] In England nude sun- and air bathing had also been practised informally for decades, but in 1923 the classically named English Gymnosophist Society opened a sunbathing lodge in Upper Norwood, followed by the more obvious Sunbathing Society in 1927; French and Scandinavian naturist lodges were opened in the 1930s. In the United States the American Sunbathing Association was formed in 1923 with lodges in Cleveland and New York State, while Bernarr Macfadden's American League for Physical Culture was started in 1929, with its own sunbathing lodge at Sky Farm, New Jersey.[29] Macfadden was a vocal supporter of 'physical culture' and the *freikorperkultur* ('free-body') movement in America, and promoted the accompanying eugenic–Aryan ideals of physical beauty and fitness for men and women as progenitors of a fit race: 'Strength through Joy... Weakness is a Crime'.

The rise of physical culture and body-building magazines complemented the commercial sports of boxing and wrestling, encouraged all other athletic feats of strength and endurance, and brought on a new generation of brawny record-breakers in tennis, yachting, cricket, athletics, cycling, and all other sports—especially swimming.[30] In its heyday in the inter-war

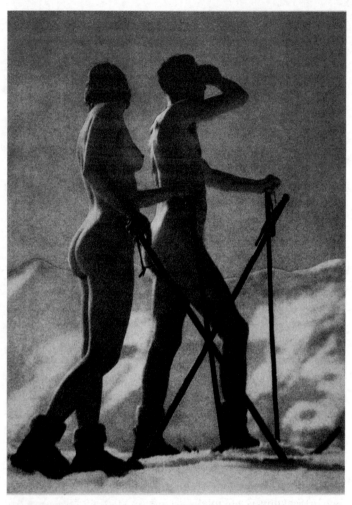

21 The ultimate test of naturist hardiness (and its love affair with photography): naked air-bathing in the European Alps in 1930.

years, swimming was considered to be the most physical and most beautiful of all outdoor sports; and was a gift to the new media of photography. In the last decades of the nineteenth century, especially after 1875, when Captain Matthew Webb swam the English Channel and became an international hero, endurance and 'display' swimmers had become popular celebrities. During the 1920s and 1930s competition diving and synchronized swimming were developed, and the new Australian overarm racing crawl developed ever-faster leg-beats and competition times. Local rivers and pools ('swimming holes') were developed, and ardent swimmers travelled long distances to find secluded, classically inspired, or challenging sheets of water all over the world, with their cameras in their packs. Cameras and film also brought the first pictures of night-swimming parties, common since Byronic days among gilded youth, now often lit by low electric lights around the nouveau riche private pool, set near the house.[31]

By the 1930s Joy of Light pure naturism had gone far beyond the remit of medical therapeutics and had become increasingly enmeshed in socialist and fascist body-politics. For dedicated political radicals, naturist nude swimming and sunbathing in large mixed groups was absolutely de rigueur. At Progressive League summer schools in Britain (and Fabian Society summer retreats), the rambles, picnics, swimming, sunbathing, and barefoot early-morning country dancing that accompanied the political discussions were strong bonding occasions. In America, Progressives went into summer seclusion to Asheville in North Carolina, or to the island of Martha's Vineyard off Cape Cod in Massachusetts.[32] But the dark cloud of eugenics was fast approaching in Europe. Socialist ramblers on German mountainsides were harried by the emerging right-wing *naturheil* Nazi Youth organizations; and groups such as the pacifist and anti-racist radical Christian Bruderhof communes were forced to emigrate in the early 1930s—at about the same time that Jews were being banned from German gymnastic clubs.[33] In 1933 Hitler banned nudism in Germany—more for its 'freethinking' philosophy than for reasons of morality, since the Nazis also laid full claim to physical culture, nature worship, and hygienic public health, including vegetarianism, naturopathy, anti-smoking campaigns, and cancer screening. The details of Heinrich Himmler's carefully constructed neo-pagan Nazi religious cult are now very well known: the shrines, the Ark, the myths, the purificatory rules and initiations, the physically perfect specimens, the marriage laws, the naturism and pure diet, the flags, the songs. Hitler took on additional sacred authority as the Master, or Führer, of this patriotic and purist nature cult; and his sober personal habits and vegetarianism were an integral part of Nazi propaganda.[34] In the longer term, Nazi eugenics and appropriation of the term 'social hygiene' undoubtedly brought the (previously unquestioned) morality of hygiene into disrepute, and so played a considerable role in the intellectual avoidance, or downgrading, of the word 'hygiene' in the post-war era.

Post-1945 Hard Sell

The visual image of the 1950s is that of an exceptionally sanitized decade. Post-1945 was above all the era of a new *americaine*, which exported—largely through film and television—the hygienic ideals of the affluent American suburbs, including a fervent nouveau riche obsession with domestic and personal cleanliness. New colour film not only emphasized the toilette of the stars but threw light into domestic interiors that had never been so glamorized before. A huge American consumer market developed the all-electric 'white goods' sector, and a booming advertising industry sold housework as effortless, even chic. Women consumers, advertisers, and manufacturing suppliers colluded in a fragrant revolution. The first ever television advert was

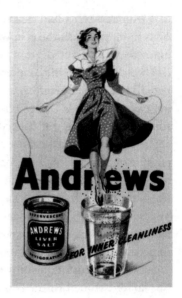

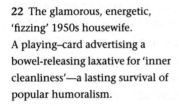

22 The glamorous, energetic, 'fizzing' 1950s housewife. A playing–card advertising a bowel-releasing laxative for 'inner cleanliness'—a lasting survival of popular humoralism.

for soap; and laundry in the 1950s was made 'whiter than white' with 'blues' and bleaches, with its 'fresh' smell always heavily emphasized. Well-packaged cleansing products such as liquid detergents, spray polish, bathroom cleaners, air fresheners, liquid soaps, and shower gels began to fill the post-war house with perfume—a stunning array, compared to the 1900s house. Scenting its quarry accurately, household advertising abandoned the medical hard sell of the inter-war years and went over to pastel-coloured soft sell from the 1970s; the old 'antiseptic' scents were slowly replaced by floral essences and (latterly) by a new range of powerful herbal, spice, and fruit scents.[35] Household cleaners are not quite the staple of TV advertising budgets that they were, and it is noticeable that cosmetic adverts (including even menstrual products) have largely taken over their slot.

Wartime austerity had created a pent-up urge to spend money on beautification. In the post-war period, 'glamour' was in, and cosmetic sales rocketed. From America came the concept of 'BO' (body odour) and the use of underarm deodorants, spread through a large advertising campaign in the 1950s—and which accompanied the American habit of showering. The history of twentieth-century personal hygiene could easily be written as the rise of the cheap and convenient domestic shower, and the small efficient domestic washing machine, which made the laundering of underlinen easier than ever before and banished the now unwelcome smell of bacterial decomposition. The male toilette generally was given a fresh start in the 1950s with hair creams, electric and safety razors, and ruggedly perfumed aftershave (notably the US world brand leader Old Spice). The cosmetics historian Jim Obelkevich has suggested that it was largely women who transformed the male toilette: 'It was women, not ads, who got men to change . . . Women bought aftershave, gave it to their husbands and boyfriends, kept after them to use it, complimented them when they did, bought more when it ran out—and so on, year after year. Fathers, husbands, sons, brothers, cousins, uncles, in-laws—no male relative was spared.'[36] For all men, bodily 'self-presentation' was an additional selling point in an increasingly competitive labour market, whose main twentieth-century feature had been the arrival of women—strongly encouraged by the continuing spread of progressive, free-body philosophies.

Flower Power and Multiculturalism

There was a distinctly pagan, non-Western approach to the good life in the last third of the century, that was not nearly so puritanical and clean-cut as it was even in the 1930s or 1950s. For this, multiculturalism was largely responsible. Many radical activists of the 1960s and 1970s spent their formative years living in what they saw as the 'alternative society' to worldwide consumer capitalism, and their political and social networks were as intense (and as internationalist) as those of the 1790s, 1840s, 1890s, or 1930s. Some activists found to their great surprise that, although their grandparents or parents could not actually become 'hippies', they were more than capable of becoming 'Greens' or tree-savers, or protesting against world war, apartheid, or nuclear power. It was the ecological puritans of the 1960s who were the first to point out that there was a global environmental pollution problem. Their bible was Rachel Carson's *Silent Spring* (1962), which not only exposed the extent of the man-made chemical contamination of the environment, but warned of possible long-term consequences for human genetic mutation and destruction of chromosomes. At the same time the ecology-inspired principle of 'intermediate technology' and the 'Gaia' philosophy of a self-sustaining planet, originally proposed by James Lovelock, was being developed within the alternative 'green' student movements of the 1960s and 1970s; ten years later it had moved into international aid organizations and colonized university academic departments. Ecology conquered the United Nations and 'greened' many global economists in the 1980s–1990s.[37]

Another hidden link with older radicals was through pure food movements, and the campaign for 'real' and organic foods. Alternative food reform was accompanied by 'purist' cookery using authentic recipes and ingredients from the world's peasant cuisines (also peasant or traditional beauty receipts), and took over the marketing of naturopathic macrobiotic foods in a surge of small 'health food' producers and cooperative outlets selling yoghurt, muesli, lentils, wholemeal bread, brown rice, organic vegetables, and natural cosmetics— older naturopathic outlets were often saved from extinction.[38] Starting in the 1980s, ethnic cuisines, organic products, and an unprecedented array of fresh vegetables and fruit have been successfully mass marketed by globalized supermarket chains, feeding growing numbers of healthy-lifestyle consumers.

It was pre-1945 naturopaths who had begun to experiment with yoga, meditation, acupuncture, and other forms of multicultural medicine. Their moral stand against orthodox medicine had never slackened, and was quietly picked up by activists from the 1960s onwards. 'Flower power', 'ethnic', or non-Christian multicultural moral philosophies and therapies played a large part in the late-century surge of holistic health care—an 'alternative' (or 'fringe') medicine that included many things that Granny might have tried, while sharing the same rooted distrust of doctors.

Self-Help and Holistic Medicine

During the 1950s, when scientific hospital-based medicine became widely accessible (and freely used the new wonder-drug penicillin and a whole range of new antibiotics), many people had thrown out their array of home remedies with apparent relief.[39] After 1945 in Britain and elsewhere, what had remained of the old medical categories of the 'Institutes of Hygiene' were split administratively between scores of different government and university departments and sciences. Public health problems were now largely tracked by epidemiologists and social welfare analysts; welfare agencies were hived off into separate departments of Social Services; and layers of hospital-based regional and district health authorities were put into place. Other so-called 'ancillary' body services such as dentistry, chiropody, ophthalmology, midwifery, diet and nutrition, psychology, and physical and occupational therapy, slowly re-organized their professions and expanded their publicly funded work in separate niches within the hospital system.[40]

But by the 1970s patients were starting to vote with their feet again, in both Europe and the United States. The complaint voiced by 1970s radical authors such as Ivan Illich, Fritjof Capra, and René Dubos was that orthodox medicine was still too uncaring and 'invasive', too narrow and mechanistic, and still far too drug-based. It was failing to cope with chronic disease, and it was certainly failing to deal with the 'whole person': the six- to seven-minute average consultation time was a particular complaint. At the same time women's liberation groups were pioneering medical 'self-help' through feminist medical advice books, self-help videos, classes, and communal group analysis; which all proved very effective in launching the widespread natural birth movement (which included the use of massage and warm-water birthing pools, a throwback to ancient Methodist techniques).[41] Progressive doctors responded quickly to these critiques. In the United States a pressure group of doctors working within the profession, the American Holistic Medicine Association, was set up in 1978; the British Holistic Medical Association followed in 1981 (its motto: 'Physician heal thyself'). Fringe medicine was often now more gracefully called 'complementary medicine', with the idea that it should work alongside orthodox medicine—or better still, change it. In Britain consultation rates with 'lay' holistic practitioners rose steadily during the 1970s at a rate of 10–15 per cent per year: by 1983 there were an estimated 28,000 self-trained therapists of hypnosis, herbalism, homoeopathy, manipulation, yoga, acupuncture, and other alternative therapies, in addition to 2,000 or so associate-trained therapists. This was in total almost as many as Britain's 29,000 general practitioners combined (and in one sample no less than 80 per cent of GPs wanted to learn their techniques). These consultation rates certainly increased during the 1980s–2000s.[42]

The grass-roots revival of self-help strategies attracted the attention of late twentieth-century sociologists, and gradually forced a revision of state health policies. In Britain the fragmentation of public medical services came under criticism, and was to some extent reversed in new multidisciplinary departments of 'health policy, biology, and environmental science'. Moreover, the old sociological model of overlapping medical 'sectors' radiating out from a professional 'hub' was found inadequate to describe the real, anthropological parameters of welfare: localized, decentralized, professionally based, cross-disciplinary 'primary care' became the new buzzword in health administration. So little was known about the history of domestic medical care generally that it came as something of a surprise for medical sociologists to discover that professional medical help is normally only sought for roughly 1 in 10 medical episodes—or even less (for depression 1 in 74; for headache 1 in 60; backache 1 in 38; sleeplessness 1 in 31; muscle and joint aches 1 in 18; cold or flu 1 in 12; a sore throat 1 in 9). By the 1990s popular medical self-help groups covered almost every condition and ailment, meeting and communicating and sharing common experiences of self-diagnosis, new techniques, and remedies, a process made even easier by the Internet. With medical self-help groups apparently becoming a permanent feature of the medical scene, patient power moved up the political agenda and entered government health policies on both sides of the Atlantic; helping citizens to help themselves is now thought to be very cost-effective. In Britain the small Health Education Council (originating in the 1920s) became the much larger Health Development Agency, with a brief to raise health awareness, change health 'risk' behaviour, and ameliorate health inequalities.[43] New Internet technology was also used to set up a new government diagnostic and advice service, and the first page of NHS Direct online (one of the last in our long list of health advice texts) opens thus:

- Want to find out more?—our health encyclopaedia covers a wide range of topics.
- Not feeling well?—try our self-help guide for advice.
- Want to stay healthy?—we have advice in the healthy section.[44]

The healthy section, of course, contains most of the old positive precepts of hygienic care, but never uses the word 'hygiene'. But a modern terminology of need has slowly been devised. We find that while industrial executives, advertisers, health administrators—and the public—may know nothing about the philosophy of hygiene, they know all about the new 'well-being sector'. The well-being sector (organic products, vitamins and minerals, spas, beauty salons, and gymnastic products and services) is a recognized late twentieth-century market phenomenon.

Modern Well-Being

In the 1960s and 1970s naturism and wealth coincided on the warm and sunny Pacific coast of California, and produced a luxurious 'New Age' theology of body culture that ultimately became the 'well-being sector'. 'Hippie' teenagers who grew up in the 1970s and 1980s formed the core group of affluent health enthusiasts who rediscovered multicultural medicine in the 1980s and 1990s; and in the United States, where personal health insurance was expensive or simply not affordable, and individual preventive health care strategies were even more essential, New Age holism was rapidly adopted and mass-marketed as a new moral 'wellness' crusade: 'Your health is your responsibility... don't just sit there, do something,' as one American best-seller energetically put it.[45]

Therapeutically speaking, modern holistic medicine is a revival of ancient humoralism, and starts from the premiss of a holistic physical interconnection between mind, body, and the universe, derived from both eastern Asian and Western classical–vitalist cosmologies. It pays close attention to the action of primary elements (earth, air, fire, water, metal, and wood), and to the old existential or environmental categories such as air, food and drink, exercise, sleep and work, the evacuations, and passions of the mind. The body is seen as existing in a biological envelope through which the cosmic physical forces of 'bio-energy' (or ying and yang) flow with a transcendent psychic energy that can be either harmful or benign. There is a particular interest in the tonic therapeutic actions and reactions of the five senses (acting not only through the nose, but through the eyes, the hands, the ears, and the voice) and in psychosomatic medicine generally; the term favoured by progressive holistic GPs is 'biopsychosocial medicine'.[46] The techniques used to control bio-energy are mainly those preserved and developed in the ancient practical-medicine traditions of eastern Asia, such as reflexology, aromatherapy, aerobics, Shiatsu, astrology, colour therapy, crystal dowsing, hot-stone massage, laughter therapy, and, more recently, Reiki, Shen Qi, Tui-Na, Feng Shui, and Qi Gong.[47] Aromatherapy, deep breathing and meditation, and massage are considered particularly good for easing psychic blocks of energy flow, and overworked or 'stressed-out' individuals (rather like Roman citizens) are urged to cool down, 'chill out', lie back, unwind, relax. The famous cleansing or purging 'detox' regime starts with full 'colonic irrigation' of the bowels, followed by fasting and a planned dietary programme of pure foods and liquids, gentle exercises, meditation, aromatherapy, massage, and skin-cleansing, taken straight from the naturopathic textbooks. The much-desired 'state of relaxation and health' that these therapies enshrined also eventually led to a re-examination of the old non-natural category of 'work and rest'—now popularly called 'work–life balance'. But any references to ancient Western medical therapeutics are rare.

Meanwhile, on the other side of the Pacific Ocean, humoral medicine itself has developed and moved on, but in harmony with ancient traditions. The dual Western–Eastern medical policy of Chinese state medicine is well known. Japanese engineers, on the other hand, have taken several ancient diagnostic procedures to their ultimate conclusion with their technical redesign of the toilet. Japanese electronic toilets are famous for their water-washing and air-drying facilities; less well known perhaps is the so-called 'smart toilet', which not only weighs you, but analyses your stools. Based on these readings, it can tell you whether or not you have had too much alcohol, too much protein, or too much of anything harmful, and can inform and act as your doctor. It can prescribe a special diet, order it from the supermarket, and have it delivered to your home, ready to be microwaved.[48]

Beauty care has made a big comeback. Glowingly healthy, attractive self-presentation knows no social or geographical boundaries. The beautiful people who flit through the pages of late-century health texts are self-empowered, strong, and pure, inside and out. A 'Gaia philosophy' advice book from 1995 told its readers:

> In a state of relaxation and health, the body is perfectly designed to be self-cleansing, self-regulating and self-healing. But the toxic overload in the air we breathe, the water we drink, our food, our work places, and our homes undermines our health and immunity... *Body Tonic* is a practical handbook for everybody in our polluted world. It features unique questionnaires to assess your own level of toxicity, and suggests appropriate programmes of diet, exercise, cleansing and meditation for detoxification and long-term well-being.[49]

Diet, exercise, and a good spiritual attitude are essential for producing the holistically perfect beautiful body, which lives in spotlessly clean, white, natural, and minimalist surroundings (not unlike a virgin's or monk's cell). The virginal theme reappears in a new ethic of intensive grooming. Total cleansing and a purist attitude towards cosmetic care has replaced the 'killer glamour look' in certain elite circles: skin moisturizers instead of foundation paint, tinted lashes instead of mascara, expensively pedicured feet and manicured hands, organically treated glossy hair, scrupulous depilation, and a understated dress code that is modest, even severe, yet wildly expensive. As one fashion stylist put it, 'My clothes are quite minimal...the main attention goes on body maintenance—facials, saunas, nail upkeep. I don't drink and I try to keep a balanced diet. Virtuous? Maybe, but it's not until I've done my exercise that I feel balanced and clean.'[50]

These higher standards of personal hygiene seem in fact to have come about incrementally in the wider population, in the last fifty years. In 2001 British cosmetic and toiletry sales totalled £4,115 million (up 18 per cent over four years)—a sharp contrast to 1949, when the total was £120 million, with an average personal 'spend' of 3s. 10d. a month. In 1949 British women apparently did a hair-wash 'on average between once a week and once a fortnight'.[51] By 1965 over half were using underarm deodorants daily, and shaving their underarms; and recently it was found that 'more than four-fifths of the population change their underwear every day...One in 10 women carries a spare pair of knickers everywhere. Almost all of them change every day. More than half shower daily.' Shaving, waxing, plucking, and moisturizing the body became a general habit during the 1980s, while full-body depilation (beyond the 'bikini line') is an old *ganika* art that re-emerged as a fashion accessory in the 1990s, to complement the all-over tan; tanning machines (and fake tanning lotions) are available in every high street or shopping mall.

Retail analyst figures provide some graphic insights into the modern history of cosmetics and toiletries, on a global scale. The 'well-being' industries have soared faster than any other retail sector; private gyms and health clubs took off in

the 1980s; artificial 'spa bathing' has undergone a parallel economic resurgence (up 25 per cent in the United States) and the
world's natural spas have recently become elite holiday destin-
ations.[52] Meanwhile, global cosmetics retailers are already
charting their course for years ahead. The so-called 'mature'
markets in the United States and Europe have been heavily
'segmented' into niche markets by age, gender, and income,
but are apparently showing signs of market saturation; while
the 'undeveloped' markets in Asia–Pacific, South America, and
central Europe, on the other hand, are filled with new potential
and contributed largely to the 9 per cent growth in the world
market in 2004. As global urbanization continues and increasing numbers of women enter paid work, these regions are
being targeted through direct 'home selling' (Avon, Oriflame),
the Internet, local celebrity endorsement, sustained television
campaigns, and buyouts of local or national companies. America and France are still the global market leaders—the United
States with Procter & Gamble–Gillette, France with L'Oréal—
and over the last ten years they and other companies have
poured research and development into three new sectors:
high-income older women, men's cosmetics, and the teenage
market.[53]

Women still dominate the cosmetics market in all countries,
buying mostly skin care and hair care products, followed by
fragrances and colour cosmetics; but women in developed markets now prefer high-end 'value-added' goods. Organic and
natural products showed the biggest (11 per cent) increase in
the US and French markets, selling 'wellness products' that
make an explicit connection between beauty products, diet,
and vitamins—or 'cosmeceuticals', as they are now known in
the trade. In the United States this 'cross-over' also spread into
expensive organic baby care products, as women 'baby
boomers' from the 1960s and 1970s had their children at a
later age. Any sharp distinction between the male and female

toilette has been blurred by the recent phenomenal rise of commercial cosmetic surgery for both sexes, correcting supposed bodily imperfections and signs of ageing, at middle-class prices.[54] It was mainly older women (and 'metrosexual' men) in Europe and the United States who brought about the boom in anti-ageing dermatological products marketed by cosmetic surgeons and global companies—like Elizabeth Arden's half-strength botox Prevage Anti-Ageing Treatment and L'Oréal's vitamin C skin-serum 'skinceuticals'. Another potentially lucrative market has opened up with high-end 'ethnic' cosmetics scientifically developed to suit the different skin types and demands of black, Hispanic, and Chinese women (and men), especially after it was noticed that although African Americans made up 12 per cent of the US population, they accounted for 25 per cent of the total spend on cosmetics and toiletries.

The sales of men's cosmetics have shot up everywhere in Europe and the United States, kick-started in France, where male skin care products showed an extraordinary 67 per cent rise between 2000 and 2005; sales also clearly show there is an untapped market among men elsewhere in the world. Men may eventually start buying toiletries en masse, like women, but retail surveys of their current grooming habits suggest that there are many hurdles to overcome—not least the super-confident 'Retrosexual Groomer' (the majority, 57 per cent), whose body is adequately showered and washed, but whose grooming routine takes a swift ten minutes—twenty at most—and who refuses to use fragrances or expensive extras of any kind. Researchers have managed to find some groups of slightly more fastidious 'Practical Groomers', who will at least use deodorants; and some groups of older 'Natural Groomers', who use fragrances, skin care, and anti-ageing products, and who, like their younger counterparts, the 'Metrosexual Groomers', are 'clearly in no hurry to leave the bathroom', spending

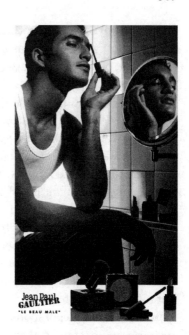

23 *Le Beau Male*—masculine narcissism (*c.*2006). The French cosmetic and fashion industries worked together in developing the current niche market revival of male beauty products.

well over half an hour a day on a full range of grooming routines. Narcissus, of course, was a male god; and the cosmetics industry has faithfully mirrored the rise of the well-groomed, affluent, gay male economy, and the power of the so-called 'pink' pound/dollar/euro/yen. But the proportion of intensive male groomers is small (15 per cent) and studies show that boys, unlike girls, are generally 'taught to believe that what they do is more important than how they look or smell'; fathers still pass on the traditional male right to perspire without embarrassment: 'sweat is a sign of hard work, nothing to be ashamed of, a fact of life'. In one deodorant survey it was often the more socially confident boys (or young men) who actually washed and groomed themselves less—alpha males in the making—which may explain why another survey found that it was frequently 'the bosses who are smellier, with manual workers and the unemployed changing their underwear more frequently: 82 per cent wear clean smalls every day, compared with 78 per cent of the middle classes'.[55]

But things may change in the future. Affluent young teenagers have become an ever larger part of the late-century personal hygiene market. The 'Afro' haircut of the 1960s was one of the first symbols of Western youth's liberation from its own culture. It was part of a youth fashion rebellion against everything that Western bourgeois hygiene represented, in youth groups ranging from the 'Beats', Hell's Angels, and hard-rockers, through to punk, 'grunge', and Green 'crusties'. Since the 1960s virtually all the ancient ethnic body-arts (nail art, hair art, facepainting, ring-piercing, tattooing, pomades, foot jewellery, thongs, etc.) have been rediscovered by young multiculturalists, and have lodged firmly in European and US teenage bedrooms. But today's teenage boys, by and large, prefer to wear American global brands or styles of sportswear that emancipate them from their past and/or connect them to their peers around the world, with a casual, pristine, 'locker-room look' that also requires that they use quantities of deodorants (Lynx, Axe), shower frequently, change their underwear, and care very deeply about the cleanliness of their face, breath, feet, and hair. Boys will never catch up on the girls, though. Between the ages of 7 and 10, girls are already treating grooming as a fun play activity— 'dressing up'—complete with cheap and cheerful body sprays, flavoured lipsticks, and glitter nail varnish; between 11 and 14 they go in for more sophisticated fragrances, deodorants, heavy showering, skin moisturizers, complex hairstyling, and a broader repertoire of make-up. By ages 15 to 19 girls already have established grooming routines, at a time when boys are just beginning to grapple with shaving. As a group, however, modern teenagers fully realize that smelliness is now socially unacceptable (you can even lose your job) and that personal cleanliness is a required norm. But the old primate grooming display urges lie close beneath the surface. In one 1980s teenage survey, 'wanting to have friends and to attract the opposite sex were cited as the main reasons for concentration on hygiene. All agreed that it gives you more confidence knowing that you are clean.'[56]

It is what the retail analysts say about the consumer lifestyles of their target 'undeveloped' rural markets that really brings the history home—the places where the old and ancient ways are still fully operational, and which so closely resemble the relatively recent past in Europe and the United States. So it is with a thrill of recognition that we read that rural classes in India prefer to use bar soap for 'head-to-toe body washing' (the strip wash); that many 'even use home preparations'—or purchase local 'generic products'; or that there is a large trade in smuggled high-class cosmetics from overseas, as well as cheap local 'counterfeit' copies; or that 'rural consumers typically visit an outdoor barber' for shaving and haircuts—which is what most British men also did in 1949 (only the local barber was of course indoors), while many of them also bought all their toilet necessities there as well. (The majority still go out for a haircut, but shaving has been made easier at home, and supermarkets provide most of the products.) The consumer lifestyle in Turkmenistan is equally revealing. Turkmenistan is still a predominantly rural peasant economy (53.9 per cent) with very few 'premium outlets', and most of its population use traditional means of grooming.[57] The men are always crisply turned out, even though all laundering is done by hand, without washing machines; the women use home preparations such as olive oil and locally produced fragrances to dress their hair, but generally do not use beauty products at all 'except on special occasions'. However, even in Turkmenistan things are changing, and these changes are illuminating. One key event has been that 'love marriages' were made legal in

2000: sales of cosmetic depilatories immediately shot up by a staggering 1,408 per cent, and cosmetic sales rose by over 200 per cent. Another (universal) trend is that many young Turkmenistan men and women are now moving into office work, where good daily grooming is essential. The message from the retail analysts is clear and very familiar: it is the new urban and suburban classes that are forcing cosmetic demand worldwide; and these upwardly mobile people are driven by personal ambition and the need to succeed in an expanded global marketplace.

The search for the body beautiful is truly relentless. Narcissism (the 'tendency to self-worship, absorption in one's own physical perfections') seems to occur among privileged groups during every period of prosperity; and the mind inevitably drifts to Ovid, and to all those exquisite gallants of courtly life, male and female, clothed or semi-clothed, and all those other keen gymnasts and self-improvers, throughout the centuries. The human body has undoubtedly been caught up in the twentieth-century celebration of godless technical materialism—this beauty is skin deep, and proud of it—but the twentieth- and twenty-first-century evidence gives us just a hint of what a powerful social force beauty is and always has been.[58] If love, luxury, and leisure are the key determinants of successful health and beauty care, then rising global affluence has done the most of all to promote it. It requires only a few well-known changes in habits and manners for social aspirants to gentrify now within a single generation. At this point in time in advanced industrial countries, decades of increased personal hygiene and cosmetic awareness have finally paid off. Teeth are better, feet are rarely deformed, and gross skin diseases, and particularly gross facial deformities, have become almost non-existent; as one cosmetic surgeon put it, 'we catch them all much earlier now'. There are, quite literally, many more beautiful and unblemished people around.

Epilogue: Future Trends

There is a little bit of this whole history in all of us. We are, when all is said and done, merely biological animals with a special tendency to sensuous pursuits such as sex, beautification, and pleasure—all of which roused such contrary human passions, and ascetic forms of self-control. Greek hygiene is still with us, transformed into a global industry (or rather, many industries). We still adore Roman-style bathing and pampering—and we still like to do it in crowds, like medieval communities. Early modern puritans continued the religious healing mission, and transformed our attitudes to personal and public hygiene; a process which was facilitated by the long and steady rise in disposable income, throughout the nouveau riche eighteenth and nineteenth centuries. The health crusaders of the nine-teenth century helped cope with a crisis and built the world as we know it; and the continuing affluence of the twentieth and twenty-first centuries has preserved these gains, and greatly extended human longevity. Yet still we are worried about the future. We always are worried—it seems to be a necessary part of the human condition. It is how we adapt and survive. There are two complementary themes in this book: the material empiri-cism of 'personal hygiene', and the immaterial imagination of 'purity'. We are still worried on both fronts—but especially now about global environmental pollution.

We are slowly realizing that urban civilization is a very thin veneer, and that longevity and luxury are fragile commodities. When Greenpeace and various other ecological protest move-ments merged under the 'green' umbrella, stung into action by a whole series of rusty oil tanker disasters, global pollution became global news. A scenario unfolded which exposed the growing pollution of the earth, air, and water through human activity and its various by-products and 'evacuations', and set in motion the long-term scientific analysis of the phenomenon of global warming. Like the nineteenth-century sanitarians before them, the international ecologists and their scientific supporters found that they could only warn and influence, and that the process of reform took much longer than anticipated.

Clean water for urbanites had been a steady policy throughout the twentieth century, but it came at a price. Domestic water demand for bathing and cleaning is at an all-time high, and large water-borne sewage systems are in place; but we find we have polluted seas and coastlines with our liquid evacuations, while the building of dams, reservoirs, and embankments along major rivers has destroyed ancient habitats and flood plains, and aggravated the politics of water rights. Clean air has been another twentieth-century hygienic fetish, and Clean Air legislation was successfully introduced in the 1970s. Coal smoke was banished at low atmospheric levels, but not the chemical fumes or 'plumes' from industrial products that went into the upper atmosphere; the existence of the 'ozone layer'—and its decay—has only recently been observed. Toxic residues from industrial smoke stacks continue to destroy tree cover downwind for thousands of miles with acid rain; and the old sanitary belief in trees as the 'lungs' of the city is now projected in global terms, as satellite photography shows how commercial logging has decimated the world's oxygenating virgin forests. Clean fuels are now a hotly debated topic. The worldwide nuclear industry was hailed in the 1960s as a new source of clean electrical energy replacing the dirty coal-run power stations; but has proved to be the source of virtually indestructible contamination. 'Clean' oil reserves are finite, and have passed their peak. 'Clean' fuel from low-tech sustainable energy technology— wave, wind, and solar power, and biomass fuels—was put on the back burner for over fifty years, but is now beginning to attract 'ethical' private investment and state support. Meanwhile, we attend to our health by buying 'pure' bottled mineral water in vast quantities, and drink it out of oil-based plastic containers. By inventing new trouble-free materials, new cleaning machines, and layers of extra wrappings, we banished many germs—and efficiently swept, buried, burned, or shipped our discarded refuse clean out of sight. Or so we thought until recently, when the vast piles of indestructible rubbish mounting annually in the world's largest conurbations suddenly became a visible problem, and the scavenging or recycling industry was reborn.

We are still especially careful of what we put into our mouths—and it must be clean and pure food. Our primitive disgust responses are still very much alive. A few years ago BSE (mad cow disease) emerged on British farms, and by a short but unsuspected route (cattle feed) infected European and other herds, and entered the human food chain. Within a few weeks of BSE being discovered, a significant proportion of consumers of all classes worldwide had stopped buying and eating beef—though others 'took a risk' and limited themselves to 'organic' beef certified as untainted. The political and economic fallout was immediate: Britain was called 'the leper of Europe', the 'dirty man of Europe', 'an island of sick animals', 'the whore of an England', and probably many other unprintable things, for having generated these poxes. It certainly did not go unnoticed either, during the later foot and mouth epidemic of 2001, that the horrific piles of burning carcasses, the mattresses soaked with disinfectant washes, the specially clothed operatives, the closing of footpaths and public parks, and the enforced incarceration of farmers and their families on their land and within their houses, resembled nothing so much as a seventeenth-century plague scene.[59] Meanwhile, the public image of meat butchery declines still further, and yet more children lean towards ethical vegetarianism and green politics.

There was another sharp shock for 'agri-business' in the 1990s when the European public was alerted by an international public campaign on the Internet, and rose up in moral indignation against the genetic pollution of the world's natural food stocks through genetically modified (GM) crops (not to mention a corporate plan for 'introducing' sterile GM seeds to the world's farmers) and refused to buy genetically modified foods. 'Green', or pro-nature, agricultural reformers now call for the deglobalization of agricultural trading by shortening the international food supply chains, and returning to local, mixed, traditional organic farming without chemicals—a move strongly supported by chefs, animal welfare campaigners, and industrialized farmers trying desperately to 'clean up their act', many of whom have turned both organic and 'humane'. But so long as global air transport is economic, 'ethical development' will have to live with modern technology. And so it has. To green, multicultural food reformers, small is beautiful wherever it exists. The 'ethical consumer' who will charitably pay extra cash to small Third World farmers (or indeed even their own small farmers) directly, through buying organic 'fair trade' products, is the latest green bombshell in food retailing. Along with all this is the rise of the Rousseauian 'ethical mother'. Organic reform has touched many areas where women are in control, not only in personal cosmetic regimes, but in family food-shopping and children's diet. In 2004–5 the young chef Jamie Oliver shook the British public with his exposé of the heavily processed food (and health effects) contained in cheap school dinners; while Morgan Spurlock's film *Super Size Me* caused a market crash in McDonald's 'fast food' meals (and a prompt corporate revision of nutritional content and portions).

Children's health has led to another future worry—the so-called 'hygiene hypothesis', which suggests we have possibly all become too clean for our own good; and that this may be the cause of the disturbing rise in allergic and auto-immune diseases (hay fever, asthma, and nut and other food allergies) in industrialized urban societies with high standards of hygiene. The sneezing and wheezing diseases were always thought to come from polluted air; but the 'hygienic' immune phenomenon was first noticed in Germany, when an asthma study of East German and West German families found that the children in the dirtier and less hygienic East had significantly fewer cases of asthma than children from the cleaner and more modern West. The hypothesis was further tested; it was found that country children, or indeed children who have been around animals from an early age, or even those who had attended crowded day care centres, or who had larger families, had a stronger immune system response than children in towns who lived in clean and disinfected homes and streets. The immune system had been challenged at an early age, and stimulated into action. The same contrasts can be found in the immune systems of 'dirty' wild and 'clean' captive animals, such as rats. The problem, if the hypothesis stands up, is what to do about it. Unfortunately, our bodies need only the right kind of dirt: feces-contaminated dirt, or chemically contaminated dirt, can be fatal. It has got to be wholesome dirt. Meanwhile, it may be best to play safe and hold off from the 700 new antibacterial cleansing products that apparently hit the market between 1992 and 1998.[60]

Further problems have arisen over the last thirty years in connection with the many man-made chemicals or biological weapons used in or around the human body, as broadly predicted in *Silent Spring*. The very rapid fraying of the microbiological medical safety net, however, was not predicted. Antibiotics have already been redeveloped many times, as resistant strains have endlessly mutated. The most recent problem has been the rapid biological development of penicillin-resistant MRSA (methicillin-resistant staphylococcus aureus) in many different forms. In the United Kingdom, MRSA-related deaths rose from thirteen in 1993 to over 1,600 in 2004; and cross-infection is only controlled through strict and old-fashioned hygienic measures: thorough hospital ward cleaning, hand-washing, asepsis, and quarantine.[61] Meanwhile, other potential physiological problems (for example, the problem of sperm count decline), possibly due to ingesting man-made chemical trace elements in food and water supplies, packaging materials, or cleaning materials, still lie in the future.

'Puritanism' in all its forms, good or bad, has to be considered a deep-seated part of our physiological and psychological make-up, and a major historical continuity. Globally, the darker side of the psychology of puritanism has also been very much in evidence in the twentieth and twenty-first centuries. On every continent warring groups have used the language of the political purge, and 'ethnic cleansing' genocides have been distressingly common. Extreme religious puritanism is currently being used worldwide as a political instrument by a new wave of evangelical ascetics, whose extremely conservative world-view abhors the gleaming façade of modern urban materialism. Like the ancient Jews and Christians, for people who feel they lack everything in the present world, religious millenarianism and perfection in a future world still holds a real significance.[62] As one historian of technology points out (with a little exaggeration), even in the twentieth century, 'we have never been modern...the modern world permits scarcely anything more than small extensions of practices, slight accelerations in the circulation of knowledge, a tiny extension of societies, minuscule increases in the number of actors, small modifications of old beliefs'.[63] Perhaps Hegel was right, and there is a semi-closed system at work: the environmental, social, and biologically determined limitations imposed on the body often make it seem so.

But the past continues to exist on many polytemporal levels. We all have our Neolithic moments, although (when adults) we are often reluctant to acknowledge them. The idea of the simultaneity of time-frames in our everyday existence is a theory almost without the possibility of proof; but one particularly poignant final story seems to illustrate something very like it. The story comes from the Holocaust and involves a puzzled male doctor and a consignment of red lipsticks arriving in Belsen concentration camp immediately after the Second World War. The internees were people surviving like trapped animals, whose bio-hygienic clocks and human grooming codes had been almost—but not quite—totally destroyed:

> piles of corpses, naked and obscene, with a woman too weak to stand propping herself against them . . . men and women crouching down just anywhere in the open relieving themselves of the dysentery which was scouring their bowels, a woman standing stark naked washing herself with some issue soap from a tank in which the remains of a child floated . . .

To the doctor's astonishment, they clung with extraordinary ferocity to a single talisman of their former human lives:

> I don't know who asked for lipstick. I wish so much that I could discover who did, it was the action of genius, sheer unadulterated brilliance. I believe nothing did more for those internees than the lipstick. Women lay in bed with no sheets and no nightie but with scarlet lips, you saw them wandering about with nothing but a blanket over their shoulders, but with scarlet lips. I saw a woman dead on the post mortem table and clutched in her hand was a piece of lipstick. At last someone had done something to make them individuals again, they were someone, no longer merely the number tattooed on the arm. At last they could take an interest in their appearance. That lipstick started to give them back their humanity.[64]

In extreme conditions humans still revert to their old animal survival skills, and we should perhaps take some comfort from the continued survival of our ancient coping mechanisms. Many of these are socially trained; but the most innate live continually inside us. We are probably 'right' to let instinct guide us when confronting the microbiological world that we cannot normally see. But as one immunologist recently pointed out, what is really astounding is how few micro-organisms actually cause human disease, and how peacefully they have coexisted with the very recent species *Homo sapiens sapiens*. A world without bacteria, says Gerald Callahan, would be a poorer world:

> This is not a war, as it has often been described, even though we have mustered an impressive array of weapons—bactericidal cribs and mattresses, toilet cleaners and counter tops, blankets, deodorants, shampoos, hand soap, mouthwashes, toothpastes. This is not a war at all. If it were, we would have lost long ago, overpowered by sheer numbers and evolutionary speed. This is something else, something like a lichen, something like a waltz. This waltz will last for all of human history. We must hold our partners carefully, and dance well.

What cannot change either, in the near or far future, is the strong human need for being touched and groomed and generally cleansed and cared for in a close physical sense. The holistic issues surrounding health inequalities and social 'well-being' are steadily turning into a future political conundrum. Social inequalities and the sense of 'unfairness' (a lack of love or respect) can create great stress and anxiety in the human animal; and too much stress and thankless labour can eventually kill as surely as poor diet or poisoned water or air. In today's world it is apparently the more egalitarian societies, with fairer income distribution, that have the highest life expectancies and 'happiness levels'—not the richest ones.[65] Despite the great edifices of modern medicine, classic technology, ancient religion, and modern capitalism, perhaps the core image that might be taken away from this history is of compact family and kin groups quietly and mindlessly grooming, feeding, and otherwise looking after themselves, in their own homes and shelters, for their own purposes, day after day, year after year, generation after generation. 'Well-being' is ultimately neither a fad nor a luxury, but a necessary mental and physical state.

notes

Introduction

1. P. E. Razzell, 'An Interpretation of the Modern Rise of Population in Europe', *Population Studies*, 28: 5–17 (1974), 13; W. Reyburn, *Flushed with Pride: The Story of Thomas Crapper* (London: Macdonald, 1969); Lawrence Wright, *Clean and Decent: The History of the Bath and Loo, and of Sundry Habits, Fashions and Accessories of the Toilet Principally in Great Britain, France and America* (London: Routledge & Kegan Paul, 1960). See also Lucinda Lambton, *Temples of Convenience and chambers of Delight* (London: Pavillion, 1995). The standard text for most occasions when referring to the history of hygiene was Henry Sigerist's elegant essay *Landmarks in the History of Hygiene*, Heath Clark Lectures (London: Oxford University Press, 1956); this superseded his previous survey article 'The Philosophy of Hygiene', *Bulletin of the Institute of the History of Medicine*, 1 (1933), 323–32.

2. Wright, *Clean and Decent*, 1.

3. William Morris, *News from Nowhere; or, An Epoch of Rest*, ed. James Redmond (London, 1890; London: Routledge & Kegan Paul, 1970), 6. See also the classic 19th-century text by Sir John Simon, *English Sanitary Institutions, Reviewed in the Course of their Development, and in Some of their Political and Social Relations* (London, 1890), 142.

4. F. Braudel, 'The History of Civilisations: The Past Explains the Present', in Braudel, *On History* (*Écrits sur l'histoire*), trans. Sarah

Matthews (London: Weidenfeld & Nicolson, 1980); Norbert Elias, *The Court Society*, trans. Edmund Jephcott (1st German edn., 1969; Oxford: Blackwell, 1983), 13: 'biological evolution, social development, and history, form three distinct layers . . . the speed of change being different at each level . . . In the contexts of different rates of change, phenomena in the slower current are apt, from the position of the faster current, to seem immutable, and eternally recurrent.' See also Elias, *Time: An Essay*, trans. Edmund Jephcott (Oxford: Blackwell, 1993), 96–7.

5. The chess analogy is usually cited for malarial disease, not hygiene; but the analogy arguably still holds true. See L. W. Hackett, *Malaria in Europe: An Ecological Study* (London: Oxford University Press, 1937); cited in Mary J. Dobson, *Contours of Health and Disease in Early Modern England* (Cambridge: Cambridge University Press, 1997). See also W. H. McNeill, *Plagues and Peoples* (London: Penguin, 1979), 15–16.

6. Robert Boyle, quoted in A. C. Crombie, *Augustine to Galileo: Science in the Later Middle Ages and Early Modern Times, 13th–17th Century*, 2 vols. (New York: Doubleday, 1959), ii. 297; see also *Robert Boyle's 'Heads' and 'Inquiries'*, ed. Michael Hunter, Robert Boyle Project (London: University of London, 2005).

Chapter 1 **Bio-physicality**

1. See e.g. Kenneth Jon Rose, *The Body in Time* (New York: Wiley, 1988).

2. As in Frank Macfarlane Burnet, *The Integrity of the Body* (Cambridge: Cambridge University Press, 1962); id., *Self and Not-Self: Cellular Pathology* (Cambridge: Cambridge University Press, 1969). See also A. I. Tauber, *The Immune Self: Theory or Metaphor?* (Cambridge: Cambridge University Press, 1994); Ian Burkitt, 'The Shifting Concept of the Self', *History of the Human Sciences*, 7 (1994), 7–28.

3. Quoted from Günter von Hagens, *Autopsy: Life and Death*, Lesson III: 'Poison', Channel Four TV, 18 Jan. 2006.

4. Diane Ackerman, *A Natural History of the Senses* (London: Phoenix, 1990), 10–11; Bartolomeus Anglicus, *De Propriatibus Rerum* ('On the Properties of Things'), trans. John Trevisa (Oxford: Clarendon Press, 1975), ii. 1296–7. For historical views on smell, see the pioneer anthropologist Dan Mackenzie, *Aromatics and the Soul: A Study of Smells* (London: Heinemann, 1923); Alain Courbin, *The Foul and the Fragrant* (Cambridge, Mass.: Harvard University Press, 1986).

5. What is happening in the brain here is as yet not fully understood. See generally Susan Greenfield, *The Private Life of the Brain* (London: Allen Lane, 2000); ead., *Brain Story: Unlocking our Inner World of Emotions, Memories, Ideas and Desires* (London: BBC, 2000); and more specifically William Ian Miller, *The Anatomy of Disgust* (Cambridge, Mass.: Harvard University Press, 1997).

6. Robin Dunbar, *Grooming, Gossip, and the Evolution of Language* (London: Faber & Faber, 1996), 36–8; see also B. M. Spruijt, J. A. R. A. M. van Hoof, and W. H. Gispen, 'Ethology and Neurobiology of Grooming Behaviour', *Physiological Review*, 72/3 (1992), 834–9.

7. Lyall Gordon, 'The Sweet Stench of Success', *Independent on Sunday*, 12 Sept. 1999, 18–20; see also id., *Jacobson's Organ and the Remarkable Nature of Smell* (London: Allen Lane, 1999); *London Evening Standard*, 5 Aug. 1999, 22.

8. For a recent overview, see Matt Ridley, *Nature via Nurture: Genes, Experience and What Makes Us Human* (London: Harper Perennial, 2004); also Steven Pinker, *The Language Instinct: The New Science of Language and Mind* (London: Allen Lane, 1992).

9. Constance Classen, *Worlds of Sense: Exploring the Senses in History and Across Cultures* (London: Routledge, 1993), introd., 1–3, and *passim*; see also D. Howes (ed.), *The Varieties of Sensory Experience: A Sourcebook in the Anthropology of the Senses* (Toronto: Toronto University Press, 1991), and L. Vinge, *The Five Senses: Studies in a Literary Tradition* (Lund: C. W. K. Gleerup, 1975).

10. Many further examples are raised in T. McLaughlin, *Coprophilia, or, A Peck of Dirt* (London: Cassell, 1971); and in R. Reynolds, *Cleanliness and Godliness* (London: Allen & Unwin, 1943). An Internet

trawl of the word 'disgust' brings up the subjects of food, sex, racial politics, referees, dirty clothing, and (in one experiment) being asked to kiss a stranger—most people had a disgust reaction at that.

11. Paul Rozin, *Towards a Psychology of Food Choice* (Brussels: Institut Danone, 1998); see also Miller, *Anatomy of Disgust*.

12. Mary Douglas, *Purity and Danger: An Analysis of the Concepts of Pollution and Taboo* (1966; London: Routledge & Kegan Paul/Ark, 1984), p. viii.

13. Norbert Elias, *The Civilising Process: Sociogenetic and Psychogenetic Investigations*, trans. Edmund Jephcott (1939; Oxford: Blackwell, 2000), 68–72; an additional note on cleanliness appears at 530–1 n. 124.

14. On ethology, see P. J. Bowler, *The Environmental Sciences* (London: Fontana, 1972); Desmond Morris, *The Naked Ape: A Zoologist's Study of the Human Animal* (London: Jonathan Cape, 1967); id., *Manwatching: A Field Guide to Human Behaviour* (London: Jonathan Cape, 1977); William McGrew, *Chimpanzee Material Culture: Implications for Human Evolution* (Cambridge: Cambridge University Press, 1992); Frans de Waal, *The Ape and the Sushi Master: Cultural Reflections by a Primatologist* (London: Allen Lane, 2001).

15. Dunbar, *Grooming, Gossip, and the Evolution of Language*, 35.

16. Robert Barton, 'Grooming Site Preferences in Primates and their Functional Implications', *International Journal of Primatology*, 6/5 (1985), 519–32.

17. The classic work on body techniques is Marcel Mauss, *Sociology and Psychology Essays*, trans. Ben Brewster (1950; London: Routledge & Kegan Paul, 1979), pt. IV: 'Body Techniques'; see esp. p. 104.

18. On relic gestures, see Morris, *Manwatching*, 47–52.

19. As with Frank McCourt's father—'sucking the bad stuff out of Michael's head . . . that's what we did in Antrim long before there were doctors riding their horses' (Frank McCourt, *Angela's Ashes: A Memoir of a Childhood* (London: Flamingo, 1997), 112–13).

20. See M. D. Murray, 'Effects of Host Grooming on Louse Populations', *Parasitology Today*, 3/9 (1987), 276–9.

21. Francis Beckett interviewing Rosa Rust, 'Unsentimental Education', *Independent on Sunday Review*, 19 Mar. 1995, 2.

22. See Dunbar, *Grooming, Gossip, and the Evolution of Language, passim*; but see also id., *Primate Social Systems* (London: Croom Helm, 1988); W. G. Runciman, J. Maynard Smith, and R. Dunbar (eds.), *Evolution of Social Behaviour Patterns in Primates and Man* (Oxford: Oxford University Press, 1996); Frans de Waal (ed.), *Tree of Origin: What Primate Behaviour Can Tell Us About Human Social Evolution* (Cambridge, Mass.: Harvard University Press, 2001).

23. One female Tanzanian chimpanzee once gave a fascinating display of grooming and nursing care. As chief allo-groomer she particularly liked grooming teeth, laying the patient on his or her back, using the thumb to groom the upper teeth and the forefinger to groom the lower teeth, and using a twig for close work. These dental grooming bouts were exceptionally long-lasting, particularly for a young male losing his early molars; but she also regularly performed dental care during normal grooming sessions (W. C. McGrew and C. E. G. Tutin, 'Chimpanzee Tool Use in Dental Grooming', *Nature*, 24 (16 Feb. 1973), 477–8).

24. For an excellent short description of the Neolithic domestic healing context, see Guenter B. Risse, 'Medical Care', in W. F. Bynum and Roy Porter (eds.), *Companion Encyclopedia of the History of Medicine* (London: Routledge, 1993), esp. 'The Healing Framework', 47–51; see also the early anthropologist Daniel Mackenzie, *The Infancy of Medicine: An Enquiry into the Influence of Folk-Lore upon the Evolution of Medicine* (London: Macmillan, 1927). On food-gathering and the extra time provided by the 'grandmother revolution', see Richard Rudgley, *Secrets of the Stone Age* (London: Century, 2000).

25. Dunbar, *Grooming, Gossip, and the Evolution of Language*, 1. See also J. Sparks, 'Allo-Grooming in Primates: A Review', in D. Morris (ed.), *Primate Ethology* (London: Weidenfeld & Nicolson, 1967); C. Goosen, G. Mitchell, J. Erwin (eds.), *Social Grooming in Primates* (New York: Arliss, 1987).

26. Spruijt *et al.*, 'Ethology and Neurobiology of Grooming Behaviour', 830 and *passim*.

27. See generally Clive Ponting, *World History: A New Perspective* (London: Chatto & Windus, 2000); Andrew Sherratt, *Economy and Society in Prehistoric Europe: Changing Perspectives* (Edinburgh: Edinburgh University Press, 1997); Richard Rudgley, *Lost Civilisations of the Stone Age* (London: Century, 1998); Paul G. Bahn (ed.), *The Story of Archaeology* (London: Weidenfeld & Nicolson/Phoenix Illustrated, 1997).

28. See the classic text by Bernard Rudofsky, *Architecture without Architects: A Short Introduction to Non-Pedigreed Architecture* (1964; New York: Academy Editions, 1973), preface; see also contributions to the Sixth International Theriological Congress, 'Perspectives in Mammalian Environmental Physiology', Sydney, Australia, 1994, *Australian Journal of Zoology*, 24/1. The term 'habitus' was first used by the anthropologist Marcel Mauss, but was greatly extended by Pierre Bourdieu, *Outline of a Theory of Practice*, trans. Richard Nice (Cambridge: Cambridge University Press, 1977). The phrase 'customs, habits and manners' was commonly used by 18th-century ethnographers.

29. Robert Parker, *Miasma: Pollution and Purification in Early Greek Religion* (Oxford: Clarendon Press, 1983), 18 and *passim*. See also the range of psychologies discussed in Margaret Horsfield, *Biting the Dust: The Joys of Housework* (London: Fourth Estate, 1998).

30. T. Darvill and J. Hawes, *Neolithic Houses in North West Europe and Beyond* (Oxford: Oxbow, 1996); see also M. Parker Pearson and C. Richards (eds.), *Architecture and Order: Approaches to Social Space* (London: Routledge, 1994).

31. V. Gordon Childe, *Skara Brae* (Edinburgh: HMSO, 1983); see photographs in Bahn (ed.), *The Story of Archaeology*, 76–7.

32. The classic description of the 'string revolution' is Elizabeth Wayland Barber, *Women's Work: The First 20,000 Years. Women, Cloth, and Society in Early Times* (New York: Norton, 1994).

33. UK Association of Housebuilders, *Model Schedule of Works*, courtesy of Cityshape plc (London, 1997). The majority of references to

cleanliness on the Internet come from the industrial cleaning sector.

34. 'Cleanliness': *Oxford English Dictionary on Historical Principles* (Oxford: Clarendon Press, 1893), 475–9. The *OEDHP* contextual definitions (actually full of later 12th-century Middle English words) describe *clene* as 'clear—free from anything that dims lustre or transparency... Pure—undefiled, unsullied, free from dirt or filth, unstained, chaste, innocent... Fine—comely, neat, clever, trim, smart... Clear of obstruction or unevenness—clear, bare, void, clean-cut... Nothing left behind—complete, perfect, total, a clean sweep, get clean away...'. On *genus* words and those categorized as 'achievements of the imagination', see G. Lakoff, *Women, Fire and Dangerous Things* (Chicago: University of Chicago Press, 1987), 1–38; David Crystal, *The Cambridge Encyclopedia of the English Language* (Cambridge: Cambridge University Press, 1995), pt. I, ch. 3: 'Old English', 22–3 and *passim*; see also id., *Language Play* (London: Penguin, 1998).

35. See generally Uno Winblad and Wen Kilama, *Sanitation without Water* (Basingstoke: Macmillan, 1985), 1 and *passim*.

36. This particular *ger* is in the collection of tents held by the Horniman Museum of Natural History, Dulwich, London.

37. Quotation from a Berber woman in a refugee camp in the Sahara. Older refugees had built solidly sculpted mud huts, but with their original tent still pitched beside them—a sign of their eventual return to their homelands; see *Michael Palin in the Sahara*, BBC TV, 13 Oct. 2002; see also Michael Palin, *Sahara* (London: Weidenfeld & Nicolson, 2002).

38. The traditional 'Table of Opposites' used by the Greek Pythagoreans, and Aristotle, were left–right, female–male, below–above, back–front, cold–hot, wet–dry, heavy–light, dense–rare. See G. E. R. Lloyd, *Polarity and Analogy* (Cambridge: Cambridge University Press, 1966), 64–6; Jansheed K. Chosky, *Purity and Pollution in Zoroastrianism: Triumph over Evil* (Austin: University of Texas Press, 1989).

39. The full list of thirty-six demons is described in William R. Lafleur, 'Hungry Ghosts and Hungry People', in Michel Feher, Ramona Nadeff, Nadia Tazi, and E. Alliez (eds.), *Fragments for a History of the Human Body* (New York: Zone; Cambridge, Mass.: MIT Press, 1989), 270–303.

40. P. P. Jensen, 'Graded Holiness: A Key to the Priestly Conception of the World', *Journal for the Study of the Old Testament*, NT Supplement Series, 106 (1992), 80–2. Zoroastrianism was especially hylozoic (i.e. worshipping of matter): 'The use of water to wash away dirt and impurities, or to purify a polluted body, is regarded as a heinous sin, for through such action water is exposed to demonic impurities...The *Vendidad* states that anyone who pollutes water with carrion becomes ritually impure forever' (Chosky, *Purity and Pollution in Zoroastrianism*, 11–12; Mary Boyce, *Zoroastrianism: Their Beliefs and Practices* (London: Routledge & Kegan Paul, 1979)).

41. E. N. Fallaize, 'Purification (Introductory and Primitive)', quoting Pitt-Rivers, in J. Hastings (ed.), *The Encyclopaedia of Religion and Ethics* (Edinburgh: T. & T. Clark; New York: Charles Scribner's Sons, 1913), 455–66, 461. Mary Douglas thought that a comprehensive categorization of purity rules was 'utterly beyond the scope of objective scholarship...The formal ritual of public occasions teaches one set of doctrines. There is no reason to suppose that its message is necessarily consistent with those taught in private rituals, or that all public rituals are consistent with one another, nor all private rituals. There is no guarantee that the ritual is homogeneous...' (*Purity and Danger*, 166).

42. Douglas, *Purity and Danger*, 165.

43. Jacob Neusner, *The Idea of Purity in Ancient Judaism* (Leiden: E. J. Brill, 1973), 1.

44. Douglas, *Purity and Danger*, 176–9.

45. *Kumbh Mela: The Greatest Show on Earth*, Channel Four TV, 8–12 Jan. 2001.

46. Louis Dumont, *Homo Hierarchicus: The Caste System and its Implications* (1966; Chicago: Chicago University Press, 1981).

47. 'Purdah indicates that a family can do without the income of its women' (Santi Rozario, *Purity and Communal Boundaries: Women*

and *Social Change in a Bangladeshi Village* (London: Allen & Unwin, 1992), 94); see also Douglas, *Purity and Danger*, 140.

48. As described by a prince of the South African Xhosa, Nelson Mandela, in Nelson Mandela, *Long Walk to Freedom* (London: Little, Brown/Abacus, 1995), 30–6.

49. N. Soderblum, 'Holiness (General and Primitive)', in Mircea Eliade (ed.), *Encyclopedia of Religion* (London: Macmillan, 1987), 731, on the perceived 'absurdity' of total holiness, which also requires that there be profanity.

50. Mary Douglas, 'Purity and Danger: Leviticus—a Retrospective', seminar at Clare College, Cambridge, 21 Oct. 1997.

51. See Claudia Benthien, *Skin: On the Cultural Borderline between Self and the World*, trans. Thomas Dunlop (New York: Columbia University Press, 2002); Mark Lappé, *The Body's Edge: Our Cultural Obsession with Skin* (New York: H. Holt, 1996); Steven Connor, *The Book of Skin* (London: Reaktion, 2004).

52. M. Gompper and A. M. Hoylman, 'Grooming with Trattinnickia Resin: Possible Pharmaceutical Plant Use by Coatis in Panama', *Journal of Tropical Ecology*, 9 (1993), 533–7; see also Cindy Engel, *Wild Health* (London: Weidenfeld & Nicolson, 2002).

53. Leo Kanner, *The Folklore of the Teeth* (London: Macmillan, 1928).

54. Bruce M. Knauft, 'Bodily Images in Melanesia: Cultural Substances and Natural Metaphors', in Feher *et al.* (eds.), *Fragments for a History of the Human Body*, 253; Victoria Ebin, *The Body Decorated* (London: Thames & Hudson, 1979), 81. The main body parts were usually named earliest; see Stanley R. Witowski and Cecil H. Brown, 'Climate, Clothing, and Body-Part Nomenclature', *Ethnology*, 24/3 (1985), 197–214.

55. Karl Gröning, *Decorated Skin: A World Survey of Body Art*, trans. Lorna Dale (London: Thames & Hudson, 1997); see also Ebin, *The Body Decorated*, *passim*.

56. W. D. Hambley, *The History of Tattooing and its Significance: With Some Account of Other Forms of Corporal Marking* (London: H. F. & G. Witherby, 1925), 806–7 and *passim*. On Melanesian dress code, see Knauft, 'Bodily Images in Melanesia', 240.

57. Description of Dolní Věstonice by the historian Richard Rudgley in *The Secrets of the Stone Age*, Channel Four TV, 15 Dec. 2001; see also Rudgley, *Secrets of the Stone Age: A Prehistoric Journey* (London: Century, 2000), *passim*. Castelmerle in France had three main sites (Abri de la Souquette, Abri Castanet, and Abri Blanchard) where intensive bead-making was carried out *c*.35,000 BC.

58. John Hoffecker, 'Ice Age Art and Burials in Eastern Europe', in Bahn (ed.), *The Story of Archaeology*, 64–5.

59. Sherrat, *Economy and Society in Prehistoric Europe, passim*.

60. See e.g. Bahn (ed.), *The Story of Archaeology*, 156–7; and the archaeologist Natalya Polosmak in *Ice Mummies* (2), BBC TV, 30 Jan. 1997.

61. P. and J. Read (eds.), *Long Time, Olden Time: Aboriginal Accounts of Northern Territory History* (Alice Springs: Institute for Aboriginal Development Publications, 1991), 120, 145–6; Paul G. Bahn, 'Water Mythology and the Distribution of Paleolithic Parieta Art', *Proceedings of the Prehistoric Society*, 44 (1978), 125–34.

62. Alfred Martin, 'The Bath in Japan', *Ciba Symposia*, 1/5 (1939), 156–62 and *passim*.

63. See the 17th-century description of an Indian sweat-bath and river-sluice in G.R. [George Rosen], 'Early Observations on Sweatbaths', *CIBA Symposia*, 1/5 (1939), 163.

64. Herodotus, *The Histories*, trans. Aubrey de Sélincourt (London: Penguin, 1996), book IV, paras. 73–4, pp. 238–9. See also Richard Rudgley, *Essential Substances: A Cultural History of Intoxicants in Society* (London: British Museum Press, 1993).

65. Pietro Querini, quoted by Leslie Plommer, 'In Cod They Trust', *Guardian Weekend*, 25 Jan. 1997, 40–2.

66. One thinks especially of flood, wartime conditions—and rock festivals. For a general introduction to body sociology, see Chris Shilling, *The Body and Social Theory* (London: Sage, 1993), 12, 100–6; B. S. Turner, *Regulating Bodies: Essays in Medical Sociology* (London: Routledge, 1992).

Chapter 2 **The Cosmetic Toilette**

1. See generally Geoffrey Barraclough (ed.), *The Times Atlas of World History* (London: Times Books, 1979), *passim*; Clive Ponting, *A Green History of the World: The Environment and the Collapse of Great Civilisations* (London: Penguin, 1992), 295–314; id., *World History: A New Perspective* (London: Chatto & Windus, 2000), 109–37, 195.

2. The rough figure of a 10 per cent elite is an acceptable estimate for ancient societies (and seems remarkably modern), i.e. in the planned city of Ahkentaten, 7–9 per cent of the population was elite royal retinue; 40 per cent middle-rank craftsmen, tradesmen, and administrators; the remaining 50 per cent rural labourers and craftsmen. See Eugen Strouhal, *Life in Ancient Egypt* (Cambridge: Cambridge University Press, 1992), 67, recording the findings of Christian Tietze.

3. Louis Dumont, *Homo Hierarchicus: The Caste System and its Implications* (1966; London: Paladin, 1972), 106–7 and *passim*.

4. W. H. McNeill, *Plagues and Peoples* (London: Penguin, 1979), 64. Half a million bodies are required to keep measles in circulation in modern urban communities—the size of the capital of ancient Sumeria.

5. Herodotus, *The Histories*, trans. A. Selincourt (London: Penguin, 1972), 198.

6. Cynthia Wright Shelmerdine, *The Perfume Industry of Mycenan Pylos* (Göteborg: Astroms, 1985), 131–2.

7. Dioscorides, quoted in Lise Manniche, *An Ancient Egyptian Herbal* (Austin: University of Texas; London: British Museum Press), 51.

8. Maurizio Forte (ed.), *Virtual Archaeology: Great Discoveries Brought to Life through Virtual Reality* (London: Thames & Hudson, 1997), 75.

9. This cosmetic case is held in the British Museum. See also Alan Gardiner, *The Egyptians: An Introduction* (Oxford: Oxford University Press; London: Folio Society, 1962), 383–7; and J. R. Partington, *Origins and Development of Applied Chemistry* (London: Longmans, Green, 1935), 5–6, 143.

10. Partington, *Origins and Development of Applied Chemistry*, 135–43; Julia Samson, *Nefertiti and Cleopatra: Queen–Monarchs of Ancient Egypt* (London: Rubicon, 1985), cataloguer of the Armana Palace Collection. Washtub dowry sets recorded in Amy Tan, *The Kitchen God's Wife* (London: Fontana, 1992), 148.

11. Perishability is discussed in Michael Vickers and David Gill, *Artful Crafts: Ancient Greek Silverware and Pottery* (Oxford: Clarendon Press, 1994).

12. Moti Chandra, *Costumes, Textiles, Cosmetics and Coiffure in Ancient and Medieval India* (Delhi: Oriental Publishers, Indian Archaeological Society, 1973), 185.

13. Kunda B. Patkar and P. V. Bole, *Herbal Cosmetics in Ancient India: With a Treatise on Planta Cosmetica* (Mumbai: Bharatiya Vidya Bhavan, 1997), 45.

14. Crito, summarized in Florence E. Wall, 'Historical Development of the Cosmetic Industry', in Edward Sagarin (ed.), *Cosmetics, Science and Technology* (New York: Interscience Publishers, 1957), 11.

15. See generally H. S. F. Saggs, *The Babylonians: A Survey of the Ancient Civilisation of the Tigris–Euphrates Valley* (London: Folio Society, 1999); Ernst H. Kantorowicz, *The King's Two Bodies: A Study in Mediaeval Political Thought* (1957; Princeton: Princeton University Press, 1981), 3–5.

16. Philip Peter Jensen, 'Graded Holiness: A Key to the Priestly Conception of the World', *Journal for the Study of the Old Testament*, NT Supplement Series (Apr. 1992), 37 and *passim*.

17. Saggs, *The Babylonians*, 282, 283–4, 288–90.

18. Dimitri Meeks and Christine Faroud-Meeks, *Daily Life of the Egyptian Gods*, trans. G. M. Gasgherian (Ithaca, NY: Cornell University Press, 1997), 126–9.

19. *Shorter Oxford English Dictionary on Historical Principles* (Oxford: Oxford University Press, 1933), 401; on *ellu*, see E. Jan Wilson, *'Holiness' and 'Purity' in Mesopotamia* (Kevelaer: Butzon & Bercker, 1994), esp. ch. 2: 'Holy Objects', 67. *The Kama Sutra of Vatsyayana*, ed. Kenneth Walker, trans. Richard Burton and F. F. Arbuthnot

(London: Luxor Press, 1964), chs. 2 and 3; see also Alain Daniélou, *Kama Sutra: Le Breviare de l'amour. Traité d'érotisme de Vatsyayana*, trans. Alain Daniélou (Monaco: Éditions du Rocher/Jean-Paul Bertrand, 1992), 7–18.

20. Sagg, *The Babylonians*, 271–2; Jensen, 'Graded Holiness', 37 and *passim*; Bahn (ed.), *The Story of Archaeology*, 146.

21. Chandra, *Costumes, Textiles, Cosmetics and Coiffure in Ancient and Medieval India*, 207.

22. Ganges water is also held to behave, taste, and look unusually 'clean' (Eric Newby, *Slowly Down the Ganges* (London: Hodder & Stoughton, 1966), 212–18 and *passim*). Thanks to Dennis Herbstein for observations on contemporary ear-cleaning services.

23. Herodotus, *Histories*, 99.

24. A. M. Blackman, 'Purification (Egyptian)', in J. Hastings (ed.), *The Encyclopaedia of Religion and Ethics* (Edinburgh: T. & T. Clark; New York: Charles Scribner's Sons, 1913), 476–82.

25. Saggs, *The Babylonians*, 302.

26. Homer, *The Iliad*, trans. E. V. Rieu (London: Penguin, 1950), book 14, lines 261–2.

27. Homer, *The Odyssey*, trans. Walter Shewring (Oxford: Oxford University Press, 1998), 72. See also Jean-Pierre Vernant, 'Dim Body, Dazzling Body', in Michel Feher, Ramona Nadeff, Nadia Tazi, and E. Alliez (eds.), *Fragments for a History of the Human Body* (New York: Zone; Cambridge, Mass.: MIT Press, 1989), 30–1; on religious beauty contests, see Richard Hawley, 'The Dynamics of Beauty in Classical Greece', in Dominic Montserrat (ed.), *Changing Bodies, Changing Meanings: Studies on the Human Body in Antiquity* (London: Routledge, 1998), 37–9.

28. Alain Daniélou, *Shiva and Dionysus*, trans. K. F. Hurry (London: East/West, 1982).

29. Burgo Partridge, *A History of Orgies* (London: Spring Books, 1958), 19, 20–4.

30. Sagg, *The Babylonians*, 154; Sosso Logiadou-Platanos, *Knossos: The Palace of Minos. A Survey of the Minoan Civilisation*, trans. David

Hardy (Athens: private publication, 1999). It is suggested that the angle of drainage in the queen's suite was too shallow to be used for sewage, but does suggest a shower run-off.

31. Richard Hakluyt, *Voyages and Documents*, ed. Janet Hampden (Oxford: Oxford University Press, 1958), 88–9.

32. Homer, *Odyssey*, 19. 235.

33. Johan Huizinga, *Homo Ludens: A Study of the Play Element in Culture* (1944; London: Routledge & Kegan Paul, 1980).

34. Morris, *Manwatching: A Field Guide to Human Behaviour* (London: Jonathan Cape, 1977), 230–6; Camille Paglia, *Sexual Personae: Art and Decadence from Nefertiti to Emily Dickinson* (London: Penguin, 1991), 62–4.

35. Shelmerdine, *The Perfume Industry of Mycenan Pylos*, 129.

36. i.e. bear-grease or beef-fat; A. V. Lucas, 'Cosmetics, Perfumes, and Incense in Ancient Egypt', *Journal of Egyptian Archaeology*, 16 (1930), 41–53. It was also noted in the 17th century that 'the [wild] Irish have a custom of standing naked before the fire, and rubbing and as it were pickling themselves with old salt butter' (Francis Bacon, *Historia Vitae et Mortis*, book 3, vol. iv, in *The Collected Works of Francis Bacon*, ed. J. Spedding, R. Ellis, and D. Heath (London: Routledge/Thoemmes, 1996), 285.

37. Chandra, *Costumes, Textiles, Cosmetics and Coiffure in Ancient and Medieval India*, 211. A list of twenty-four rules of the toilette was laid down by the Vedic commentator Susruta sometime between 10 BC and AD 150; see ibid. 202–8.

38. A famous passage from the Roman author Diodorus Siculus on the physical appearance of the Celts, popularly quoted, as, for example, in J. Anthony Delmege, *Towards National Health; or, Health and Hygiene in England from Roman to Victorian Times* (London: Heinemann, 1931), 4.

39. *The Kama Sutra*, 14.

40. Chandra, *Costumes, Textiles, Cosmetics and Coiffure in Ancient and Medieval India*, 208.

41. Samson, *Nefertiti and Cleopatra*, 42. See also the less well-known but elegant tomb paintings of Queen Nefertari.

42. Elizabeth Wayland Barber, *Women's Work: The First 20,000 Years. Women, Cloth, and Society in Early Times* (New York: Norton, 1994), 130–1, 194, and *passim*.

43. Jack Goody, *The Culture of Flowers* (Cambridge: Cambridge University Press, 1993), 12, 18–19. See Chandra, *Costumes, Textiles, Cosmetics and Coiffure in Ancient and Medieval India*, 212, 223–5, in which at least 133 regional hairstyles are counted and illustrated.

44. Leslie P. Pierce, *The Imperial Harem: Women and Sovereignty in the Ottoman Empire* (Oxford: Oxford University Press, 1993), 5.

45. Hakluyt, *Voyages and Documents*, 80–1.

46. Lise Manniche, *Sexual Life in Ancient Egypt* (London: Kegan Paul International, 1987), 88.

47. *Kama Sutra*, 12, 62; see also John Jakob Meyer, *Sexual Life in Ancient India: A Study in the Comparative History of Indian Culture* (London: George Routledge & Sons, 1930), 269–72 and *passim*.

48. *Kama Sutra*, 161.

49. Public women and courtesans do not fit neatly into the status divisions historians have identified in the classical Greek period; see Sarah B. Pomeroy, *Goddesses, Whores, Wives and Slaves* (1975; London: Pimlico, 1994). The concept of the 'whore' in particular is anachronistic, since the word is linked to the Christian concept of sex as a sin; the word 'prostitute' also carries the same overtones of self-violation. On Cleopatra, see the excellent book by Lucy Hughes-Hallett, *Cleopatra: Histories, Dreams, Distortions* (London: Bloomsbury, 1990).

50. Norman Davies, *Europe: A History* (London: Pimlico, 1997), 90–4; J. M. Roberts, *History of the World* (London: Penguin, 1990), 98–9; Ponting, *A Green History of the World*, 71 and *passim*.

Chapter 3 **Greek Hygiene**

1. The current standard of living index is the Human Development Index, which measures longevity (sanitation and health services),

knowledge (education), and income (a certain standard of domestic life). See Sudhir Anand, *Human Development Index: Methodology and Measurement*, Human Development Report Office Occasional Papers, 12 (United Nations Development Programme, 1994). Public health impacts are notoriously difficult to assess, since all ancient-world demographic statistics are necessarily constructed from relatively slight evidence; but see Mirko Grmek, *Diseases in the Ancient Greek World*, trans. M. and L. Muellner (Baltimore: Johns Hopkins University Press), 91–2 and *passim*. See also Robin Osborne, *Greece in the Making, 1200–479 BC* (London: Routledge, 1996).

2. R. E. Wycherley, *How the Greeks Built Cities* (London: Macmillan, 1962), 198–204.

3. George Ryley Scott, *The Story of Baths and Bathing* (London: T. W. Lawrie, 1939), 30.

4. Serge Lancel, *Carthage: A History*, trans. A. Nevill (Oxford: Blackwell, 1995). On the Greek public fountains, and balneology, see René Ginouvès, *Balaneutikē: Recherches sur le bain dans l'antiquité grecque* (Paris: Éditions E. de Boccard, 1962).

5. Wycherley, *How the Greeks Built Cities*, 177; David M. Robinson and J. Walther Graham, *Excavations at Olynthus*, pt. VIII: *The Hellenic House: A Study of the Houses Found at Olynthus with a Detailed Account of those Excavated in 1931 and 1934* (Baltimore: Johns Hopkins University Press, 1938), 199–201.

6. Jean-Nicolas Corvisier, *Santé et société en Grèce ancienne* (Paris: Economica, 1985), 68–9.

7. Inge Nielson, *Thermae et Balnea* (Aarhus: Aarhus University Press, 1990), 7.

8. Henry E. Sigerist, 'Religious Medicine: Asclepius and his Cult', in Sigerist, *A History of Medicine*, ii: *Early Greek, Hindu, and Persian Medicine* (Oxford: Oxford University Press, 1961); for a modern study, see Robert Parker, *Miasma, Pollution and Purification in Early Greek Religion* (Oxford: Clarendon Press, 1996); and id., *Athenian Religion: A History* (Oxford: Clarendon Press, 1996), 175.

9. On temple baths, see Ginouvès, *Balaneutikē, passim*.

10. Parker, *Miasma, Pollution and Purification in Early Greek Religion*, 307.

11. Walter Burkert, *The Orientalising Revolution: Near Eastern Influence on Greek Culture in the Early Archaic Age* (Cambridge, Mass.: Harvard University Press, 1992); on fragmentation, Parker, *Miasma, Pollution and Purification in Early Greek Religion*, 210, 304–7.

12. Parker, *Miasma, Pollution and Purification in Early Greek Religion*, app. 2: 'The Cyrene Cathartic Law', 332–51, 335, 339.

13. Ibid. 322–3. The translation of the word 'honest' comes from 'to have *hosia*'.

14. See generally E. Norman Gardiner, *Athletics of the Ancient World* (Oxford: Clarendon Press, 1930); Mark Golden, *Sport and Society in Ancient Greece* (Cambridge: Cambridge University Press, 1998); David Sansone, *The Genesis of Sport* (Los Angeles: University of California Press, 1988).

15. See also Harold D. Evjen, 'The Origins and Functions of Formal Athletic Competition in the Ancient World', in William Coulson and Helmut Kyrileis (eds.), *Proceedings of an International Symposium on the Olympic Games, 5–9 September 1988* (Athens: Aohna, 1992); Roland Renson, Pierre Paul de Nay, and Michel Ostyn (eds.), *The History, the Evolution and Diffusion of Sports and Games of Different Cultures*, Proceedings of the International Association for the History of Physical Education and Sport, Apr. 1975 (Brussels, 1976).

16. Lucian, 'Anacharsis, or Athletics', in *Lucian*, trans. A. M. Harmon (London: Heinemann; New York: G. P. Putnam's Sons, 1925), iv. 11, 13–15, 19.

17. But girls and young women (in Sparta especially) did participate in public games. See Golden, *Sport and Society in Ancient Greece*, 128–9; Allen Guttmann, *Women's Sports: A History* (New York: Columbia University Press, 1991), 23–4. For Amazonian sports, see Lyn Webster Wilde, *On the Trail of the Women Warriors* (London: Constable, 1999).

18. Golden, *Sport and Society in Ancient Greece*, Olympic schedule table 2, p. 20.

19. Wycherley, *How the Greeks Built Cities*, 175–97, 143, ch. vi and *passim*.

20. Corvisier, *Santé et société en Grèce ancienne*, 54–5; Nielson, *Thermae et Balnea*, 1, 9–10.

21. Golden, *Sport and Society in Ancient Greece*, 65–9.

22. N. J. Richardson, 'Panhellenic Cults and Panhellenic Poets', in D. M. Lewis, John Boardman, J. K. Davies, and M. Ostwald (eds.), *The Cambridge Ancient History*, 2nd edn. (Cambridge: Cambridge University Press, 1992), v: *The Athletes: Background and Careers*, 232–6.

23. *The Dialogues of Plato*, v: *The Republic*, trans. Benjamin Jowett (London: Sphere Books, 1970), 175; Jacques Jouanna, *Hippocrates*, trans. M. B. DeBevoise (Baltimore: Johns Hopkins University Press, 1999), 166–7. See also G. E. R. Lloyd, *The Revolutions of Wisdom: Studies in the Claims and Practises of Ancient Greek Science* (Berkeley: University of California Press, 1987), 19–20; satirical comments by Philostratus on the art of gymnastics, in Robert Brophy and Mary O'Reilly Brophy, 'Medical Sports Fitness: An Ancient Parody of Greek Medicine', in K. A. Rabuzzi and R. W. Daley (eds.), *Literature and Medicine*, viii (Baltimore: Johns Hopkins University Press, 1989).

24. Lucian, 'Anacharsis, or Athletics', 3, 5, 7.

25. Golden, *Sport and Society in Ancient Greece*, 68.

26. The 2001 Australian cricket team had large dustbins of iced water provided after the game for all players when on tour—'some of us spend half an hour "in the bin", the body feels great after it'—and travel with a dietitian, masseur, psychologist, and coach. Interview in *The Ashes*, BBC TV, 15 Aug. 2001.

27. H. A. Harris, *Sport in Greece and Rome* (London: Thames & Hudson, 1972), 112–32; Gardiner, *Athletics of the Ancient World*, *passim*.

28. Grmek, *Diseases in the Ancient Greek World*, 92, 99; see generally Mark Nathan Cohen, *Health and the Rise of Civilisation* (New Haven: Yale University Press, 1989).

29. See G. E. R. Lloyd, 'The Hot and the Cold, the Dry and the Wet in Greek Philosophy', *Journal for Hellenic Studies*, 84 (1964), 92–106; Vivian Nutton, 'Humoralism' (1), in Bynum and Porter (eds.), *Companion Encyclopedia of the History of Medicine*, 283, 286.

30. Donald J. Harper, *Early Chinese Medical Literature: The Mawangdui Medical Manuscripts* (London: Kegan Paul International, 1998), 110–12 and *passim*. Recently discovered Mawangdui and Zhangjishan medical manuscripts from around 400–200 BCE found in aristocratic tombs at Hubei and Hunan in central north-eastern China revealed a body of macrobiotic hygiene literature that was 'far more extensive' than previously thought. I am indebted to Dr Vivienne Lo for this reference.

31. Jouanna, *Hippocrates*, 156–7; Kenneth G. Zysk, *Asceticism and Healing in Ancient India: Medicine in the Buddhist Monastery* (Oxford: Oxford University Press, 1991), 5–6. G. E. R. Lloyd discusses the crucial concept of 'semantic stretch' for words such as *katharsis*, *pharmaka*, *therapeia*, and *hygieia* in his *In the Grip of Disease: Studies in the Greek Imagination* (Oxford: Oxford University Press, 2003), 9–11 and *passim*.

32. See the classic description by L. J. Rather, 'The Six Non-Naturals: The Origins of a Doctrine and the Fate of a Phrase', *Clio Medica*, 3 (1968), 337–47; see also Harold J. Cook, 'Physical Methods', in Bynum and Porter (eds.), *Companion Encyclopedia of the History of Medicine*, 940.

33. 'A Regimen for Health', in *Hippocratic Writings*, ed. Lloyd, trans. J. Chadwick and W. N. Mann (London: Penguin, 1987), 272–6.

34. On temperance, see especially Aristotle, *Nicomachean Ethics*, ed. J. L. Ackrill and J. O. Urmson, trans. David Ross (Oxford: Oxford University Press, 1998), book 10 and *passim*.

35. *Hippocratic Writings*, Aphorisms, 211–12.

36. Ibid. 161. See also Andrew Shail and Gillian Howie (eds.), *Menstruation: A Cultural History* (Basingstoke: Palgrave Macmillan, 2005), esp. Luigi Arata, 'Menses in the Corpus Hippocraticum', and Monica H. Green, 'Flowers, Poisons and Men: Menstruation in Medieval Western Europe'.

37. For *miaino* (and all other Greek translations given here), see H. W. and F. G. Fowler (eds.), *The Concise Oxford Dictionary of Current English* (Oxford, 1964); see also 'Airs, Waters, Places', in *Hippocratic Writings*. On miasma, see Owsei Temkin, 'An Historical Analysis

of the Concept of Infection', in Temkin, *The Double Face of Janus, and Other Essays in the History of Medicine* (Baltimore: Johns Hopkins University Press, 1977); and more generally Margaret Pelling, 'Contagion/Germ Theory/Specificity', in Bynum and Porter (eds.), *Companion Encyclopedia of the History of Medicine.*

38. *Hippocratic Writings*, 168–9.

39. T. P. Wiseman, *Clio's Cosmetics: Three Studies in Greco-Roman Literature* (Leicester: Leicester University Press, 1979), 8.

40. Anne Carson, 'Putting her in her Place: Women, Dirt, and Desire', in D. Halperin, J. J. Winkler, and F. I. Zeitlin (eds.), *Before Sexuality: The Construction of the Erotic Experience in the Ancient Greek World* (Princeton: Princeton University Press, 1990), 154–5; Camille Paglia, *Sexual Personae: Art and Decadence from Nefertiti to Emily Dickinson* (London: Penguin, 1991), 6–28, 54–5; Helen King, *Hippocrates' Women: Reading the Female Body in Ancient Greece* (London: Routledge, 1998).

41. Plato, *Gorgias*, trans. Walter Hamilton (London: Penguin, 1981), 465 (pp. 46–7).

42. Hesiod, *Theogony and Works and Days*, ed. M. L. West (Oxford: Oxford University Press, 1988), pp. 52–3, lines 496–563.

43. Plato, *The Republic*, 401 (p. 169), 431 (p. 203).

Chapter 4 **Roman Baths**

1. More than matched by the 50 million living under the Han Empire in China between 206 BCE and AD 220 (Colin McEvedy and Richard Jones, *Atlas of World Population in History* (London: Penguin, 1978), 126 and *passim*); Mark Nathan Cohen, *Health and the Rise of Civilisation* (New Haven: Yale University Press, 1989), 140. See generally V. Hope and E. Marshall, *Death and Disease in the Ancient City* (London: Routledge, 2000).

2. E. M. Winslow, *A Libation to the Gods: The Story of Roman Aqueducts* (London: Hodder & Stoughton, 1963), 26–32 and *passim*; Ray

Laurence, *The Roads of Roman Italy: Mobility and Cultural Change* (London: Routledge, 1999), 1–10, 15–21; Inge Nielson, *Thermae et Balnea* (Aarhus: Aarhus University Press, 1990), 13.

3. O. F. Robinson, *Ancient Rome: City Planning and Administration* (London: Routledge, 1992), 47.

4. Quoted in Winslow, *A Libation to the Gods*, 7.

5. Jerome Carcopino, *Daily Life in Ancient Rome: The People and the City at the Height of the Empire*, trans. E. O. Lorimer (1941; London Penguin, 1991), 51.

6. Ibid. 52–4.

7. Nielson, *Thermae et Balnea*, 2; Richard Duncan-Jones, *Structure and Scale in the Roman Economy* (Cambridge: Cambridge University Press, 1990), 178–84; Garret G. Fagan, *Bathing in Public in the Roman World* (Ann Arbor: University of Michigan Press, 1999), 343, with an inscription from Serjilla, Syria, AD 473.

8. Garret G. Fagan, 'The Physical Environment: Splendor and Squalor', in Fagan, *Bathing in Public in the Roman World*.

9. Stephen Inwood, *A History of London* (London: Macmillan, 1998), 23–4.

10. Samuel S. Kottek, *Medicine and Hygiene in the Works of Flavius Josephus* (Leiden: E. J. Brill, 1994), 61–8; Stephen T. Newmeyer, 'Public Health in the Holy Land: Classical Influence and its Legacy', in Manfred Wiserman and Samuel S. Kottek (eds.), *Health and Disease in the Holy Land* (Lewiston, Me.: Edwin Mellen, 1996), 89.

11. On Baiae and the Campanian coast generally, see Fikret Yegül, *Baths and Bathing in Classical Antiquity* (New York: Architectural History Foundation; Cambridge, Mass.: MIT Press, 1992), 93–110; Nielson, *Balnae et Thermae*, 21–6; Ralph Jackson, 'Waters and Spas in the Classical World', in Roy Porter (ed.), *The Medical History of Waters and Spas*, Medical History Supplement 10 (London: Wellcome Institute for the History of Medicine, 1990).

12. Burgo Partridge, *A History of Orgies* (London: Spring Books, 1958), 67.

13. Jackson, 'Waters and Spas in the Classical World', 1–3.

14. Yegül, *Baths and Bathing in Classical Antiquity*, 93.

15. Partridge, *A History of Orgies*, 59.

16. Lucian, 'Hippias, or, The Bath', in *Lucian*, trans. A. M. Harmon (London: Heinemann; New York: G. P. Putnam's Sons, 1925).

17. Otto Kiefer, *Sexual Life in Ancient Rome* (1934; London: Constable, 1994); Seneca, Epistles 86 and 171.

18. See Fik Meijer and Otto van Nijf, *Trade, Transport and Society in the Ancient World: A Sourcebook* (London: Routledge, 1992).

19. Ovid, *Ars Amatoria*, book III, in *The Love Poems*, trans. A. D. Melville (Oxford: Oxford University Press, 1990), 131.

20. See generally A. J. Cooley, *The Toilet in Ancient and Modern Times* (London: Robert Hardwick, 1866); Carcopino, *Daily Life in Ancient Rome*, 161–90.

21. Ovid, *Ars Amatoria*, 129–30.

22. Only 100 lines of 'Cosmetics for Ladies' have survived; it breaks off abruptly after fifty lines of recipes. Ovid, *Love Poems*, 83–5.

23. Ibid. 84–5. Ovid's recipes did not come cheap: 'take two pounds of ground barley, 10 eggs, two ounces of ground antler horn, twelve narcissus bulbs, two ounces of gum and Tuscan seed. Mix with honey nine times that quantity... [for a cream for a fresh complexion] take incense, nitre, gum, myrrh, honey, fennel, rose petals, frankincense... then pour some barley-liquor on the lot.'

24. Ovid, *Ars Amatoria*, 129–32; 'Cosmetics for Ladies', 83. For an excellent fictional account of a pupil of Ovid, see the character Helena Justina in Lindsey Davis's Didius Falco detective series.

25. *Ars Amatoria*, 133–5.

26. Ibid. 100–1.

27. Carcopino, *Daily Life*, 179, 183, 138. 'The Maiden' was the Virgo Aqueduct.

28. Roy Porter, *The Greatest Benefit to Mankind: A Medical History of Humanity from Antiquity to the Present* (London: HarperCollins, 1997), 66–86; Harold J. Cook, 'Physical Methods', in W. F. Bynum

and Roy Porter (eds.), *Companion Encyclopedia of the History of Medicine* (London: Routledge, 1993), 942–5.

29. Celsus, *De Medicina*, trans. W. G. Spencer, 3 vols. (London: Heinemann; Cambridge, Mass.: Harvard University Press, 1935), i. 7. See also Elizabeth Rawson, 'The Life and Death of Asclepiades of Bythnia', *Classical Quarterly*, 32/2 (1982), 358–79; Vivian Nutton, *Ancient Medicine* (New York: Routledge; London: Taylor & Francis, 2004), ch. 13: 'Methodism'.

30. Rawson, *Life and Death*, 359–60, 7, 175.

31. See Henry Sigerist, *Landmarks in the History of Hygiene*, Heath Clark Lectures (London: Oxford University Press, 1956); and Ludwig Edelstein, 'The Methodists', in Owsei Temkin and C. Lilian Temkin (eds.), *Ancient Medicine: Selected Papers of Ludwig Edelstein* (Baltimore: Johns Hopkins University Press, 1987), 184 and *passim*.

32. Edelstein, 'The Dietetics of Antiquity', in Temkin and Temkin (eds.), *Ancient Medicine*, 308.

33. Celsus, *De Medicina*, 43, 45, Proemium, 41.

34. Galen, *Galen's Hygiene (De Sanitate Tuenda)*, trans. Robert Montraville Green (Springfield, Ill.: Charles C. Thomas, 1951); Porter, *The Greatest Benefit to Mankind*, 73; Cook, 'Physical Methods', 944–5.

35. See Heinrich von Staden, 'Body, Soul, Nerves: Epicurus, Herophilus, Erasistratus, the Stoics, and Galen', in John P. Wright and Paul Potter (eds.), *Psyche and Soma: Physicians and Metaphysicians on the Mind–Body Problem from Antiquity to Enlightenment* (Oxford: Clarendon Press, 2000), 80, 106–7, 110, and *passim*. The tag *mens sana in corpore sano* is found in Juvenal, *Satires*, 10. 356.

36. Galen, *Hygiene*, 47. See also L. J. Rather, ' "The Six Things Non-Natural": A Note on the Origins and Fate of a Doctrine and a Phrase', *Clio Medica*, 3 (1968), 337–47; Peter H. Niebyl, 'The Non-Naturals', *Bulletin of the History of Medicine*, 45 (1971), 486–92; Nutton, 'Humoralism', in Bynum and Porter (eds.), *Companion Encyclopedia of the History of Medicine*, 289.

37. Galen, *Hygiene*, 12, 5.

38. Ibid. 57–8. The difficulty of transmitting practical skills was only one reason for the overall decline of massage therapy in western Europe after the fall of Rome, though it survived elsewhere in Eurasia (India, the Middle East).

39. Peter Brown, *The Making of Late Antiquity* (Cambridge, Mass.: Harvard University Press, 1978), 2–8; Norman Davies, *Europe: A History* (London: Pimlico, 1997), 210–14 and *passim*.

40. Winslow, *A Libation to the Gods*, 56–7, 36. See generally Nielson, *Thermae et Balnea*; Yegül, *Baths and Bathing in Classical Antiquity*.

41. Yegül, *Baths and Bathing in Classical Antiquity*, 317–29.

Chapter 5 **Asceticism**

1. See generally Michel Foucault, *The History of Sexuality*, i: *An Introduction*, ii: *The Use of Pleasure*, iii: *The Care of the Self*, trans. Robert Hurley (London: Penguin, 1986); on *askesis*, ii. 72–7. See also generally Peter Brown, *The Making of Late Antiquity* (Cambridge, Mass.: Harvard University Press, 1978), and id., 'Asceticism: Pagan and Christian', in Averil Cameron and Peter Garnsey (eds.), *The Cambridge Ancient History*, xiii: *The Late Empire, AD 337–425* (Cambridge: Cambridge University Press, 1998).

2. William James, *The Varieties of Religious Experience*, ed. Martin E. Marty (London: Penguin, 1985), 392–9.

3. Ilana Friedrich Silber, *Virtuosity, Charisma and Social Order* (Cambridge: Cambridge University Press, 1995), 80–6, 211–22.

4. Jean Levi, 'The Body: The Daoists' Coat of Arms', in Michel Feher, Ramona Nadeff, Nadia Tazi, and E. Alliez (eds.), *Fragments for a History of the Human Body* (New York: Zone; Cambridge, Mass.: MIT Press, 1989), pt. iii, pp. 114–17. See also the comments of Marcel Mauss, *Sociology and Psychology Essays*, trans. Ben Brewster (1950; London: Routledge & Kegan Paul, 1979), 122; and the sociological studies of his friend the religious historian Marcel Granet, *The Religion of the Chinese People*, trans. Maurice Freedman (1922; Oxford: Blackwell, 1975). See also Francesca Bray, 'Chinese Medicine', in

W. F. Bynum and Roy Porter (eds.), *Companion Encyclopedia of the History of Medicine*, 2 vols. (London: Routledge, 1993), i. 728–54; Philip S. Rawson, 'The Body in Tantra', in J. Benthall and T. Polhemus (eds.), *The Body as a Medium of Expression* (London: Penguin/Allen Lane, 1975).

5. Marcus Aurelius, *Meditations*, trans. Maxwell Staniforth (London: Penguin, 1964), 93; see also Michel Foucault, *Technologies of the Self: A Seminar with Michel Foucault*, ed. L. H. Martin, H. Gutman, and P. H. Hutton (London: Tavistock, 1988), 22–30.

6. Arnobius, *The Case against the Pagans*, trans. George E. McCracken (Westminster, Md.: Newmans; London: Longmans Green, 1949), *Attack on Philosophy: The Mortality of the Soul*, book ii, paras. 4 and 10, pp. 116–17, 121–2.

7. See Brown, *The Making of Late Antiquity*, 7–9; Jacob Neusner, *Judaism, Christianity and Zoroastrianism in Talmudic Babylon* (Lanham, Md.: University Press of America,1986), p. x; W. T. Whitley, 'Sects (Christian)', in J. Hastings (ed.), *The Encyclopaedia of Religion and Ethics* (Edinburgh: T. & T. Clark; New York: Charles Scribner's Sons, 1913); see also Henry Wace and William Coleman Piercy, *A Dictionary of Christian Biography and Literature to the End of the Sixth Century AD; with an Account of the Principal Sects and Heresies* (London: John Murray, 1911). The sectarian history of these regions is extraordinarily dense; among the Judaic Christian sects alone, main groups included the Gnostics, Manichaeans, Nazarenes, Copts, Nestorians, and Ebionites, with smaller groups of Marcosians, Monarchians, Melchizedekites, Montanites, and Novationists.

8. Luke 5: 12–39; Ezekiel 36: 25–6.

9. Amos 5: 10–23, 6: 1–6.

10. Jacob Neusner, 'The Idea of Purification in Ancient Judaism', Haskell Lectures 1972–3, with a critique by Mary Douglas, repr. in Neusner, *Studies in Judaism in Late Antiquity from the First to the Seventh Century*, i (Leiden: E. J. Brill, 1973), 535, 7; Peter Brown, *Body and Society: Men, Women, and Sexual Renunciation in Early Christianity* (New York: Columbia University Press, 1988), 35–6.

11. Leviticus 19: 27–8, 21: 5.

12. Isaiah 3: 16–24.

13. The belief that their martyred prophet had been miraculously revived from the dead, and deified, has been described as a 'stunning suspension of the inflexible laws of the normal', especially in an era when the sciences were apparently so dominant; see Brown, *Body and Society*, 38–9, 44. Celsus, for example, roundly attacked Christianity for its belief in miracles; see the line-by-line rebuttal of this (lost) work in Origen, *Contra Celsum*, trans. H. Chadwick (Cambridge: Cambridge University Press, 1953), 31 and *passim*.

14. Lloyd P. Gerson (ed.), *The Cambridge Companion to Plotinus* (Cambridge: Cambridge University Press, 1996); J. A. M. Guckin, 'Christian Asceticism and the Early School of Alexandria', in W. J. Shiels (ed.), *Monks, Hermits and the Ascetic Tradition* (Oxford: Ecclesiastical History Society/Blackwell, 1985), 30–1.

15. St Augustine, *Confessions*, trans. R. S. Pine-Coffin (London: Penguin, 1961), book vi, pp. 129–30 and *passim*. See also Henry Chadwick, *Augustine: A Very Short Introduction* (Oxford: Oxford University Press, 1986), 17–26; Peter Brown, *Augustine of Hippo* (London: Faber & Faber, 1967); Brown, 'Asceticism', 602, 605–8, 614. Augustine died quoting Plotinus.

16. St Athanasius, 'On Sickness and Health', in David Brakke, *Athanasius and the Politics of Asceticism* (Oxford: Clarendon Press, 1995), 310–11, app. D. See also Michael Williams, 'Divine Image—Prison of Flesh: Perceptions of the Body in Ancient Gnosticism', in M. Feher *et al.* (eds.), *Fragments for a History of the Human Body*, 128–47.

17. Elizabeth Abbott, *A History of Celibacy* (Cambridge: Lutterworth Press, 2001), 104–5. The verdict of Edward Gibbon, that they were 'horrid and disgusting', has remained; but though their skin was unwashed, since they ate and drank very little, their evacuations were probably not very great.

18. Caroline Walker Bynum, 'The Female Body and Religious Practice in the Late Middle Ages', in Feher *et al.* (eds.), *Fragments for a History of the Human Body*, 162–3; Brown, *Body and Society*, 441–2.

19. Including the so-called 'libertine sects'; see Henry C. Lea, *A History of Sacerdotal Celibacy*, 2 vols. (London: Williams & Norgate, 1907), i. 20–1.

20. Abbott, *A History of Celibacy*, 102–4.

21. On the 'democracy' of asceticism, see Brown, 'Asceticism', 614 and *passim*; as far as I know, he does not address anarchism.

22. Ibid. 616 and *passim*.

23. Colin Spencer, *The Heretics Feast: A History of Vegetarianism* (London: Fourth Estate, 1993), 128–9.

24. See St Athanasius, 'Second Letter to Virgins', in Brakke, *Athanasius and the Politics of Asceticism*, app. B, p. 299; Lea, *A History of Sacerdotal Celibacy*, 56. See also Joyce E. Salisbury, *Church Fathers, Independent Virgins* (London: Verso, 1991); Elizabeth Schussler Fiorenza, *In Memory of Her: A Feminist Theological Reconstruction of Christian Origins* (Oxford: Oxford University Press, 1992).

25. St Ambrose, *Concerning Virginity*, in Henry Wace and Philip Schaff (eds.), *A Select Library of Nicene and Post-Nicene Fathers of the Christian Church: A New Series*, 14 vols. (Oxford: Parker, 1890–1900), vol. x, book I, ch. VII, pp. 32, 39. The easiest way to access this text is via the Catholic site <http:// www.newadvent.org/fathers/34071.htm>. See also Mary Laven, *Virgins of Venice: Enclosed Lives and Broken Vows in the Renaissance Convent* (London: Penguin, 2002).

26. St Jerome, Letter 45, in Wace and Schaff (eds.), *A Select Library of Nicene and Post-Nicene Fathers of the Christian Church*, vi. 3–5, <http://newadvent.org/fathers/3001.htm>.

27. Ambrose, *Concerning Virginity*, book III, chs. II–III, <http://newadvent.org/fathers/34073.htm>; id., *On the Duties of the Clergy*, book I, ch. XVIII, <http://newadvent.org/fathers/34011.htm>; Brakke, *Athanasius and the Politics of Asceticism*, app. B, p. 294.

28. Ambrose, *Concerning Virginity*, book I, pp. 37, 39.

29. Abbott, *A History of Celibacy*, 96; Brown, *Body and Society*, 157–8.

30. Augustine's statement of his washing habits in *De Sermone Domini in Monte* is noted by Henry Chadwick, 'The Ascetic Ideal in the

History of the Church', in Shiels (ed.), *Monks, Hermits, and the Ascetic Tradition*, 16 n. 70; Brown, *Body and Society*, 283–4.

31. Ambrose, *Duties of the Clergy*, 77–80; Exodus 28: 42.

32. Jerome, see esp. Letters 45 and 125; see also J. N. D. Kelley, *Jerome: His Life, Writings and Controversies* (London: Duckworth, 1975).

33. St Athanasius, 'Dangers of the Public Bath', in 'Second Letter to Virgins', 297–8.

34. William Popper, 'Purification (Muslem)', in Hastings (ed.), *The Encyclopaedia of Religion and Ethics*, 497.

35. On Olympias, see Brown, *Body and Society*, 283; Porter, *The Greatest Benefit to Mankind*, 88–91; Dorothy Porter, *Health, Civilisation and the State: A History of Public Health from Ancient to Modern Times* (London: Routledge, 1999), 20–3; Ralph Jackson, *Doctors and Diseases in the Roman Empire* (London: British Museum Press, 1988), 133–6; on local hospitals in Egypt, see Peter von Minnen, 'Medical Care in Late Antiquity', in P. J. van der Eijk, H. F. Horstmanhoff, and P. H. Schrijvers (eds.), *Ancient Medicine in its Socio-Cultural Context*, i (Amsterdam: Rodopi, 1995).

36. The Christian Church 'had become, in effect, an institution possessed of the ethereal secret of perpetual self-reproduction', and as such was an entirely new type of public institution (Brown, *Body and Society*, 120–1). See also Richard Fletcher, *The Conversion of Europe: From Paganism to Christianity, 371–1386 AD* (London: HarperCollins, 1997).

Chapter 6 **Medieval Morals**

1. See generally Fernand Braudel, *Civilisation and Capitalism, 15th–18th Century*, 3 vols., trans. Sian Reynolds (London: Collins, 1981–4), i: *The Structures of Everyday Life*; Raffaella Sarti, *Europe at Home: Family and Material Culture 1500–1800* (New Haven: Yale University Press, 2002). The celebrated twenty-seven volumes of Alfred Franklin, *La Vie privée d'autrefois: Arts, métiers, mode, mœurs, usage des parisiens du XIIe au XVIIIe siècle* (Paris: Plon, 1887–1902) have

recently been superseded by Philippe Ariès and George Duby (eds.), *A History of Private Life*, i–v (Cambridge, Mass.: Belknap Press, 1987–94).

2. Einhard and Notker the Stammerer, *Two Lives of Charlemagne*, trans. Lewis Thorpe (London: Penguin, 1969), 133, 77; Henry Maguire (ed.), *Byzantine Court Culture from 829 to 1204* (Washington, DC: Dumbarton Oaks, 1997).

3. M. A. Manzalaoui (ed.), *Secretum Secretorum: Nine English Versions* (Oxford: Oxford University Press, 1977), introd. and 'Regimen Sanitatis: The Booke of Good Governance and Guyding of the Body', 3–9 and *passim*. See generally C. Stephen Jaeger, *The Origins of Courtliness: Civilising Trends and the Formation of Courtly Ideals* (Philadelphia: University of Pennsylvania Press, 1985), 113–75, 179, and *passim*; Aldo Scaglione, *Knights at Court: Courtliness, Chivalry, and Courtesy from Ottonian Germany to the Italian Renaissance* (Berkeley: University of California Press, 1991).

4. As for example in the many editions of Hugh Rhodes's *The Book of Nurture for Menservants and Children (with Stans puer ad mensam)* (London: Abraham Veale, 1550?). See generally Norbert Elias, *The Civilising Process: Sociogenetic and Psychogenetic Investigations*, trans. Edmund Jephcott (1939; Oxford: Blackwell, 2000), pt. 2 and *passim*.

5. Sarti, *Europe at Home*, 151.

6. Notker the Stammerer, *Two Lives of Charlemagne*, introd., 30, 131.

7. See Notker, 'Shaving the Devil', in Notker, *Two Lives of Charlemagne*: 'The bishop who broke the Lenten fast and then made penance by washing the poor, including the Devil' (introd., 30, 115–17).

8. John Julius Norwich, *The Normans in Sicily: The Normans in the South 1016–1130 and, The Kingdom in the Sun 1130–1194* (London: Penguin, 1992), 464, 599–602, 765–7.

9. Francois Boucher, *A History of Costume in the West*, trans. John Ross (London: Thames & Hudson, 1987), 171–6; David Jacoby, 'Silk in Western Byzantium before the Fourth Crusade', report VII, in Jacoby, *Trade, Commodities, and Shipping in the Medieval*

Mediterranean (Aldershot: Variorum, 1997), 462; Norwich, *The Normans in Sicily*, 492.

10. On bards, see John Mathews (ed.), *The Bardic Source Book: International Legacy and Teachings of the Ancient Celts* (London: Blandford, 1988), esp. 26–42; Daniel Corkery, 'The Bardic Schools', see also David Crystal (ed.), *The Cambridge Encyclopedia of the English Language* (Cambridge: Cambridge University Press, 1995), 34–9.

11. *The Owl and the Nightingale: Cleanness. St Erkenwald*, trans. Brian Stone (London: Penguin, 1977), 77–8, 84, 100.

12. French tapestry *La Dame à licorne* embroidered at the end of 15th century, now at the Musée des Thermes, Paris. See Georges Vigarello, *Concepts of Cleanliness: Changing Attitudes in France since the Middle Ages*, trans. Jean Birrell (Cambridge: Cambridge University Press/Éditions de la Maison des Sciences de l'Homme, 1988), 28; Wilhelm Rudeck, *Geschichte der Öffentlichen Sittlichkeit in Deutschland* (Jena, 1897; Berlin: H. Barsdorf, 1905), 12–13; believed trans. as the *History of Public Morality in Germany* (Jena, 1906) (no copies found). I am very grateful to Hedi Stadlen for translating the German used here.

13. Sir Nicholas Harris Nicholas, *History of the Orders of Knighthood of the British Empire*, 3 vols. (London: William Pickering & John Rodwell, 1842), iii. 5–7, 11–15; John Anstis, *Observations Introductory to an Historical Essay upon the Knighthood of the Bath* (London, 1725). The ceremonial sequence is painted in full in a medieval Garter Book reproduced in Anthony Wagner, Nicolas Barker, and Ann Payne (eds.), *Medieval Pageant: Writhe's Garter Book: The Ceremony of the Bath and the Earldom of Salisbury Roll* (London: Roxburghe Club/Quaritch, 1997). Actual bathing ceased in 1815, when the mature officers of Waterloo were made companions en masse, and was not revived (personal communication, Garter Herald at Arms).

14. Francis Packard, 'Note on the History of the School of Salerno', in Humphrey Mitford (ed.), *The School of Salernum: Regimen Sanitatis Salernitanum* (London: Humphrey Mitford, 1922), 14–15; Fielding H. Garrison, 'The History of the *Regimen Sanitatis*', ibid. 56–7. On Salerno hydraulics, see *The Trotula: An English Translation of the*

Medical Compendium of Women's Medicine, ed. and trans. Monica Green (Philadelphia: University of Pennsylvania Press, 2001), 6 and nn. 18, 19; also Paulo Squatriti, *Water and Society in Early Medieval Italy, AD 400–1000* (Cambridge: Cambridge University Press, 1998).

15. Porter, *The Greatest Benefit to Mankind*, 106–9. In the 1840s medical historians reported that there was nothing left in the town of Salerno—no remains, no library, and only one doctor, who did not even own a copy of the Salerno Regimen (Mitford (ed.), *The School of Salernum*, 39–40).

16. Macbeath, *Regimen Sanitatis*, trans. H. Cameron Gillies (Glasgow: Robert Maclehose, 1911), col. IX, pp. 38–9; Luis García-Ballester, Roger French, Jon Arrizabalaga, and Andrew Cunningham, *Practical Medicine from Salerno to the Black Death* (Cambridge: Cambridge University Press, 1994), 1–29, 274. See generally Miriam Usher Chapman, *Lay Culture, Learned Culture: Books and Social Change in Strasbourg, 1480–1599* (New Haven: Yale University Press, 1982); Michael McVaugh and Nancy G. Siraisi (eds.), *Renaissance Medical Learning: Evolution of a Tradition* (Philadelphia: University of Pennsylvania Press, 1990).

17. *Aristotle's Secrets* was still going strong in the 18th century: see Roy Porter, ' "The Secrets of Generation Display'd": Aristotle's Masterpiece in Eighteenth-Century England', in R. P. Maccubbin (ed.), *'Tis Nature's Fault': Unauthorised Sexuality during the Enlightenment* (Cambridge: Cambridge University Press, 1987), 7–21; Mary E. Fissell, 'Making a Masterpiece: The Aristotle Texts in Vernacular Medical Culture', in Charles E. Rosenberg (ed.), *Right Living: An Anglo-American Tradition of Self-Help Medicine* (Baltimore: Johns Hopkins University Press, 2003).

18. Nicholas Orme, *From Childhood to Chivalry: The Education of the English Kings and Aristocracy 1066–1530* (London: Methuen, 1984), 88–90 and *passim*. A Vienna tacuinum thought to be of Arabic origin, reproduced with tacuinums from Liège, Paris, and Rouen, in Luisa Cogliati Arano, *The Medieval Health Handbook: Tacuinum Sanitatis* (London: Barrie & Jenkins; New York: George Braziller, 1976), fo. 4.

19. Mitford (ed.), *The School of Salernum*, 78. On *iocunditas, hilaritas*, and *affabilitas*, see Jaeger, *The Origins of Courtliness*, 116–18.

20. Garrison, 'The History of the *Regimen Sanitatis*', 60–1. For plague regimens, see Jon Arrizabalaga, 'Facing the Black Death: Perceptions and Reactions of University Medical Practitioners', in García-Ballester *et al.*, *Practical Medicine from Salerno to the Black Death*.

21. Glenn Hardingham, 'The *Regimen Sanitatis* in Late Medieval England', unpub., Cambridge, 2003; I am grateful for his assistance, and English regimens are starting to be surveyed. But see Paul Slack, 'Mirrors of Health and Treasures of Poor Men: The Use of Vernacular Medical Literature in Tudor England', in Charles Webster (ed.), *Health, Medicine and Mortality in the 16th Century* (Cambridge: Cambridge University Press, 1979); see also Virginia Smith, 'Cleanliness: The Development of Idea and Practice in Britain, 1770–1850', Ph.D. thesis, University of London, 1985.

22. W. G. Hoskins, *The Making of the English Landscape* (London: Penguin, 1978); Montague Fordham, *The Rebuilding of Rural England* (London: Hutchinson, 1924); Christopher Dyer, *Everyday Life in Medieval England* (London: Hambledon, 1994), 139, 165; Anthony Emery, *Greater Medieval Houses of England and Wales, 1300–1500*, i (Cambridge: Cambridge University Press, 1996).

23. Guest latrines in Sir Roger Vaughan's improved hall-house at Tretower, Wales, in 1450 (C. A. Raleigh Radford and David M. Robinson (eds.), *Tretower Court and Castle* (Cardiff: Welsh Historic Monuments, 1986), 10). Edward III's two plumbed palaces were Westminster and King's Langley; my thanks to Dr Ian Mortimer for this reference from his forthcoming book *The Perfect King: The Life of Edward III*, ch. 12. See also Lawrence Wright, *Clean and Decent: The History of the Bath and Loo* (London: Routledge & Kegan Paul, 1980), 35–8.

24. A detailed survey of London legislation and practice can be seen in Mark Jenner, 'Early Modern English Conceptions of "Cleanness" and "Dirt" as Reflected in the Environmental Regulation of London', D.Phil. thesis, Oxford University, 1991. On urban water provision generally, see Squatriti, *Water and Society in Early Medieval*

Italy, 16; Roberta J. Magnusson, *Water Technology in the Middle Ages: Cities, Monasteries and Waterworks after the Roman Empire* (Baltimore: Johns Hopkins University Press, 2001), 18–24, 33; and a classic study of water technology by André Guillerme, *Les Temps de l'eau: La Cité, l'eau et les techniques. Nord de la France. Fin IIIe— début XIXe siècle* (Paris: Éditions du Champ Vallon/Presses Universitaires de France, 1983).

25. Wright, *Clean and Decent*, 28–30; Mark Girouard, *Life in the French Country House* (London: Cassell, 2000), 52; on furniture history and changing attitudes to body space, see also the classic work by Sigfried Giedon, *Mechanisation Takes Command: A Contribution to Anonymous History* (Oxford: Oxford University Press, 1948), 266 and *passim*.

26. Braudel, *Civilisation and Capitalism*, 285–90.

27. Christine de Pizan, *The Treasure of the City of Ladies, or, The Book of the Three Virtues*, trans. Sarah Lawson (London: Penguin, 1985), 148.

28. Boucher, *A History of Costume in the West*, 145–222; Françoise Piponnier and Perrine Mane, *Dress in the Middle Ages*, trans. Caroline Beamish (New Haven: Yale University Press, 1997), 22–3, 40–4, 99–102; Elias, *The Civilising Process*, 138–9.

29. Vigarello, *Concepts of Cleanliness*, 41; Emmanuel Le Roy Ladurie, *Montaillou: Cathars and Catholics in a French Village 1294–1324* (London: Penguin, 1980), 141.

30. *[The Noble Lyfe and Nature of Man, of Bestes, Serpentys, Fowles and Fissches ...] An Early English Version of Hortus Sanitatis ... 1521*, ed. Noel Hudson (London: Quaritch, 1954), 65; Françoise Piponnier, 'The World of Women', in Christiane Klapisch-Zuber (ed.), *A History of Women in the West*, ii: *Silences of the Middle Ages* (Cambridge, Mass.: Harvard University Press, 1994), 330; Eileen Power, 'The Menagier's Wife', in Power, *Medieval People* (1924; London: Folio Society, 1999), 127.

31. *The Trotula*, 54–5, 60–1, and *passim*; *Women's Secrets: A Translation of Pseudo-Albertus Magnus's 'De Secretis Mulierum' with Commentaries*, ed. and trans. Helen Rodnite Lemay (Albany: State University of New York Press, 1992), *passim*; Lynette R. Muir, *Literature and Society in Medieval France: The Mirror and the Image 1100–1500*

(London: Macmillan, 1985), 128; Montserrat Cabré, 'Cosmetics in the Middle Ages', unpub., Wellcome Unit, Cambridge, Feb. 1992.

32. See the survey of early cosmetic literature in Florence E. Wall, 'Historical Development of the Cosmetic Industry', in Edward Sagarin (ed.), *Cosmetics, Science and Technology* (New York: Interscience Publishers, 1957), 19–26 and *passim*.

33. Monica H. Green, 'The Possibilities of Literacy and the Limits of Reading: Women and the Gendering of Medical Literacy', Essay VII in Green, *Women's Healthcare in the Medieval West: Text and Contexts* (Aldershot: Ashgate, 2000).

34. 'Book on the Conditions of Women', in *The Trotula*, 73.

35. Ibid. 185 nn. 174–5; the full, uncut passage reproduced in Alexandra Barratt, *Women's Writing in Middle English* (London: Longman, 1992).

36. 'On Treatments for Women', in *The Trotula*, 91, 142.

37. Ibid. 99, 171–3.

38. Leslie G. Matthews, *The Royal Apothecaries*, Wellcome Historical Medical Library, NS 13 (London, 1967), 18–19; Aytoun Ellis, *The Essence of Beauty: A History of Perfume and Cosmetics* (London: Secker & Warburg, 1960), 11.

39. 'On Treatments for Women', 205; 'On Women's Cosmetics', 113–14. The reference to 'steambaths beyond the Alps' comes from the uncut version in Barratt, *Women's Writing in Middle English*.

40. Wall, 'Origins and Development', 27.

41. Green, 'The Possibilities of Literacy and the Limits of Reading', 36 and *passim*; see also Montserrat Cabré, 'From a Master to a Laywoman: A Feminine Manual of Self-Help', *Dynamis: Acta Hisp. Med. Sci. Hist. Illus.* (2000), 20: 391 n. 56.

42. Luis García-Ballester, Michael R. McVaugh, and Agustín Rubio-Vela, 'Medical Licensing and Learning in Fourteenth Century Valencia', *Transactions of the American Philosophical Society*, 79/6 (1989), 36–8 n. 13. On 16th-century figures, see Margaret Pelling, 'Appearance and Reality: Barber–Surgeons, the Body, and Disease

in Early Modern London', in L. Beier and R. Finlay (eds.), *London 1500–1700: The Making of the Metropolis* (London: Longman, 1986).

43. García-Ballester *et al.*, 'Medical Licensing and Learning in Fourteenth-Century Valencia', 30–3.

44. Carlo Ginzburg, *The Cheese and the Worms: The Cosmos of a Sixteenth-Century Miller*, trans. John and Anne Tedeschi (London: Routledge & Kegan Paul, 1981), 83.

45. Rudeck, *Geschichte der Öffentlichen Sittlichkeit in Deutschland*, 28–9, 9; Vigarello, *Concepts of Cleanliness*, 30.

46. Mikkel Aaland, *Sweat: The Illustrated History and Description of the Finnish Sauna, Russian Bania, Islamic Hammam, Japanese Mushiburo, Mexican Temescal and American-Indian and Eskimo Sweatlodge* (Santa Barbara, Calif.: Capra, 1978), 60.

47. There are many illustrations in Rudeck, *Geschichte der Öffentlichen Sittlichkeit in Deutschland*; and in Mitford (ed.), *The School of Salernum*; but see the larger collection in Alfred Martin, *Deutsches Badewesen in Vergangenen Tagen. Nebst einem Beiträge zur Geschichte der deutschen Wasserheilkunde* (Jena, 1906).

48. Paul B. du Chaillu, *The Land of the Midnight Sun: Journeys through Sweden, Norway, Lapland, and Northern Finland, 1882*, quoted in Wilhelm Paul Gerhard, *Modern Baths and Bathhouses* (New York: Wiley, 1908), ch. xvii, pp. 288–92.

49. Rudeck, *Geschichte der Öffentlichen Sittlichkeit in Deutschland*, 5, quoted from Guarinonius, *Die Grewel der Verwustung* (1610). See also the many German bath-books noted in Miriam Usher Chapman, *Lay Culture, Learned Culture: Books and Social Change in Strasbourg, 1480–1599* (New Haven: Yale University Press, 1982), 105.

50. Alfred Martin, 'The Bath in Japan', *Ciba Symposia*, 1/5 (1939), 135 and *passim*.

51. Pizan, *The Treasure of the City of Ladies*, 154.

52. George Ryley Scott, *The Story of Baths and Bathing* (London: T. Werner Lawrie, 1939), 77–80.

53. Henry Card, *The Reign of Charlemagne: Considered Chiefly with Reference to Religion, Laws and Literature and Manners* (London: Longman, Hurst, Rees, and Orme, 1807), 54.

54. Aaland, *Sweat*, 61–2.

55. Malcolm Letts, *Bruges and its Past* (London: A. G. Berry, 1924), quoted in Elspeth Morris (ed.), *The Dorothy Dunnett Companion* (London: Michael Joseph, 1994), 191–2 (illustrating the dramatized canal journey in Dunnett's novel *Niccolo Rising*).

56. Vigarello, *Concepts of Cleanliness*, 30, 24.

57. Francis Gagens, *Wiesbaden: Its Hot Springs, and their Efficacy and Application*, trans. Christian William Kreidel (Wiesbaden, 1851), 3–6; B. Fricker, *The Swiss Thermal Watering Places* ([1881?]), no page number.

58. Arano, 'Spring', in *Tacuinum Sanitatis*, Paris, fo. 103.

59. Elias, *The Civilising Process*, 178–9; Vigarello, *Concepts of Cleanliness*, 23–5; Jacques Rossiaud, *Medieval Prostitution*, trans. Lydia G. Cochrane (Oxford: Blackwell, 1988), ch. 8 and *passim*.

60. Rudeck, *Tractatus de Cursu Mundi* (1397), in Rudeck, *Geschichte der Öffentlichen Sittlichkeit in Deutschland*, 16–21.

61. Ibid. 22; the illustration is from Breslau.

62. Rossiaud, *Medieval Prostitution*, 5.

63. Margaret Wade Labarge, *Women in Medieval Life* (London: Hamilton, 1986), 199–201; J. B. Post, 'A Fifteenth-Century Customary of the Southwark Stews', *Journal of the Society of Archivists*, 5 (1976), 422–8.

64. The picture on the cover of Vigarello, *Concepts of Cleanliness*, and often shown elsewhere.

65. Vigarello, *Concepts of Cleanliness*, 27; Johannes Fabricius, *Syphilis in Shakespeare's England* (London: Jessica Kingsley, 1994), 81–3.

66. Rudeck, *Geschichte der Öffentlichen Sittlichkeit in Deutschland*, 39.

67. Vigarello, *Concepts of Cleanliness*, 9–11, 32–4; Rossiaud, *Medieval Prostitution*, chs. 7, 9, and *passim*. Both downplay syphilis in favour of plague.

68. Claude Quétel, *History of Syphilis*, trans. Judith Braddock and Brian Pike (London: Polity Press, 1990), 70.

69. Ibid. 13, 33.

70. Fabricius, *Syphilis in Shakespeare's England*, 25; Quétel, *History of Syphilis*, 71, 66.

71. Quétel, *History of Syphilis*, 17, 18, 27, 281.

72. Pelling, 'Appearance and Reality', 7, 196, and *passim*; Fabricius, *Syphilis in Shakespeare's England*, 72–7.

73. Fabricius, *Syphilis in Shakespeare's England*, 81, 110. See also Kevin P. Siena, *Venereal Disease, Hospitals and the Urban Poor: London's 'Foul Wards', 1600–1800* (Rochester, NY: Woodbridge, University of Rochester Press, 2004).

74. George Cross, 'Celibacy (Christian)', in Hastings (ed.), *The Encyclopaedia of Religion and Ethics*, 271–5.

Chapter 7 **Protestant Regimens**

1. Sir Francis Bacon, *Historia Vitae et Mortis*, in *Collected Works of Francis Bacon*, 12 vols., ed. J. Spedding, R. Ellis, and D. D. Heath (London: Routledge/Thoemmes, 1996), v. 215.

2. Erasmus, 'Antibarbari', in *The Collected Works of Erasmus*, i: *Literary and Educational Writings*, ed. Craig Thompson (Toronto: University of Toronto Press, 1978), 23–4. Peter Burke, 'Without Spot or Stain: Rituals of Purification in Early Modern Europe', seminar, Cambridge, Oct. 1997, highlighted the phenomenon of the political purge; see also Patrick Collinson, 'Ecclesiastial Vitriol: Religious Satire in the 1590s and the Invention of Puritanism', in John Guy (ed.), *The Reign of Elizabeth I: Court and Culture in the Last Decade* (Cambridge: Cambridge University Press, 1995). Erasmus himself supported a late medieval Catholic reform movement known as the Devotio Moderna, a Franciscan ascetic revival promoting personal piety, repentance, and active discipleship that gave rise to the influential Brethren of Common Life. He later refused to endorse Luther, or to join the Protestant

cause (Kenneth Ronald Davis, *Anabaptism and Asceticism: A Study in Intellectual Origins* (Scottdale, Pa.: Herald, 1974), 62 and *passim*).

3. Roy Porter, *Enlightenment: Britain and the Creation of the Modern World* (London: Allen Lane, 2000), 54–60; id., *Flesh in the Age of Reason: The Modern Foundations of Body and Soul* (London: W. W. Norton, 2004).

4. See generally Fernand Braudel, *Civilisation and Capitalism, 15th–18th Century*, i: *The Structures of Everyday Life*, trans. Sian Reynolds (London: Collins, 1981), *passim*; see the chapter 'Superfluity and Sufficiency: Houses, Clothes, and Fashion', in Roy Porter and John Brewer (eds.), *Consumption and the World of Goods* (London: Routledge, 1993); Lorna Wetherill, *Consumer Behaviour and Material Culture in Britain, 1660–1760* (London: Routledge, 1988); Lisa Jardine, *Worldly Goods: A New History of the Renaissance* (London: Macmillan, 1996).

5. Paulo Squatriti, *Water and Society in Early Medieval Italy, AD 400–1000* (Cambridge: Cambridge University Press, 1998); Roberta J. Magnusson, *Water Technology in the Middle Ages: Cities, Monasteries and Waterworks after the Roman Empire* (Baltimore: Johns Hopkins University Press, 2001), 31.

6. Robert J. Knecht, 'Francis I and Fontainebleau', *Court Historian*, 42 (Aug. 1999), 101. One of the most famous bath paintings of the School of Fontainebleau is the enigmatic *Gabrielle d'Estrées and One of her Sisters*; see generally the illustrations in Françoise de Bonneville, *The Book of the Bath*, trans. Jane Brenton (London: Thames & Hudson, 1998), 78 and *passim*.

7. Documents of the Great House of Easement, and Henry VIII's bathing facilities generally, still rest in the archives. Some details can be found in Simon Thurley, *Royal Palaces of Tudor England: Architecture and Court Life* (New Haven: Yale University Press, 1993). I am indebted to Dr Joanna Marschner and Dr Jonathan Foyle for information on recent finds at Hampton Court Palace.

8. Baldesar Castiglione, *The Book of the Courtier*, ed. George Bull (London: Penguin, 1967), 13. Castiglione was translated into English in 1561, and popularized in Sir Thomas Elyot's schoolroom book *The Gouvernor*, from 1564. On conduct books, see Anna Bryson, *From*

Courtesy to Civility: Changing Codes of Conduct in Early Modern England (Oxford: Clarendon Press, 1998). For a classic statement on the psychology of intimacy, see Lawrence Stone, 'The Growth of Affective Individualism', in Stone, *The Family, Sex, and Marriage in England, 1500–1800* (London: Penguin, 1979).

9. See the descriptions in J. E. Neale, *Queen Elizabeth I* (1934; London: Penguin, 1960), 216–20; more recently, see David Starkey, *Elizabeth: Apprenticeship* (London: Chatto & Windus, 2000).

10. Susan Watkins, *In Public and in Private: Elizabeth I and her World* (London: Thames & Hudson, 1998), 59–63; see also Simon Thurley, *Whitehall Palace: An Architectural History of the Royal Apartments, 1240–1698* (New Haven: Yale University Press, 1999).

11. There is a large historical literature on childbirth; for more unusual visual representations, see Jacqueline Marie Mosocchio, *The Art and Ritual of Childbirth in Renaissance Italy* (New Haven: Yale University Press, 1999).

12. Neville Williams, *Powder and Paint: A History of the Englishwoman's Toilet, Elizabeth I–Elizabeth II* (London: Longmans, Green, 1957), 6–7; Margaret Pelling, 'Trimming, Shaping and Dyeing: Barbers and the Presentation of Self in Early Modern London', seminar, Social History Society, Jan. 1993, 7. See generally Margaret Pelling, 'Appearance and Reality: Barber–Surgeons, the Body, and Disease in Early Modern London', in L. Beier and R. Finlay (eds.), *London 1500–1700: The Making of the Metropolis* (London: Longman, 1986); ead., 'Occupational Diversity: Barbersurgeons and the Trades of Norwich, 1550–1640', *Bulletin of the History of Medicine*, 56 (1982), 484–511.

13. Johannes Fabricius, *Syphilis in Shakespeare's England* (London: Jessica Kingsley, 1994), 167–8; Sara F. Matthews Grieco, 'The Body, Appearance, and Sexuality', in Natalie Zemon Davies and Arlette Farge (eds.), *A History of Women*, iii: *Renaissance and Enlightenment Paradoxes* (Cambridge, Mass.: Belknap Press, 1993), 55–63; Michael Walzer, *The Revolution of the Saints: A Study in the Origins of Radical Politics* (London: Weidenfeld & Nicolson, 1966), 254.

14. Williams, *Powder and Paint*, 14, 46–7. Soap-smuggling dominated parliamentary reports on soap until 1852, when the tax was abolished. On the tax on 'necessities' as precursor to income tax, see W. Kennedy, *English Taxation, 1640–1799: An Essay on Policy and Opinion* (London: G. Bell, 1913), 83 and *passim*; see also Virginia Smith, 'Soap', unpub., 1985.

15. Georges Vigarello, *Concepts of Cleanliness: Changing Attitudes in France since the Middle Ages*, trans. Jean Birrell (Cambridge: Cambridge University Press/Éditions de la Maison des Sciences de l'Homme, 1988), 62–9, 78, 60.

16. De Bonneville, *The Book of the Bath*, 84–5 and *passim*.

17. Vigarello, *Concepts of Cleanliness*, 16, 69.

18. Margaret Spufford, *The Great Reclothing of Rural England: Petty Chapmen and their Wares in the Seventeenth Century* (London: Hambledon, 1984), 112–13; Vigarello, *Concepts of Cleanliness*, 71–2; Raffaella Sarti, *Europe at Home: Family and Material Culture 1500–1800* (New Haven: Yale University Press, 2002), 196–201.

19. See Gregory King's scheme, among others, in Peter Laslett, *The World We Have Lost* (London: Methuen, 1965), 32–3 and *passim*; see also Peter Earle, *The Making of the English Middle Classes: Business, Society and Family Life in London, 1660–1730* (London: Methuen, 1989), 80–1; David Underdown, *Revel, Riot and Rebellion: Popular Politics and Culture in England 1603–1660* (Oxford: Oxford University Press, 1987), 20, 24–8.

20. Earle, *The Making of the English Middle Classes*, 14–15 and *passim*; see also Lorna Weatherill, *Consumer Behaviour and Material Culture in Britain, 1660–1760* (London: Routledge, 1988).

21. On the English evidence of 'disorder' in towns of this period, see Peter Clark and Paul Slack (eds.), *Crisis and Order in English Towns 1500–1700* (London: Routledge & Kegan Paul, 1972); Anthony Fletcher and John Stevenson, *Order and Disorder in Early Modern England* (Cambridge: Cambridge University Press, 1985); Norman Davies, *The Isles: A History* (London: Macmillan, 2000), 386.

22. For example, the Anabaptist sects of the lower Rhine valley, the Mennonites, were proselytized by English Quakers (who also maintained contacts with the German Pietists), and later settled in America on land given by the Quaker William Penn. See John L. Ruth, *Maintaining the Right Fellowship: A Narrative Account of the Oldest Mennonite Community in North America* (Scottdale, Pa.: Herald, 1984).

23. Walzer, *The Revolution of the Saints*, x. 254–5. Pepys served as an officer of the Navy Board, which had acquired discipline under Cromwell; see Claire Tomalin, *Samuel Pepys: The Unequalled Self* (London: Penguin, 2002), 111–18, 139–48, and *passim*.

24. Thomas Hall, *The Beauty of Holinesse . . . or a Description of the Excellency, Amiableness, Comfort, and Content which is to be Found in the Ways of Purity and Holiness* (London, 1653), 93.

25. Daniel Defoe, *A Journal of the Plague Year* (1722; London: Dent Dutton, 1966), 17–19; see also Paul Slack, *The Impact of Plague in Tudor and Stuart England* (London: Routledge & Kegan Paul, 1985), 23–5, 242–3.

26. Andrew Wear, *Knowledge and Practice in English Medicine, 1550–1680* (Cambridge: Cambridge University Press, 2001), 41. See also Miriam Usher Chrisman, *Lay Culture, Learned Culture: Books and Social Change in Strasbourg, 1480–1599* (New Haven: Yale University Press, 1982), 170–1, and accompanying volume *Bibliography of Strasbourg Imprints, 1480–1599*, esp. pie charts S.1, 2, and 3, pp. 229–50 for full outputs; H. S. Bennett, *English Books and Readers, 1475 to 1557, 1558 to 1603*, 2 vols. (Cambridge: Cambridge University Press, 1970). English market figures estimated by Paul Slack, 'Mirrors of Health and Treasures of Poor Men: The Use of Vernacular Medical Literature in Tudor England', in Charles Webster (ed.), *Health, Medicine and Mortality in the 16th Century* (Cambridge: Cambridge University Press, 1979).

27. [Humphrey] Lloyd, *The Treasuri of Helth contayning Many Profitable Medicines, gathered out of Hippocrats, Galen and Avicen by one Petrus Hyspanus and translated into English by Humfre Lloyd* (London, [c.1556]), introd., no page numbers.

28. Thomas Moulton, *The Myrrour or Glasse of Helth* (London, n.d. [1545?]), no page numbers; Vigarello, *Concepts of Cleanliness*, 9–15.

29. Thomas Elyot, 'The Proheme', in Elyot, *The Castel of Helth corrected, & in some places augmented, by the first author* (1539; London, 1541), no page number; with editions almost every decade in the second half of the century. See also Thomas Cooper, *Bibliotheca Eliotae* (London, 1548–52).

30. See the Stuart monarchy's policy in their *Book of Sports* (London: J. Baker, 1633), issued by James I in 1618 and enacted in 1633. See also Nicolas Orme, *Early British Swimming, 55 BC–AD 1719* (Exeter: University of Exeter Press, 1983), 64 and *passim*; Wear, *Knowledge and Practice in English Medicine*, 160–1.

31. Elyot, *Castel of Helth* (1539), 51–2, 49–50, 53.

32. Leonard Lessius, *Hygiasticon: or, The Right Course of Preserving Life and Health unto Extream Old Age* (London, 1636), 13, 201–2; see also Gerald G. Gruman, 'Ideas about the Prolongation of Life', *American Philosophical Society*, 56 (1966), 68–73 and *passim*. The word 'health' rather than 'hygiene' was preferred in Britain, up until the late 19th century.

33. Sanctorius Sanctorius (Santorio), *Medicina Statica: or, Rules of Health, in eight sections of aphorisms. English'd by J.D.* (1614; London, 1676); see also J. Mackenzie, *The History of Health, and the Art of Preserving It, etc.* (Edinburgh: W. Gordon, 1758), chs. xv–xvii. On mechanical Methodism, see Walter Pagel, 'Religious Motives in the Medical Biology of the XVIIth Century', *Bulletin for the History of Medicine*, 3/4 (1935), 272, describing Robert Fludd on expansion and contraction as the key explanation of the world.

34. E. T. Renbourne, 'The Natural History of Insensible Perspiration: A Forgotten Doctrine of Health and Disease', *Medical History* (1960), 4: 135–52. A surprising number of Sanctorean-style diary records are turning up from the 17th and 18th centuries; see also the urine-measuring efforts of 17th-century spa-goer Michel Montaigne, famously recorded in his *Travel Diary*, for example in E. S. Turner, *Taking the Cure* (London: Michael Joseph, 1967), 35–7; and Michel

Jaltel, *La Santé par les eaux: 2000 ans de thermalisme* (Orléans: L'Instant Durable, 1983), 28–9.

35. Thomas Junta, *De Balneis Omnia quae extant apud Graecos, Latinos et Arabas... In quo Aquarium et Thermarium Omnium* (Venice, 1553).

36. William Turner, *A Book of the Natures and Properties as well as of the Bathes in England as of Other Bathes in Germanye and Italye* (1562; Collen: Arnold Birkman, 1568), 97–8. Mixed bathing was also the custom at the warm springs in Buxton, described by John Jones in *The Bathes of Bathes Ayde: Wonderful and Most Excellent against Manie Sicknesses* (London, 1572). On the subsequent rise of English bath-books, see Charles F. Mullett, 'Public Baths and Health in England, 16th–18th Century', *Bulletin for the History of Medicine*, suppl. 5 (1946), 56–80.

37. Patrick Madan, *A Philosophical and Medicinal Essay of the Waters of Tunbridge* (London, 1687), quoted in Turner, *Taking the Cure*, 45 and *passim*.

38. Rudeck, *Geschichte der Öffentlichen Sittlichkeit in Deutschland*, 35–9. The regulations mostly forbade naked bathing and segregated men and women, and were still in force for schoolchildren in the 1930s, according to Hedi Stadlen (private communication). See also de Bonneville, *The Book of the Bath*, 40–1.

39. If there had been anything in Britain like the mainland European urban bathing culture, we would have discovered at least some hard evidence of it by now. *Tittle-Tattle* (1603), a well-known picture satirizing the idleness and gossip of women AT THE CHILDBED, AT THE CONDUITE, WASHERS AT THE RIVER, and AT THE HOTTE-HOUSE, was probably taken from a reused Dutch printing-block; repr. in Philippa Pullar, *Consuming Passions: A History of English Food and Appetite* (London: Penguin, 2001). C. J. S. Thompson, 'Bagnios and Cuppers', in Thompson, *The Quacks of Old London* (London: Brentano's, 1928), 263–75; Lawrence Wright, *Clean and Decent: The History of the Bath and Loo* (London: Routledge & Kegan Paul, 1980), 64.

40. *The Autobiography of Francis Place*, ed. M. Thale (Cambridge: Cambridge University Press, 1972), 213–14. Place went on to refurbish

his bathhouse lodgings, cheerfully ripping out 'the very old pan-
elled wainscoating' and marble slabs to get rooms that were 'all
modern, all neat and good in a very plain stile', and triumphantly
installing 'a capital water-closet on the first floor'.

41. Peter Chamberlen, *A Vindication of Publick Artificial Bathes and Bath-
stoves* (London, 1648); id., *To the Honourable Committee for Bathes
and Bath-Stoves: A Paper* (London, 1648), 2, 5 (Royal College of
Physicians Collection, London).

42. *The Christian Householder* (London, 1607), 8.

43. Simon Schama, *The Embarrassment of Riches: An Interpretation of
Dutch Culture in the Golden Age* (London: Fontana, 1991), 375–400
and *passim*. See also Hannah Wooley, *The Accomplish'd Ladies
Delight, in Preserving, Physick, Beautifying and Cookery* (London,
1675); and more generally Caroline Davidson, *A Woman's Work Is
Never Done: A History of Housework in the British Isles 1650–1950*
(London: Chatto & Windus, 1986), 115–20.

44. J. A. Comenius [Jan Amos Komenský], *The School of Infancy: An
Essay on the Education of Youth, during their First Six Years* (London,
1633), 15–16, 52–3.

45. John Woolman, *The Journal of John Woolman*, in William James,
The Varieties of Religious Experience, ed. Martin E. Marty (London:
Penguin, 1985), 294–6: while observing cloth-dyeing, it raised 'a
longing in my mind that people might come into cleanness of
spirit, cleanness of person, and cleanness about their houses and
garments'. See generally on collars, cuffs, and lace, Vigarello, *Concepts of Cleanliness*, 69–72 and *passim*.

46. Edward Topsell, *The Reward of Religion* (London, 1596); Philip
Stubbes, *An Anatomie of Abuses: Containing a Discoverie and Brief
Summary of Such Noble Vices and Imperfections as now Raigne in Many
Countries of the World* (London, 1583). See also Keith Thomas,
'Cleanliness and Godliness in Early Modern England', in Anthony
Fletcher and Peter Roberts (eds.), *Religion, Culture and Society in
Early Modern Britain: Essays in Honour of Patrick Collinson* (Cam-
bridge: Cambridge University Press, 1994), 62–3.

47. George Herbert, 'The Church-Porch', LXII, in *The English Works of George Herbert*, ed. G. H. Palmer, 3 vols. (London: Hodder & Stoughton, 1905), ii. 214.

48. William Bullein, *The Government of Health* (London, 1558), 24.

49. Thomas Hall, *Loathsomeness of Long Hair... with an appendix against Painting, Spots, Naked Breasts, etc.* (London, 1654), 24–49 and *passim*. Francis Bacon acknowledged the legitimacy of cosmetics as a branch of health: 'The good of man's body is of four kinds: health, beauty, strength, and pleasure. So the knowledges are, medicine, or the art of cure; the art of decoration, which is called cosmetic; the art of activity, which is called athletic; and art voluptuary, which Tacitus truly calleth "Eruditas luxus"' (*On Life and Death*, repr. in Sir John Sinclair, *The Code of Health and Longevity*, 4 vols. (Edinburgh, 1807), iv. 258–9, 267).

50. J. A. Comenius, *Janua Linguarum Reserata* ('The Gates of Language Unlocked'), trans. Thos. Horne and J. Rowbotham, 6th edn. (London, 1643), ch. 53: 'Of Bathing and Cleanliness'; Arthur Dent, *The Plain Man's Pathway to Heaven* (1590; London, 1831), 41–4.

51. Stubbes, *An Anatomie of Abuses*, 32–3, 40–1; Hall, *The Beauty of Holinesse*, 3, 90–1.

52. Christopher Hill, *The World Turned Upside Down: Radical Ideas during the English Revolution* (London: Penguin, 1972), 155–9.

53. See G. Winstanley, *The Law of Freedom in a Platform: or, True Magistracy Restored* (London: for the author, 1652), and, for example, the empiric practitioner and disciple William Westmacott, *Historia Vegetabilium Sacra: or, A Scriptural Herbal* (London: T. Salusbury, 1694), cited by Peter Krivatsy, 'William Westmacott's Memorabilia: The Education of a Puritan Country Physician', *Bulletin for the History of Medicine*, 49 (1975), 331–8; see also Margaret Pelling, 'Knowledge Common and Acquired: The Education of Unlicensed Medical Practitioners in Early Modern London', in V. Nutton and R. Porter (eds.), *The History of Medical Education in Britain* (Amsterdam: Rodopi, 1995).

54. Hill, *The World Turned Upside Down*, 145–50, 317–18. The heresies of Anabaptists and others are described in J. Taylor, *A Swarme of*

Sectaries and Schismatiques (London, 1641); see also Charles Webster, *The Great Instauration: Science, Medicine and Reform 1626–1660*
(London: Peter Lang, 2002), p. xxiii and *passim*.

55. Sir John Floyer, *An Enquiry into the Right Use and Abuse of Hot, Cold,
and Temperate Baths in England* (London, 1697), preface.

56. Keith Thomas, *Man and the Natural World: Changing Attitudes in
England 1500–1800* (London: Penguin, 1984), 289–92; Stubbes, *An
Anatomie of Abuses*, 59–60; Tristram Stuart, *The Bloodless Revolution:
Radical Vegetarians and the Discovery of India* (London: HarperCol-
lins, 2006), 15–59 and *passim*.

57. *The English Hermite, or, Wonder of this Age: Being a Relation of the Life
of Roger Crab* (London, 1655), no page numbers.

58. Katherine Gillespie, *Domesticity and Dissent in the Seventeenth Century* (Cambridge: Cambridge University Press, 2004), 182–3, 203–5;
Jane Shaw, 'Religious Experience and the Formation of the Early
Enlightenment Self', in Roy Porter (ed.), *Rewriting the Self: Histories
from the Renaissance to the Present* (London: Routledge, 1997), 65–7.

59. Thomas Taylor 'the Platonist' was a Cambridge usher and secretary
who dedicated his life to translating Plato; see W. E. Axon, *Thomas
Taylor the Platonist: A Biographical and Bibliographical Sketch* (London, 1890); Henry More, *The Immortality of the Soul, So Farre Forth
as is Demonstrable from the Knowledge of Nature and the Light of
Reason* (London, 1659), 258; Richard Ward, *The Life of the Learned
and Pious Henry More* (London, 1710), 229–30. The British Library
copy of More's *Opera Omnia, the Theological Works of H. More, etc.*
(London, 1708), Preface General: 'Temper of Body and Mind', has
MS notes by S. T. Coleridge. See also Virginia Smith, 'Physical
Puritanism and Sanitary Science: Material and Immaterial Beliefs
in Popular Physiology, 1650–1840', in W. F. Bynum and Roy Porter
(eds.), *Medical Fringe and Medical Orthodoxy, 1750–1850* (London:
Croom Helm, 1987).

60. Thomas Tryon, *A Treatise of Cleanness in Meats and Drinks…
Good Airs…Clean Sweet Beds* (London, 1682), 14. Tryon was later
described as 'one of the most extraordinary self-taught geniuses,
and original writers, that ever existed in this country, particularly

on the subjects of health and temperance, to which all his writings allude': Sinclair, *The Code of Health and Longevity*, ii. 297, including a complete list of Tryon's works 'some of which are very scarce', notably T. Tryon, *A Discourse of Waters, shewing the particular virtues, wonderful operations, and various uses, both in food and physic, the all-wise Creator hath endued this cleansing element with* (n.d.). See also Ginnie Smith, 'Thomas Tryon's Regimen for Women: Sectarian Health in the Seventeenth Century', in London Feminist History Group (ed.), *The Sexual Dynamics of History: Men's Power, Women's Resistance* (London: Pluto, 1983), 56; Stuart, *The Bloodless Revolution*, 60–77.

61. T. Tryon, *Wisdom's Dictates, or, Aphorisms and Rules for Preserving Health of Body, and Peace of Mind* (London, 1696), 67, 71–3.

62. T. Tryon, *Pythagoras his Mystick Philosophy Reviv'd; or, The Mystery of Dreams Unfolded* (London, 1691), 243, 246–7.

63. Aphra Behn's poem on Tryonism, handwritten on a flyleaf of Thomas Tryon's *The Way to Health, Long Life, and Happiness* (London, 1683), was published in *Miscellany, Being a Collection of Poems by Several Hands. Together with Reflections on Morality* (London, 1685); see Maureen Duffy, *The Passionate Shepherdess* (London, 1977). Hill, *The World Turned Upside Down*, 411, notes G. Woodcock, *The Incomparable Aphra* (New York: T. V. Boardman, 1948), aligning her with the Quakers and Diggers. Biographical details in T. Tryon, *Knowledge of a Man's Self, or, The Surest Guide to the True Worship of God, and Good Government of Mind and Body, or the second part of the way to long life, health and happiness, with portrait* (London, 1704), 131; see also Smith, 'Thomas Tryon's Regimen for Women: Sectarian Health in the Seventeenth Century', *passim*.

64. William Vaughan, *Approved Directions for Health* (1600; London, 1612), 3–4; Thomas Willis, *A Plaine and Easie Method for Preserving those that are Well from the Infection of the Plague, or any Contagious Distemper in City, Camp, Fleet, etc. . . . written in the year 1666* (London, 1692), no page numbers. See also J.E. Esq [John Evelyn], *Fumifugium: or, The Inconvenience of the Aer and Smoak of London*

Dissipated. Together with Some Remedies Humbly Proposed (London, 1661), preface and *passim*.

65. *The Whole Works of that Excellent Practical Physician, Dr Thomas Sydenham*, ed. John Pechey (London, 1696), 183–4; first pub. as *Observationes Medicae* (London, 1676), with emendations by John Locke; see G. G. Meynell, 'John Locke and the Preface to Thomas Sydenham's *Observationes Medicae*', *Medical History*, 1/50 (1 Jan. 2006), 93–110.

66. *The Whole Works of Sydenham*, 174, 180–1.

67. Tryon, *A Treatise of Cleanness in Meats and Drinks*, 1–16.

68. John Hancocke, *Febrifugium Magnum* (London, 1723–4), 5.

69. Sir John Floyer, *The History of Cold Bathing: Both Ancient and Modern* (London, 1706), A5, 133–4.

70. Royal Commission on the Historical Monuments of England, *An Inventory of the Historical Monuments of the City of Cambridge*, pt. 1 (London: HMSO, 1959), 37, 71; I am indebted to Rodney Smith for this reference. On the (unexcavated) Moor Barns Bath next to Aristotle's Well, see Roger Deakin, *Waterlog: A Swimmer's Journey through Britain* (London, 1999), 48–52.

71. Floyer, *An Enquiry into the Right Use and Abuse of Hot, Cold, and Temperate Baths in England*, 54–5; see also Joseph Brown, *An Account of the Wonderful Cures Performed by Cold Baths. With Advice to Water Drinkers at Tunbridge, Hampstead, Astrope, Nasborough and All Other Chalibeate Spaws . . . To which is prefixed a letter from Sir John Floyer* (London, 1707).

72. Richard Mead, *A Short Discourse concerning Pestilential Contagion*, 5th edn. (London, 1720), 46–8, 38.

73. John Locke, *Some Thoughts concerning Education* (1693; London, 1800), 13–14.

74. John Locke, *An Enquiry concerning Human Understanding* (1706), ed. John W. Yolton (London: Dent, 1977), 175 n. 176, and introd., pp. xii–xv; *The Educational Writings of John Locke*, ed. James L. Axtell (Cambridge: Cambridge University Press, 1968), 341, letter to

Edward Clark, 1684; see also Locke, *Some Thoughts concerning Education*, 7.

75. Locke, *Some Thoughts concerning Education*, 9, 14, 20, 30.

76. Ibid. 31.

77. Ibid., pp. iv, 8–9, 14–16.

78. Ibid. 10–11, 14.

79. Communication from Mr Duncan Smith, at the age of 94, on sea-bathing at Holt School, Norfolk, in the 1920s, attributing his own longevity in part to this rigorous regime.

Chapter 8 **Civil Cleanliness**

1. Adam Dickson, *Essay on the Causes of the Present High Prices of Commodities* (London, 1773), 22–4, written three years before Adam Smith's *An Inquiry into the Nature and Causes of the Wealth of Nations* (London, 1776).

2. E. L. Jones and M. E. Falkus, 'Urban Improvement and the English Economy in the Seventeenth and Eighteenth Centuries', in Peter Borsay (ed.), *The Eighteenth Century Town, 1688–1820: A Reader in English Urban History* (London: Longman, 1990), table 1: 'New Bodies of Improvement Commissioners, 1725–1799', 139, and *passim*; Norman Davies, *The Isles: A History* (London: Macmillan, 2000), 646 and *passim*. A 1718–29 survey of Dissenters showed they made up 6.2 per cent of the population; see Michael Watts, *The Dissenters: From the Reformation to the French Revolution* (Oxford, Oxford University Press, 1985), 263–70.

3. See Fernand Braudel, *Civilisation and Capitalism, 15th–18th Century*, i: *The Structures of Everyday Life*, trans. Sian Reynolds (London: Collins, 1981), 311–25 and *passim*.

4. Sir John Sinclair, *Essay on Health and Longevity* (London, 1802), 10–11.

5. Sir John Sinclair, *The Code of Health and Longevity; or, A Concise View of the Principles Calculated for the Preservation of Health and Attainment of Long Life*, 4 vols. (Edinburgh, 1807–8), i. 20–4.

6. H. Morley (ed.), *The Spectator* (London: Routledge, 1887), Essay 631 (1714), 878–9; (1711), 182, 312.

7. John Wesley, 'On Dress', in *The Works of John Wesley*, ed. Albert C. Outler (Nashville, Tenn.: Abingdon, 1986), 249; A. W. Hill, *John Wesley amongst the Physicians* (London: Epworth Press, 1958), Letters, v. 133, 118–19. For a discussion of Wesley's fastidiousness, see Keith Thomas, 'Cleanliness and Godliness in Early Modern England', in Anthony Fletcher and Peter Roberts (eds.), *Religion, Culture and Society in Early Modern Britain: Essays in Honour of Patrick Collinson* (Cambridge: Cambridge University Press, 1994), 65–6. Cleanliness was, fifthly, also a preserver against 'several Vices destructive of both mind and body [that] are inconsistent with the habit of it'. This must be a reference to sexual uncleanness, probably the pox—or possibly 'onanism' or masturbation, a new 'vice' discovered by the anonymous English clergyman who wrote *Onania, or, The Heinous Sin of Self-Pollution, and All its Frightful Consequences, in Both Sexes, Considered* (1710); later rewritten by Samuel Auguste Tissot as *De l'onanisme* (1758), and much used by 19th-century purity crusaders. The story is told in Peter Gay, *The Bourgeois Experience: Victoria to Freud*, 5 vols. (Oxford: Oxford University Press, 1984–98), ii: *The Tender Passion*, 296 and *passim*.

8. Philip Dormer Stanhope, 4th Earl of Chesterfield, *Letters to his Son*, ed. Charles Sayle (London: Camelot, 1919), Letter LVII, 12 Nov. 1750, pp. 182–5.

9. Ibid. 184; see also his letter of 6 July 1749.

10. See Norbert Elias, *The Court Society*, trans. Edmund Jephcott (1st German edn., 1969; Oxford: Blackwell, 1983), *passim*; on boudoir intimacy, see Mark Girouard, *Life in the French Country House* (London: Cassell, 2000), 111–28, 147–62; on baths and bathing places, pp. 221–35; for illustrations crossing all periods, see the excellent Françoise de Bonneville, *The Book of the Bath*, trans. Jane Brenton (London: Thames & Hudson, 1998).

11. Alexander Pope, *The Rape of the Lock* (1712); see Neville Williams, *Powder and Paint: A History of the Englishwoman's Toilet, Elizabeth I–Elizabeth II* (London: Longmans, Green, 1957), 35–6 and *passim*.

12. De Bonneville, *The Book of the Bath*, 93–6.

13. Colin Jones, 'Dentistry and the Smile Tradition in Eighteenth-Century Paris', seminar, European Association for the History of Medicine and Health Conference, Paris, 2005. The surgical work of Pierre Fouchard (1678–1761) had revolutionized dentistry; see Roy Porter, *The Greatest Benefit to Mankind: A Medical History of Humanity from Antiquity to the Present* (London: HarperCollins, 1997), 384.

14. John Hunter, *The Natural History of the Human Teeth; Explaining their Structure, Use, Formation, Growth, and Diseases* (London, 1771); see also C. G. Crowley, *Dental Bibliography: A Standard Reference List of Books on Dentistry Published throughout the World from 1526–1885* (1885; Amsterdam: Liberac, 1968); Roy Porter and Dorothy Porter, *In Sickness and in Health: The British Experience 1650–1850* (London: Fourth Estate, 1988), 36 and n. 89, 41.

15. See Sharra L. Vostral, 'Masking Menstruation: The Emergence of Menstrual Hygiene Products in the United States', in Andrew Shail and Gillian Howie (eds.), *Menstruation: A Cultural History* (Basingstoke: Palgrave Macmillan, 2005), 243, 250.

16. B. R. Mitchell and Phyllis Deane, *Abstract of British Historical Statistics* (Cambridge: Cambridge University Press, 1962), 177–8; see also Beverley Lemire, *Fashion's Favourite: The Cotton Trade and the Consumer in Britain 1660–1800* (Oxford: Oxford University Press, 1992). Muslin cloth is an extraordinary fifty threads per centimetre instead of twenty-five or less. Information courtesy of Dr Philip Sykas; I am indebted to Dr Clare Brown and Dr Sykas for information on English textiles.

17. See the story of the overnight sensation of the *chemise à la reine* in Amanda Foreman, *Georgiana, Duchess of Devonshire* (London: HarperCollins, 1998), 176. The artist Vigee Le Brun's painting *Self Portrait in a Straw Hat* (*c*.1782), which started the craze, is in the National Gallery, London.

18. On English servants, see Theresa McBride, *The Domestic Revolution: The Modernisation of Household Service in England and France 1820–1920* (London: Croom Helm, 1976), 120–2, 14. See also Pamela

A. Sambrook, *The Country House Servant* (Stroud: Sutton Publishing/ National Trust, 1999).

19. Raffaella Sarti, *Europe at Home: Family and Material Culture 1500– 1800* (New Haven: Yale University Press, 2002), 141–2 and *passim*; Mark Girouard, *Life in the English Country House: A Social and Architectural History* (New Haven: Yale University Press, 1978), 138–42 and *passim*.

20. John Brewer and Roy Porter (eds.), *Consumption and the World of Goods* (London: Routledge, 1993); John Brewer, *The Pleasures of the Imagination: English Culture in the Eighteenth Century* (London: HarperCollins, 1997); Maxine Berg, *Luxury and Pleasure in Eighteenth-Century Britain* (Oxford: Oxford University Press, 2005).

21. William Buchan, *Domestic Medicine: or, A Treatise on the Prevention and Cure of Diseases by Regimen and Simple Medicines* (1769; London, 1803), 484–93. See also *Several Letters between Two Ladies, Wherein the Lawfulness and Unlawfulness of Artificial Beauty in Point of Conscience Are Nicely Debated* (1701), a pro-cosmetics essay which Neville Williams regarded as a 'milestone in the history of the Englishwomen's toilette'; quoted in Williams, *Powder and Paint*, 50–1.

22. There are no references to bathing-dresses in Queen Caroline's accounts, suggesting that she may have bathed naked. I am indebted for these references to Dr Joanna Marschner; see also Marschner, 'Baths and Bathing in the Early Georgian Court', *Furniture History*, 31 1995), 23–8. Emily J. Climenson, *Elizabeth Montagu, the Queen of Blue Stockings: Her Correspondence from 1720 to 1761*, 2 vols. (London: John Murray, 1906), 88–9.

23. Girouard, *Life in the English Country House*, 252–6, 265; id., *Life in the French Country House*, 232–9.

24. i.e. the strip wash carefully described by the medical author and sailor Peter Crosthwaite, *The Ensign of Peace: By a Friendly Traveller* (London, 1775), 136–8. Lizzie Collingham suggested that the Indian experience helped change British attitudes towards washing and cleanliness, in Collingham, 'Shower-Baths and Underwear', seminar, Emmanuel College, Cambridge, Feb. 1998;

see also E. M. Collingham, *The Physical Experience of the Raj, c.1800–1947* (Cambridge: Polity Press, 2001).

25. See Quentin Bell, *On Human Finery* (1947; London: Hogarth Press, 1976), 125 and *passim*, esp. the portrait of Brooke Boothby by Joseph Wright: 'by his side a running brook; beneath his hand a MS copy of *La Nouvelle Héloïse*. He wears the mildly amenable look of a virtuous philosopher; he also wears a suit cut by a first-rate tailor. It is a suit carefully designed for a Natural Man who is also the eldest son of a baronet . . . '.

26. On powder, see Williams, *Powder and Paint*, 86–7.

27. James Graham, *The Guardian Goddess of Health; or, The Whole Art of Preserving and Curing Diseases and of Enjoying Peace and Happiness of Body and Mind . . . Precepts for the Preservation and Exaltation of Personal Beauty and Loveliness* (London, [1780?]), 4; de Bonneville, *The Book of the Bath*, 93–4.

28. Foreman, *Georgiana*, 50–1; Allen Guttmann, 'Cricketers on the Green and Viragos in the Ring', in Guttmann, *Women's Sports: A History* (New York: Columbia University Press, 1991). See also Paul Langford, *Englishness Identified: Manners and Character 1650–1850* (Oxford: Oxford University Press, 2000).

29. The period is discussed more fully in Virginia Smith, 'Cleanliness: The Development of Idea and Practice in Britain, 1770–1850', Ph.D. thesis, University of London, 1985; see also Ginnie Smith, 'Prescribing the Rules of Health: Self-Help and Advice in the Late Eighteenth Century', in Roy Porter (ed.), *Patients and Practitioners: Lay Perceptions of Medicine in Pre-Industrial Society* (Cambridge: Cambridge University Press, 1985).

30. George Cheyney, *Essay on Regimen* (London, 1724); see also Henry R. Viets, 'George Cheyney 1673–1743', *Bulletin for the History of Medicine*, 23/5 (Sept.–Oct. 1949), 435–52; Lucia Dokome, 'Weight-Watching', seminar given at 'The History of Self-Experimentation', Wellcome Institute for the History of Medicine, London, Nov. 2000. His influential patients included Samuel Johnson, John Wesley, the Countess of Huntingdon (founder member of the

Methodist Friends' Society), Alexander Pope, David Hume, and the
Earl of Chesterfield.

31. As in the best-known European university textbooks of rational
medicine in the early century: Hermann Boerhaave's *Institutiones
Medicae*, 6 vols. (1708) (the last volume being on hygiene and
prophylaxis and its history), and Friedrich Hoffman's *A Systematic
Rational Medicine* (1718).

32. Francis Fuller, *Medicina Gymnastica: or, A Treatise concerning the
Power of Exercise, with respect to the Animal Economy* (London,
1705), pp. xxi–xxii, 68, 77. See also Jeremiah Wainewright, *A Mechanical Account of the Non-Naturals: Being a Brief Explication of the
Changes Made in Humane Bodies, by Air, Diet, etc. . . . To which is
prefixed, The Doctrine of Animal Secretion* (London, 1707); C. F.
Mullett, *Public Baths and Health in England, 16th–18th Century* (Baltimore: Johns Hopkins University Press, 1946), 57 and *passim*:
'Whereas in the sixteenth century printings were normally in the
hundreds, by the mid-eighteenth century they were in their thousands.'

33. John Armstrong, *The Art of Preserving Health* (1744; Hawick, 1811),
59–61. See generally Smith, 'Prescribing the Rules of Health', 262–
72; Roy Porter and Dorothy Porter, 'Keeping Well', in Porter and
Porter, *In Sickness and in Health: The British Experience 1650–1850*
(London: Fourth Estate, 1988); also Roy Porter, *Health for Sale:
Quackery in England 1660–1850* (Manchester: Manchester University Press, 1989); Porter, 'Lay Medical Knowledge in the Eighteenth
Century: The Case of the *Gentleman's Magazine*', *Medical History*, 29
(1985), 138–68.

34. See the diarists Samuel Johnson, Ralph Verney, Thomas Turner,
James Woodforde, Joseph Farington, etc., using the 17th-century
Protestant genre of confessional diaries which recorded daily
activities (and temptations) in Porter and Porter, *In Sickness and
in Health*, 122–3 and *passim*; on the sickness role or invalidism
deplored by Jane Austen and others, pp. 192–3.

35. Horace Walpole, *Selected Letters*, ed. W. Hadley (London: Dent,
1926), 325–6. Spartanism has a 'shadowy' history in 18th-century

Britain, though with more interest towards the end of the century;
it was considered rather extreme. See Elizabeth Rawson, *The Spartan Tradition in European Thought* (Oxford: Oxford University Press,
1969), 356–8.

36. John Wesley, *Primitive Physic: or, An Easy and Natural Method of
Curing Most Diseases* (London, 1747), 36–7, 8–9, vi–vii.

37. Buchan, *Domestic Medicine*, 27–8.

38. There are many pools (not all of which are excavated or recorded)
and bathhouses on National Trust property in Britain; but see
especially the double-storey, octagonal, stucco-and-shell Bath-
House built by Sir Charles Mordaunt in 1748 in the park at Walton
Hall, near Stratford upon Avon. On the many upper-class baths
and bathhouses in North America, see Harold Donaldson Eberlin,
'When Society First Took a Bath', in J. Walzer Leavitt and Ronald L.
Numbers (eds.), *Sickness and Health in America: Readings in the
History of Medicine and Public Health* (Madison: University of Wisconsin Press, 1978). On the use of waterfalls, see Tobias Smollett,
An Essay on the External Use of Water (London, 1752).

39. John King, *An Essay on Hot and Cold Bathing* (London, 1737), with
an illustration of Bungay Baths. Eighteenth-century hospital baths
have scarcely been researched, but see W. B. Howie, 'Finance and
Supply in an 18th Century Hospital, 1747–1830', *Medical History*, 17
(1963), 126–46. See also Rhodomonte Dominiceti, *A Dissertation on
the Artificial Medical Water Baths . . . together with a Description of the
Apparatus, Erected in Panton-Square, Haymarket* (London, 1782); id.,
*A Dissertation on the Effects of Artificial Medicated Water, Vaporous or
Dry-Baths etc.* (London, 1794); Arthur Clarke, *An Essay on Warm,
Cold, and Vapour Bathing, with Practical Observations on Sea-Bathing*
(London, 1819), pp. iv–v; R. Metcalfe, *The Rise and Progress of
Hydrotherapy in England and Scotland* (London, 1906), 21–4.

40. Eberlin, 'When Society First Took a Bath', 331–41. 'Cleaver' in
18th-century language meant brisk, alert, revived. It was not that
Elizabeth Drinker or Mrs Tucker did not wash; see Richard
L. Bushman and Claudia L. Bushman, 'The Early History of Cleanliness in America', *Journal of American History*, 74 (1988), 1215.

41. Roger Hudson (ed.), *Coleridge among the Lakes and Mountains* (London: Folio Society, 1991), 19–21.

42. J. K. Walton, *The English Seaside Resort: A Social History 1750–1914* (Leicester: Leicester University Press; New York: St Martin's Press, 1983), 10–13. See also Phyllis Hembry, *The English Spa, 1560–1815: A Social History* (London: Athlone Press; Rutherford, NJ: Fairleigh Dickinson University, 1990), 360 and *passim*, giving details of 173 spa foundations between 1558 and 1815, 113 of them after 1700.

43. A. F. M. Willich, *Lectures on Diet and Regimen* (London, 1801), 228; Eberlin, 'When Society Took a Bath', 334–5; Gore's *Liverpool General Advertiser*, 18 Aug. 1791. See also Alain Corbin, *The Lure of the Sea: The Discovery of the Seaside in the Western World, 1750–1840*, trans. Jocelyn Phelps (London: Penguin, 1995); Walton, *The English Seaside Resort*; Jim Ring, *How the English Made the Alps* (London: John Murray, 2000).

44. Jane Austen, *Sanditon* [written 1817] (1925; London: P. Davies, 1975), 5, 9–10, 23–4.

45. Smith, 'Cleanliness', 44–8, fig. 1; Bushman and Bushman, 'The Early History of Cleanliness in America', 1222–4. There were American editions of (for example) Floyer, Cheyne, Chesterfield, Wesley, Buchan, Tissot, and A. F. M. Willich.

46. James C. Riley, *The Eighteenth-Century Campaign to Avoid Disease* (London: Macmillan, 1987), 9–19 and *passim*.

47. Mark Harrison, 'Disease, Empire, and the Rise of Global Commerce: The Origins of International Sanitary Regulation in the Nineteenth Century', seminar, London School of Hygiene and Tropical Medicine, Mar. 2006; see also Peter Baldwin, *Contagion and the State in Europe 1830–1930* (Cambridge: Cambridge University Press, 1999).

48. D. McBride, *Experimental Essays* (London, 1764), 111. Sir John Pringle, *Observations on the Diseases of the Army* (London, 1752), p. vii, said he followed no theory, but 'enquired into the most general or remote causes of [diseases]—such as depend on the air, diet, and other causes usually comprehended under the head of Non-Naturals . . . And here I have ventured to assign some sources

of diseases very different from sentiments of most writers upon this subject.'

49. James Lind, *An Essay on the Most Effective Means of Preserving the Health of Seamen in the Royal Navy* (London, 1757); John Haygarth, *Letter to Dr Percival on the Prevention of Infectious Fevers* (London, 1801); C. Booth, *John Haygarth FRS (1740–1827): A Physician of the Enlightenment* (Philadelphia: American Philosophical Society, 2005).

50. Albrecht von Haller, *De Partibus Corporis Humani Sensibilibus et Irritabilibus* ['On the Sensible and Irritable Parts of the Human Body'] (1752); Porter, *The Greatest Benefit to Mankind*, 246–53; Christopher Lawrence, 'The Nervous System and Society in the Scottish Enlightenment', in Barry Barnes and Steven Shapin (eds.), *Natural Order: Historical Studies of Scientific Culture* (Beverly Hills: Sage, 1979), 25–8; Christopher Lawrence, 'Making the Nervous System', *Social Studies of Science*, 14/1 (1984), 153–8.

51. Ebenezer Sibley, *A Key to Physic and the Occult Sciences* (London, 1794); Allen G. Debus, 'Scientific Truth and Occult Tradition: The Medical World of Ebenezer Sibley (1751–1799)', *Medical History*, 26 (1982), 259–78; James Graham, *The Guardian of Health, Long Life and Happiness: or, Dr Graham's General Directions as to Regimen, etc.* (Newcastle upon Tyne, 1790); Smith, 'Prescribing the Rules of Health', 268–71; Roy Porter, 'Sex and the Singular Man: The Seminal Ideas of James Graham', *Studies on Voltaire and the Eighteenth Century*, 228 (1984), 1–24; C. J. S. Thompson, 'Beauty Specialists', in Thompson, *The Quacks of Old London* (London: Brentano's, 1928), 201–17, 327–35.

52. Jean-Jacques Rousseau, *Émile, or, Education*, trans. Barbara Foxley (London: Dent, 1911), 5–6, 218.

53. Hugh Downman, *Infancy, or, The Management of Children* (London, 1775–7), no page numbers.

54. Emily, Duchess of Leinster, in Ireland, was so impressed by *Émile* that she set up separate house for her children at Black Rock, on the coast south of Dublin, *à la* Rousseau, in 1766. (She even asked Rousseau, then exiled in England after the publication of *The Social Contract*, to be their tutor. He refused.) See Stella Tillyard, *Aristocrats: Caroline,*

Emily, Louisa and Sarah Lennox, 1740–1832 (London: Fontana/Collins, 1994), 243–51; and on late 18th-century feminism, Barbara Taylor, *Eve and the New Jerusalem: Socialism and Feminism in the Nineteenth Century* (London: Virago, 1983).

55. Kerry Walters and Lisa Portness, *Ethical Vegetarianism: From Pythagoras to Peter Singer* (Albany: State University of New York Press, 1999), 78.

56. Ibid. 10.

57. Colin Spencer, *The Heretic's Feast: A History of Vegetarianism* (London: Fourth Estate, 1993), 237–9, 245–51.

58. Buchan, *Domestic Medicine*, pt. I, pp. 1, 484–93.

59. Ibid. 95–101, xxx, 100.

60. Dorothy Porter, *Health, Civilisation and the State: A History of Public Health from Ancient to Modern Times* (London: Routledge, 1999), 57–8; George Rosen, 'The Philosophy of Ideology and the Emergence of Modern Medicine in France', *Bulletin of the History of Medicine*, 20 (1946), 328–9; id., 'Romantic Medicine: A Problem in Historical Periodization', *Bulletin of the History of Medicine*, 25 (1951), 148–58. There was no British university training in 'state medicine' until 1854, although a course on 'medical police' briefly appeared on the Edinburgh curriculum in 1809 (John Roberton, *Treatise on Medical Police, and on Diet, Regimen, etc.* (London, 1809)).

61. Timothy Lenoir, 'The Göttingen School and the Development of Transcendental *Naturphilosophie* in the Romantic Era', in W. Coleman and C. Limoges (eds.), *Studies in the History of Biology* (Baltimore: Johns Hopkins University Press, 1981), 113–14; id., *The Strategy of Life: Teleology and Mechanics in Nineteenth Century German Biology* (Dordrecht: Reidel, 1982).

62. A. F. M. Willich, *Lectures on Diet and Regimen* (London, 1801), 28–9; Alexander von Humboldt, *Kosmos. Entwurf einer physischen Weltbeschreibung* ('Cosmos: Sketch of the Physical Description of the Universe'), ed. Ottmar Ette and Oliver Lübrich (Frankfurt: Eichborn, 2005); Daniel Johnson, 'From a Lost World', *Times Literary Supplement*, 22 July 2005, 3–4.

63. *Naturphilosophie* was called 'one of the most bizarre episodes in the history of physiology' by the classic historian of physiology Karl Rothschuh (*History of Physiology*, ed. and trans. Guenter B. Risse (Huntington, NY: Re. E. Krieger, 1973), 155); see also Christopher Lawrence and George Weisz (eds.), *Greater than the Parts: Holism and Biomedicine, 1920–1950* (Oxford: Oxford University Press, 1998).

64. Thus the term 'macrobiotic' held little meaning for English-speakers until the early 20th century, when it was reimported as something vaguely German, to do with eating health foods.

65. C. W. Hufeland, *The Art of Prolonging Life*, ed. E. Wilson (London, 1852), preface, p. xixv.

66. Willich, *Lectures on Diet and Regimen*, 10; C. A. Struve, *Asthenology, or, The Art of Preserving Life* (London, 1801), ch. vii: 'National Debility', 158–71; *Introductory Lecture ... to A Familiar Treatise on the Physical Education of Children by C. A. Struve*, trans. A. F. M. Willich (London, 1801), 49–50.

67. The key works in dermatology were the systematic classifications of Joseph Plenck in 1776 and Antoine Lorry in 1777; Lorry in particular was an enthusiastic hygienist. A London group emerged at the end of the century centred on the medical studies of Dr Thomas Willan, summarized in his *Report on the Diseases of London* (1801). Dermatology is relatively under-researched; but see F. H. Garrison, 'The Skin as a Functional Organ of the Body', *Bulletin of the New York Academy of Medicine*, 9 (1933), 303–18.

68. Hufeland, *The Art of Prolonging Life*, 225–9. Willich, *Lectures on Diet and Regimen*, 61–6, 224–6: 'The most ignorant person is convinced that proper care of the skin is indispensably necessary for the existence and well-being of horses and various animals ... Such a simple idea, however, never occurs to him in respect to his child. Since we show so much prudence and intelligence in regard to animals, why not in regard to men?'

69. Willich, *Lectures on Diet and Regimen*, 233, 249–50.

70. Arthur Young, *Travels in France* (18 Jan. 1790), quoted in a classic text on 18th-century health philanthropy, M. C. Buer, *Health,*

Wealth and Population in the Early Days of the Industrial Revolution (London: Routledge, 1926), 196.

71. Eberlin, 'When Society Took a Bath', 335–8; Bushman, 'The Early History of Cleanliness in America', 1214–15.

72. Thomas Beddoes, *Hygëia: or, Essays Moral and Medical* (London, 1802), 26–7.

Chapter 9 **Health Crusaders**

1. Norman Davies, *Europe: A History* (London: Pimlico, 1997), 1294; Peter N. Stearns (ed.), *Encyclopedia of European Social History from 1350 to 2000* (New York: Charles Scribner's Sons, 2001), ii: *The Population of Europe*, table 1, p. 160; on the UK, see M. C. Buer, *Health, Wealth and Population in the Early Days of the Industrial Revolution* (London: Routledge, 1926), 122; B. R. Mitchell and Phyllis Deane, *Abstract of British Historical Statistics* (Cambridge: Cambridge University Press, 1962), 24–6; Norman Davies, *The Isles: A History* (London: Macmillan, 2000), 646–9.

2. The Society for the Suppressing of Vice (1802), described caustically by Sydney Smith as 'The Society for suppressing the Vices of Persons whose income does not exceed £500 per annum', replaced the equally disliked late 17th-century Society for the Reformation of Manners; Roy Porter, *English Society in the Eighteenth Century* (London: Penguin, 1982), 312; Richard Johnson, 'Educational Policy and Social Control in Early Victorian England', *Past and Present*, 49 (1970), 96–119: 96 and *passim*. The SBCICP itself had a powerful subcommittee—the Ladies Society for the Education and Employment of the Female Poor. The Society for Distributing Religious Tracts among the Poor (1782) was followed (among others) by the National Society for Promoting the Education of the Poor (1811), the Society for the Diffusion of Useful Knowledge (1825), and the Ladies' National Association for the Diffusion of Sanitary Knowledge of 1857 (also called the Ladies' Sanitary Association).

3. *The Metropolitan Charities, Being an Account of the Charitable, Benevo-
lent, and Religious Societies... in London and its Immediate Vicinity*
(London, 1844); A. F. C. Bourdillon (ed.), *Voluntary Social Services:
Their Place in the Modern State* (London: Methuen, 1945), including G. D. H. Cole, 'Retrospect of the History of the Voluntary
Social Services'; see also Colin Jones, 'Charity before *c.*1850', in
W. F. Bynum and Roy Porter (eds.), *Companion Encyclopedia of the
History of Medicine*, 2 vols. (London: Routledge, 1993). The wide-
scale closure of public toilets in the United Kingdom in the late 20th
century is due to the fact that town planners discovered there was
no formal legislation that actually covered their provision.

4. C. Stanger, *Remarks on the Necessity and Means of Suppressing Contagious Fever in the Metropolis* (London, 1802), 25–9.

5. E. P. Thompson, *The Making of the English Working Class* (London:
Penguin, 1968), 865–71. See also J. F. C. Harrison, *Robert Owen and
the Owenites in Britain and America* (London: Routledge & Kegan
Paul, 1969).

6. Roger Cooter, *The Cultural Meaning of Popular Science: Phrenology and
the Organisation of Consent in Nineteenth-Century Britain* (Cambridge:
Cambridge University Press, 1984), 358 n. 108.

7. [Samuel Brown], 'Physical Puritanism', *Westminster Review*, 2 (1852),
409. I am indebted to Roger Cooter (and J. F. C. Harrison) for the
reference, and for identifying Samuel Brown as the anonymous
author; see also Cooter, *The Cultural Meaning of Popular Science*,
177–9 n. 34.

8. Logie Barrow, *Independent Spirits: Spiritualism and English Plebeians,
1850–1910* (London: Routledge & Kegan Paul, 1986), 93. On Bacon,
see Charles Webster, 'The Nineteenth-Century Afterlife of Paracelsus',
in Roger Cooter (ed.), *Studies in the History of Alternative Medicine*
(London: Macmillan, 1988), 83. On the cultural role of unorthodox
science, see Cooter, *The Cultural Meaning of Popular Science*, 64 and
passim.

9. As in the career of the pioneer osteopath Andrew Taylor Still; see
Norman Gevitz, 'Andrew Taylor Still and the Social Origins of Oste-
opathy', in Cooter (ed.), *Studies in the History of Alternative Medicine*.

There is no general history of massage: but see F. C. Ireland, *Good Health, or, The Physiology of Dietetics and Massage* (Liverpool, 1827); Edward Williams, *Magnetic Masseur: The Revived Ancient Art of Massage* (London, 1887); Douglas Graham, *A Treatise on Massage*, 2nd edn. (New York, 1890); John Harvey Kellog, *The Art of Massage: Its Physiological Effects and Therapeutic Applications* (Battle Creek, Mich., 1895).

10. In 1833 the American Temperance Society reputedly had over 2 million members, and the British Temperance Society 'upwards of 30,000' (Joel Pinney, *The Alternative: Disease and Premature Death, or, Health and Long Life: Being an Exposure of the Prevailing Misconception of their Respective Sources* (London, 1838), 21–33). See also W. R. Lefanu, *British Periodicals of Medicine 1640–1899*, Research Publications, 6 (Oxford: Wellcome Institute for the History of Medicine, 1984), 8–37.

11. Colin Spencer, *The Heretic's Feast: A History of Vegetarianism* (London: Fourth Estate, 1993), 257–8; [Brown], 'Physical Puritanism', 408–9.

12. Glynis Rankin, 'Professional Organisation and the Development of Medical Knowledge: Two Interpretations of Homeopathy', in Cooter (ed.), *Studies in the History of Alternative Medicine*. The British royal family had a long connection with homeopathy, which puts Prince Charles's well-known health beliefs into perspective.

13. Barbara Griggs, *Green Pharmacy* (London: Robert Hale, 1981), 172–86 and *passim*; Samuel Thomson, *A Narrative of the Life and Medical Discoveries of Samuel Thomson, containing an Account of his System of Practise, and the Manner of Curing Diseases with Vegetable Medicine upon a Plan Entirely New; to which is added an Introduction to his New Guide to Health, or Botanic Family Physician* (Boston, Mass., 1822).

14. Ursula Miley and John V. Pickstone, 'Medical Botany around 1850: American Medicine in Industrial Britain', in Cooter (ed.), *Studies in the History of Alternative Medicine*, 146–9, 151–2. National organizations such as the People's Medico-Botanic Association, the Friendly United Medico-Botanic Sick and Burial Society, the Society of

United Medical Herbalists, and finally the National Association of Medical Herbalists, carried them through into the 20th century.

15. James Pierrepont Greaves, 'The Conditional Law' (c.1840), in A. Campbell (ed.), *Letters and Extracts from the M.S. Writings of James Pierrepont Greaves*, 2 vols. (London, 1845), ii. 81; Spencer, *The Heretic's Feast*, 260; Harrison, *Robert Owen and the Owenites in Britain and America*, *passim*. The connection with the later ideology of William Morris is evident.

16. James C. Whorton, ' "Tempest in a Flesh-Pot": The Formulation of a Physiological Rationale for Vegetarianism', *Journal of the History of Medicine and Allied Sciences*, 32 (1977), 115–39, 315. See also id., *Crusaders for Fitness: The History of American Health Reform* (Princeton: Princeton University Press, 1982); id., *Nature Cures: The History of Alternative Medicine in America* (Oxford: Oxford University Press, 2002); Spencer, *The Heretic's Feast*, 260. There was also a strong Jeffersonian tradition of political libertarianism in North America, with links to Tom Paine and William Godwin (and later claimed as anarchist forerunners; see Peter Marshall, *Demanding the Impossible: A History of Anarchism* (London: Fontana, 1993), 130–9, 182–3, 190–219); Spencer, *The Heretic's Feast*, 260.

17. Margaret Pelling, *Cholera, Fever and English Medicine, 1825–1865* (Oxford: Oxford University Press, 1978); see also Andrew Combe, *The Principles of Physiology Applied to the Preservation of Health, and the Improvement of Physical and Mental Education* (1833; London, 1837), 4–5, 24, 391–2.

18. Roy Porter, *The Greatest Benefit to Mankind: A Medical History of Humanity from Antiquity to the Present* (London: HarperCollins, 1997), 313–14; R. J. Morris, *Cholera 1832: The Social Response to an Epidemic* (London: Croom Helm, 1976), 163, 176–84, 205. The body literally evacuated itself onto the floor with the watery juices or plasma going first. The body turned blue as the blood dehydrated, and the victim died convulsively.

19. William Wadd, *Comments on Corpulency, Lineaments of Leanness* (London, 1829), 2–8, 133–4; A. Carlisle, *Practical Observations on the Preservation of Health, and the Prevention of Disease* (London, 1838),

pp. xlii–iii. On alkaloid pharmacology, see Porter, *The Greatest Benefit to Mankind*, 334. See also R. Shryock, 'Public Relations of the Medical Profession in Great Britain and the United States, 1600–1870', *Annals of Medical History*, ns 2 (1930), 308–39; John Harley Warner, *The Therapeutic Perspective: Medical Practise, Knowledge and Identity in America 1820–1885* (Cambridge, Mass.: Harvard University Press, 1986).

20. William Dale, *The State of the Medical Profession in Great Britain and Ireland* (Dublin, 1873), with a cartoon etching of *The Upas Tree of the Medical Profession*. On the social fluidity of professional medicine at this time, see Ian Inkster, 'Marginal Men: Aspects of the Social Role of the Medical Community in Sheffield 1790–1850', in J. Woodward and D. Richards (eds.), *Health Care and Popular Medicine in Nineteenth Century England* (London: Croom Helm, 1977).

21. A. Kilgour, *Lectures on the Ordinary Agents of Life, as Applicable to Therapeutics and Hygiene; or, The Uses of the Atmosphere, Habitations, Baths, Clothing, Climates, Exercise, Foods, Drinks, etc. in the Treatment and Prevention of Disease* (Edinburgh, 1834), pp. xviii–xix, 6–7.

22. The use of magazines for health advice started in the 18th century, for example in the *Ladies' Magazine*. See also William Turnbull, *The Medical Works of the Late Mr William Turnbull*, i: *A Popular Treatise on Health* (London, 1805), p. xi: 'this practice was followed at this period [1770–80] by several physicians . . . and they may be considered as the first attempt at popular medicine'.

23. *The Family Oracle of Health; Economy, Medicine, and Good Living; Adapted to All Ranks of Society, from the Palace to the Cottage; by A. F. Crell MD and W. Wallace Esq. Assisted by a Committee of Scientific Gentlemen* (London, 1824), frontispiece and title page.

24. Thomas Bull, *The Maternal Management of Children* (London, 1848), no page numbers.

25. J. S. Forsyth, *A Practical Treatise on Diet, Regimen, and Indigestion; Consisting of Rules for Eating and Drinking* (London, 1829), p. vi; Cooter, *The Cultural Meaning of Popular Science*; Porter, *The Greatest Benefit to Mankind*, 498–500.

26. Sarah Bakewell, 'Medical Gymnastics in the Library', *Friends of the Wellcome Institute Newsletter*, 12 (Spring 1997), 490. Both Ling and Jahn were 'primitivists' and strong Nordic nationalists; Jahn was prosecuted for his political activities in the 'turning' academies. German gymnasiums were the first sporting organizations to ban Jewish members during the Nazi regime. See also Guttmann, *Women's Sports*, 90–1; Catherine Beecher, *A Course of Calisthenics for Young Ladies* (1832); Donald Walker, *Exercises for Young Ladies* (1836).

27. The Revd Edward Barry MD, *The Aesculapian Monitor* (London, 1811), pp. xvi, 146–54, was an early precursor of enlightened physiological reform, insisting on 'minute cleanliness' in every part of the school. Sporting curricula were pursued at Marlborough, Uppingham, Harrow, and Loreto in particular (J. A. Mangan, *Athleticism in the Victorian and Edwardian Public School: The Emergence and Consolidation of an Educational Ideology* (Cambridge: Cambridge University Press, 1981)). Oliver Wendell Holmes quoted in John Rickards Betts, 'American Medical Thought on Exercise as the Road to Health, 1820–1860', *Bulletin of the History of Medicine*, 45 (1971), 150; see also Allen Guttmann, *A Whole New Ball Game: An Interpretation of American Sports* (Chapel Hill: University of North Carolina Press, 1988), 72–4, 101–5.

28. See generally Jean-Pierre Goubert, *The Conquest of Water: The Advent of Health in the Industrial Age* (Cambridge: Polity Press, 1989); Anthony S. Wohl, *Endangered Lives: Public Health in Victorian Britain* (London: Methuen, 1983), 234 and *passim* on river pollution. See also John Simon, *English Sanitary Institutions* (London, 1890); id., *Public Health Reports*, 2 vols. (London, 1887).

29. [Brown], 'Physical Puritanism', 439–40; he also refers to Britain's military requirements. Robert Willan, *Reports on the Diseases of London* (London, 1801), 303–5.

30. Kilgour, *Lectures on the Ordinary Agents of Life*, 103; Houses of Parliament, General Index to Bills, 1801–1852, 6 Will. IV, Sess. 1835, 16 July; 6 Will. IV, Sess. 1837, 2 Mar. The mover was James Silk Buckingham, MP for Sheffield, noted for his 'steady and

strenuous promotion of Temperance societies', later author of
Natural Evils and Practical Remedies (London, 1849). The 1844
Inquiry into the Health of Large Towns etc. made special inquiry
into the extent of provision of commercial baths. Libraries and
museums got their Act in 1850; public grounds and playgrounds
(parks) in 1857–9.

31. R. Metcalfe, *The Rise and Progress of Hydrotherapy in England and
Scotland* (London, 1906), 5–8 and *passim*. See also Virginia Smith,
'The Movement for the 1846 Act' and 'The London Parish of
Poplar', in 'Cleanliness: The Development of Idea and Practice in
Britain, 1770–1850', Ph.D. thesis, University of London, 1985;
Sally Sheard, 'Profit is a Dirty Word: The Development of Public
Baths and Washhouses in Britain 1842–1915', *Social History of
Medicine*, 13/1 (Apr. 2000), 63–85. Goulston Square Washhouse is
now the new home of the Fawcett Women's Library.

32. Wohl, *Endangered Lives*, 168–72, 142.

33. James Simpson, *Lectures on the Means of Improving the Character and
Condition of the Working Classes*, National Library of Scotland
Bound Pamphlets (Edinburgh, 1843).

34. *Baths and Wash-houses for the Million* ([1845?]), Wellcome Collection, Wellcome Institute for the History of Medicine, London.

35. Sanitary Commissioner Dr Southwood Smith, quoted in R. Metcalfe,
The Rise and Progress of Hydrotherapy in England and Scotland
(London, 1906), p. xvi; *Cleanliness* ([mid-19th century]), Wellcome
Collection, Wellcome Institute for the History of Medicine, London.
See also Dorothy Porter, *Health, Civilisation and the State: A History of
Public Health from Ancient to Modern Times* (London: Routledge,
1999), 76–8; Lawrence Goldman, *Science, Reform and Politics in Vic-
torian Britain: The Social Science Association, 1857–1886* (Cambridge:
Cambridge University Press, 2002).

36. Edwy Godwin Clayton, *Arthur Hill Hassall, Physician and Sanitary
Reformer: A Short History of his Work in Public Hygiene, and of the
Movement against the Adulteration of Food and Drugs* (London, 1908),
22 and *passim*; he opened an open-air seafront consumption hospital on the Isle of Wight in 1869, and retired to the Riviera.

Stephen Halliday, *The Great Stink of London: Sir Joseph Balzalgette and the Cleansing of the Victorian Capital* (Stroud: Sutton, 1999); Brian Abel-Smith, *A History of the Nursing Profession* (London: Heinemann, 1975), 24 and *passim*; Porter, *The Greatest Benefit to Mankind*, 377–8.

37. Wohl, *Endangered Lives*, 173–5. On monumentality, see Tristram Hunt, *Building Jerusalem: The Rise and Fall of the Victorian City* (London: Weidenfeld & Nicolson, 2004); Hazel Conway, *People's Parks: The Design and Development of Victorian Parks in Britain* (Cambridge: Cambridge University Press, 1991).

38. Jean-Pierre Goubert, *Du Luxe au confort* (Paris: Belin, 1988), 23–6.

39. J. S. Forsyth, *Practical Treatise on Diet and Regimen, and Indigestion* (London 1829), pp. xxii–xxiii. In one English country house a portable shower-bath was still in use up to 1973.

40. Sigfried Giedon, *Mechanisation Takes Command: A Contribution to Anonymous History* (Oxford: Oxford University Press, 1948), *passim*; Lawrence Wright, *Clean and Decent: The History of the Bath and Loo* (London: Routledge & Kegan Paul, 1980), 119, 152–4, and *passim*.

41. Wallace Reyburn, *Flushed with Pride: The Story of Thomas Crapper* (London: Pavilion Books, 1989); Wright, *Clean and Decent*, 132–4, 138–40, 152–9.

42. Neville Williams, *Powder and Paint: A History of the Englishwoman's Toilet, Elizabeth I–Elizabeth II* (London: Longmans, Green, 1957), 97, 101–2, and *passim*; see also A. J. Cooley, *The Toilet and Cosmetic Arts in Ancient and Modern Times; with a Review of the Different Theories of Beauty, and Copious Allied Information, Social, Hygienic, and Medical . . . and a Comprehensive Collection of Formulae and Directories* (London, 1866).

43. J. K. Walton, *The English Seaside Resort: A Social History 1750–1914* (Leicester: Leicester University Press; New York: St Martin's Press, 1983), 48–66 and *passim*.

44. James Wilson, *The Water Cure* (London, 1842).

45. *Recollections of the Late Dr Barter* (Dublin, 1873); James Wilson, *The Principles and Practice of the Water Cure and Domestic Medical Science*

(London, 1854); Kelvin Rees, 'Water as a Commodity: Hydropathy at Matlock', in Cooter (ed.), *Studies in the History of Alternative Medicine*.

46. Marshall Scott Legan, 'Hydropathy in America: A Nineteenth Century Panacea', *Bulletin of the History of Medicine*, 45 (1971), 267–80: 274–6 and *passim*.

47. William James, *The Varieties of Religious Experience*, ed. Martin E. Marty (London: Penguin, 1985), 92–3.

48. Ian Buruma, *Voltaire's Coconuts: or, Anglomania in Europe* (London: Weidenfeld & Nicolson, 1999), 174–5.

49. This overstatement of scientific opposition may have contributed to their later political decline; see Logie Barrow, 'An Imponderable Liberator: J. J. Garth Wilkinson', in Cooter (ed.), *Studies in the History of Alternative Medicine*, 92.

50. William Tibbles, 'Vegetarianism', *Journal of State Medicine*, 12/6 (1904), 343–5. See also James C. Whorton, 'Purgation', unpub., Nov. 1986, 7, 16; id., *Inner Hygiene: Constipation and the Pursuit of Health in Modern Society* (Oxford: Oxford University Press, 2000).

51. See generally, on the culture of germs, Nancy Tomes, *The Gospel of Germs: Men, Women and the Microbe in American Life* (Cambridge, Mass.: Harvard University Press, 1998). See also ead., 'The Private Side of Public Health: Sanitary Science, Domestic Hygiene, and the Germ Theory, 1870–1900', *Bulletin of the History of Medicine*, 64/2 (Winter 1990), 509–39.

52. Lloyd G. Stevenson, 'Science down the Drain: On the Hostility of Certain Sanitarians to Animal Experimentation, Bacteriology, and Immunology', *Bulletin of the History of Medicine*, 29/1 (1955), 2–3, 7–13; see also Ward Richardson, *Diseases of Modern Life* (1875); and *Biological Experimentation* (1896), an exploration of ways of avoiding animal experiments and reducing them to a minimum.

53. W. F. Bynum, 'Medical Philanthropy after 1850', in Bynum and Porter (eds.), *Companion Encyclopaedia of the History of Medicine*, ii. 1488–9. See generally James C. Whorton, 'The Hippocratic Heresy: Alternative Medicine's Worldview', in Whorton, *Nature Cures: The*

History of Alternative Medicine in America (Oxford: Oxford University Press, 2002). See also Margaret Pelling, 'Contagion/Germ Theory/Specificity', in Bynum and Porter (eds.), *Companion Encyclopaedia of the History of Medicine*, 316, 329.

54. For a detailed description of the US campaign, see Suellen Hoy, *Chasing Dirt: The American Pursuit of Cleanliness* (New York: Oxford University Press, 1995); John Clark, 'Flies in the Face of History: Babies, Troops, and Flies in Early Twentieth Century Britain', seminar, Wellcome Institute for the History for Medicine, Nov. 1999.

55. Whorton, *Crusaders for Fitness*; Hoy, *Chasing Dirt, passim*.

56. See Howard Williams, *The Pioneers of Humanity* (London: Humanitarian League, 1907).

57. E. S. Turner, *Taking the Cure* (London: Michael Joseph, 1967), 262–4.

58. Friedhelm Kirchfield and Wade Boyle, *Nature Doctors: Pioneers in Naturopathic Medicine* (Portland, Oreg.: Medicina Biologica/Buckeye Naturopathic Press, 1994). The 'Father' of naturopathy in the United States was Benedict Lust (1872–1945); in Britain, Stanley Lief (1892–1963); and in Scotland, James L. Thompson (1887–1963). The archives of the Eden Foundation at Bad Solen, catalogued by Karl Rothschuh, house the best European collection of nature cure literature; a continuing interest in *Naturheil* was carried on in exile in the United States by the German medical historian of hygiene Henry Sigerist.

59. Turner, *Taking the Cure*, 266. His first Jaeger suit, purchased in 1885, gave the young George Bernard Shaw a new social identity; see Michael Holroyd, *Bernard Shaw*, i: *The Search for Love* (London: Chatto & Windus, 1988). See also E. T. Renbourne, *Materials and Clothing in Health and Disease: History, Physiology and Hygiene, Medical and Psychological Aspects: With the Biophysics of Clothing Materials* (London: W. H. Rees, 1972); Wilhelm Paul Gerhard, *Modern Baths and Bathhouses* (New York: Wiley, 1908), 219–33.

60. Gerhard, *Modern Baths and Bathhouses*, 232–3.

61. A. J. Carter, 'A Breath of Fresh Air', *Proceedings of the Royal College of Physicians of Edinburgh*, 24/3 (1994), 397–405.

62. Whorton, *Nature Cures*, 196.

63. On Nietzsche's hardiness, see Lesley Chamberlain, *Nietzsche in Turin: The End of the Future* (London: Quartet Books, 1996), 95–101. See also the excellent swimming history by Charles Sprawson, *Haunts of the Black Masseur: The Swimmer as Hero* (London: Jonathan Cape, 1992), *passim*; Paul Delany, *The Neo-Pagans* (London: Macmillan, 1988), *passim*.

64. Turner, *Taking the Cure*, 257, 262–74; Sprawson, *Haunts of the Black Masseur*, 184–7 and *passim*; Delany, *The Neo-Pagans*. Lord Leverhulme's private habits were exposed to public view when Thornton Manor went to auction in June 2001; see Rebecca Allinson, 'Cleaning Up', *The Guardian*, 23 June 2001, 12.

65. The Revd S. A. Barnett, *The Duties of the Rich to the Poor* (1889), quoted in Wohl, *Endangered Lives*, 340–1. The same was also true in other parts of Europe; as, for example, in Nivernais, France, where washing practices were partial to non-existent, sanitation poor, and mortality high; see Guy Thuillier, 'Pour une histoire de l'hygiène corporelle. Un example regional: Le Nivernais 1860–1880', *Revue d'Histoire Économique et Social*, 46 (1968), 232–53; and on laundering, 'Pour une histoire de la lessive en Nivernais au XIX siècle', Bulletin 18, Vie Materièlle et Compartements Biologiques, *Annales*, 24/1 (1969).

Chapter 10 **The Body Beautiful**

1. Milton I. Roemer, 'Internationalism in Medicine and Public Health', in W. F. Bynum and Roy Porter (eds.), *Companion Encyclopedia of the History of Medicine*, 2 vols. (London: Routledge, 1993), ii. 1417–35; W. F. Bynum, 'Medical Philanthropy after 1850', ibid. ii. 1480–94. See also the classic work by Pyotr Kropotkin that influenced early 20th-century socialists, communists, and anarchists, *Mutual Aid: A Factor of Evolution* (London: William Heinemann, 1902).

2. M. Gorsky, J. Mohan, and T. Willis, *Mutualism and Health Care: British Hospital Contributory Schemes in the Twentieth Century* (Manchester: Manchester University Press, 2006).

3. C. E. A. Winslow, *The Evolution and Significance of the Modern Public Health Campaign* (New Haven: Yale University Press, 1923), 30. Winslow was a forceful US campaigner; Arthur Newsholme was a key figure in the United Kingdom; see John M. Eyler, *Sir Arthur Newsholme and State Medicine, 1885–1935* (Cambridge: Cambridge University Press, 1997); Newsholme, *Evolution of Preventive Medicine* (London: Balière, 1927). On public health nursing, see Christopher Maggs, 'A General History of Nursing: 1800–1900', in Bynum and Porter (eds.), *Companion Encyclopedia of the History of Medicine*, ii; and Maggs (ed.), *Nursing History: The State of the Art* (London: Croom Helm, 1987). On hygiene advertising and industry-led hygiene initiatives, see Nancy Tomes, *The Gospel of Germs: Men, Women and the Microbe in American Life* (Cambridge, Mass.: Harvard University Press, 1998), 117–23, 247–52, and Juliann Sivulka, *Stronger than Dirt: A Cultural History of Advertising Personal Hygiene in North America* (Amherst, NY: Humanity Books, 2001). The Cleanliness Institute is still maintained by the Association of American Soap and Glycerine Producers.

4. Figures from Anthony S. Wohl, *Endangered Lives: Public Health in Victorian Britain* (London: Methuen, 1983), 332–3 and *passim*.

5. Havelock Ellis, *The Task of Social Hygiene* (London, 1912), p. vi. See also Greta Jones, *Social Hygiene in Twentieth Century Britain* (London: Croom Helm, 1986), 26 and *passim*.

6. 'Housing', in *The Encyclopaedia Britannica*, 11th edn. (Cambridge: Cambridge University Press, 1911), 821–2. This excellent survey article also included a statistical housing review of 'other countries'— Austria, Belgium, France, Germany, the Netherlands, Italy, and the United States.

7. Roy Porter, *The Greatest Benefit to Mankind: A Medical History of Humanity from Antiquity to the Present* (London: HarperCollins, 1997), 510–13; Michael Burleigh, *The Third Reich: A New History* (London: Pan Macmillan, 2001), 345–8; Jones, *Social Hygiene in Twentieth Century Britain*, 28–9.

8. Agnes Campbell, *Report on Public Baths and Washhouses in the United Kingdom* (Edinburgh: Carnegie UK Trust, 1918), 10, 21–2, 28, 37;

Irene Leigh, personal communication: her grandmother Eleanor Watson used the wash-boiler to clean the children after doing the laundry.

9. The Hygiene Committee of the Women's Group on Public Welfare, *Our Towns: A Close-Up* (Oxford: Oxford University Press, 1943), pp. xiii, 4, 81–7; see also Richard Titmuss, *Poverty and Population: A Factual Study of Contemporary Social Waste* (London: Macmillan, 1938); John Stevenson, *Social Conditions in Britain between the Wars* (London: Penguin, 1977); Campbell, *Report on Public Baths and Washhouses in the United Kingdom*, 7.

10. See Alexander Kira, *The Bathroom* (London: Penguin; New York: Viking, 1976). Oral quotations from *The Rise and Spread of the Middle Classes*, pt. I, Channel Four TV, 12 Mar. 2001; there is much testimony on the novelty of bathrooms. In the 1930s George Orwell found even relatively well-off working-class neighbours almost too much for his fastidious nose and eyes to bear. This acute sense of cleanness did not, however, stop him hating the hygienic bourgeois life of the aspiring suburbs; see William Ian Miller, *The Anatomy of Disgust* (Cambridge, Mass.: Harvard University Press, 1997), 240–3.

11. See Caroline Davidson, *A Woman's Work Is Never Done: A History of Housework in the British Isles 1650–1950* (London: Chatto & Windus, 1986), 191–2; Ann Oakley, 'Four Housewives', in Oakley, *Housewife* (London: Penguin, 1974), 105–13, 127–41; Margaret Horsfield, *Biting the Dust: The Joys of Housework* (London: Fourth Estate, 1998), 123–39; on cellophane, see Tomes, *The Gospel of Germs*, 249–50.

12. Adrian Forty, *Objects of Desire: Design and Society 1750–1980* (London: Thames & Hudson, 1986), 156–81 and *passim*; and on the vacuum cleaner, pp. 175–81.

13. Bill Luckin, *Questions of Power: Electricity and Environment in Inter-War Britain* (Manchester: Manchester University Press, 1990), 29–30, 13, 53. Catherine Mills ('Clean Air, Coal and the Regulation of the Domestic Hearth', seminar, London School of Hygiene and Tropical Medicine, Mar. 2006) described the dramatic environmental impact

of the 1956 Clean Air Act 'smoke abatement zones' (on the town of Sheffield). See also Peter Thorsheim, *Inventing Pollution: Coal, Smoke, and Culture in Britain since 1800* (Cleveland: Ohio University Press, 2006).

14. Kate de Castelbajac, *The Face of the Century: 100 Years of Makeup and Style*, ed. Nan Richardson and Catherine Chermayeff (London: Thames & Hudson, 1995).

15. Tomes, *The Gospel of Germs*, 250–1; Sharra L. Vostral, 'Masking Menstruation: The Emergence of Menstrual Hygiene Products in the United States', in Andrew Shail and Gillian Howie (eds.), *Menstruation: A Cultural History* (Basingstoke: Palgrave Macmillan, 2005).

16. Joan Nunn, *Fashion in Costume, 1200–2000* (London: Herbert, 2000), 182–4; John Peacock, *20th Century Fashion: The Complete Sourcebook* (London: Thames & Hudson, 1993); Irina Lindsay, *Dressing and Undressing for the Beach* (Hornchurch: Ian Henry, 1983).

17. Like the childhood recalled by Doris Lessing, *Under My Skin*, vol. i of *My Autobiography* (London: HarperCollins, 1994); the comedian John Cleese has said that his mother did not like him to kiss her because 'she thought it would spread germs' (speaking on *Parkinson*, BBC TV, 10 Mar. 2001).

18. J. Menzies Campbell, *Dentistry Then and Now*, 3rd edn. (London: privately printed, 1981), 382–4. But preventive dentistry is still a low-status Cinderella—trained dental hygienists are not allowed to operate their own practices without the supervision of a dentist, or even put up a plaque advertising their services.

19. See Maria Montessori, *The Montessori Method*, trans. Anne E. George (London: Heinemann, 1912); Margaret McMillan, *The Nursery School* (London: Dent, 1930), with plates; also photographically illustrated in Leicester by E. Winifred Miller, *Room to Grow! The Development of the Nursery and Infant School* (London: George Harrap, 1944).

20. John Gale, *Clean Young Englishman* (London: Hogarth, 1988), 123–4.

21. Angela Rodaway, *A London Childhood* (London: Virago, 1985), 129; Roger Deakin, *Waterlog: A Swimmer's Journey through Britain*

(London, 1999), 140–4. Stroud District Council's Jubilee Leisure Park with open-air pool, sports grounds, and nursery was a typical local authority response.

22. John K. Walton, *The British Seaside: Holidays and Resorts in the Twentieth Century* (Manchester: Manchester University Press, 2000), 73–93, 122–42; see also W. W. F. Kemsley and David Ginsberg, *The Social Survey: Holidays and Holiday Expenditure* (London: Central Statistical Office, 1949), p. 13, table 10.

23. See e.g. C. E. M. Joad (ed.), *Manifesto: The Book of the Federation of Progressive Societies and Individuals* (London: Allen & Unwin, 1932). See also Joad's highly popular *Guide to Modern Thought* (London: Faber & Faber, 1933).

24. See generally Brian Inglis, 'Between the Wars', in Inglis, *Natural Medicine* (London: Fontana/Collins, 1980); id., *Fringe Medicine* (London: Faber & Faber, 1964); James C. Whorton, *Nature Cures: The History of Alternative Medicine in America* (Oxford: Oxford University Press, 2002), 131–218.

25. Phyllis Hembry, *The English Spa, 1560–1815: A Social History* (London: Athlone Press; Rutherford, NJ: Fairleigh Dickinson University, 1990); see also 'The Merits and Defects of British Health Resorts', *Proceedings of the Royal Society of Medicine*, 13, pts. I and II (1920), 1–48; and David Cantor, 'The Contradictions of Specialization: Rheumatism and the Decline of the Spa in Inter-War Britain', in Roy Porter (ed.), *The Medical History of Waters and Spas*, Medical History Supplement 10 (London: Wellcome Institute for the History of Medicine, 1990).

26. Ruth Kunz-Bircher, *The Bircher-Benner Guide*, trans. Rosemary Steed (London: Unwin, 1981), 14–17, 26, and *passim*. On vitamin science, see Porter, *The Greatest Benefit to Mankind*, 554–9.

27. Werner Zimmermann, editor of *Tao: A Monthly Magazine of Inner Consciousness and Self-Determination* (1921–4), quoted in Michael Graffenried, Harald Szeeman, and A. D. Coleman, *Naked in Paradise* (Stockport: Dewi Lewis, 1997), no page number.

28. Adam Clapham and Robin Constable, *As Nature Intended* (London: Heinemann, 1982), 8–30 and *passim*; Paul Abelman, *The Banished Body* (London: Sphere, 1982).

29. George Ryley Scott, *The Common Sense of Nudism: Including a Survey of Sun-Bathing and 'Light Treatments'* (London: T. W. Laurie, 1934), 33 and *passim*.

30. Dorothy Porter, *Health, Civilisation and the State: A History of Public Health from Ancient to Modern Times* (London: Routledge, 1999), 306–8; Whorton, *Nature Cures*, 205. Macfadden's long-running magazine *Physical Culture* (1899–) had over 100,000 subscribers in its first year. See also Julius A. Roth, *Health Purifiers and their Enemies: A Study of the Natural Health Movement in the United States with a Comparison to its Counterpart in Germany* (London: Croom Helm, 1976); John Dinan, *Sports in the Pulp Magazines* (Jefferson, NC: McFarland, 1998).

31. Kathy Watson, *The Crossing: The Curious Story of the First Man to Swim the English Channel* (London: Headline, 2000); Deakin, *Waterlog*, 206–8 and *passim*; Charles Sprawson, *Haunts of the Black Masseur: The Swimmer as Hero* (New York: Pantheon Books, 1992), 133–93 and *passim*, photographs, 84–5.

32. Some of my earliest personal memories are of Progressive League summer schools with barefoot dancing outside on the lawn before breakfast; and of inexplicably not being allowed into the high-hedged open-air swimming pool until the afternoon, i.e. after the morning nude sessions. See also Jack D. Douglas, Paul K. Rasmussen, and Carol Ann Flanagan, *The Nude Beach* (Beverly Hills, Calif.: Sage, 1977) on the nudism of 'bare-ass beaches' down the coast of California. Probably the only place in the world where nude bathing is actually obligatory by law is at the Tecopa hot springs in Death Valley, California, where nude bathing started in the 1930s and was legalized in the 1970s. There are hot springs in at least sixteen US states; see Marjorie Gersh-Young, *The Definitive Guide to Hot Springs and Hot Pools of the North-West* (Santa Cruz, Calif.: Aqua Thermal Access, 2003); ead., *Definitive Guide to Hot Springs and Pools of the South-West* (Santa Cruz, Calif.: Aqua Thermal Access, 2004).

33. The Hutterian Brethren (the Bruderhof) settled first in Britain, then Paraguay, and finally the United States. An attempt to refound the group in West Germany in the 1990s was foiled by local opposition, mobilized by a right-wing citizen's group (Yaacov Oved, *The Witness of the Brothers* (New Brunswick, NJ: Transaction, 1996), 30).

34. See e.g. Paul Weindling, *Health, Race and German Politics between Unification and Nazism, 1870–1945* (Cambridge: Cambridge University Press, 1989); Robert N. Proctor, *The Nazi War on Cancer* (Princeton: Princeton University Press, 1999), 22–57. On Nazism as a millenarian religious cult, see Burleigh, *The Third Reich*, 3–9, 193–5, 253.

35. See Horsfield, *Biting the Dust*, 153–5, 201, 257–8; David White, 'Keeping it Clean: Guilt about Dirt Remains the Adman's Great Opportunity', *New Society*, 16 Feb. 1984, 243–5; and the satiric comedy *The Thrill of It All* (1963; dir. Norman Jewison), featuring a suburban housewife, Doris Day, and her husband, Rock Hudson, caught up in the TV marketing of 'Happy Smell' soap. For a recent view on the long-term chemical effects of cleansing products, see Pat Thomas, *Cleaning Yourself to Death: How Safe Is Your Home?* (Dublin: Newleaf, 2001).

36. Jim Obelkevich, 'Men's Toiletries and Men's Bodies in Britain 1950–80', unpub., University of Warwick, Jan. 1993; White, 'Keeping it Clean', 244.

37. Rachel Carson, *Silent Spring* (Boston: Houghton Mifflin, 1962), 189–94; J. E. Lovelock, *Gaia: A New Look at Life on Earth* (Oxford: Oxford University Press, 1979); id., *Homage to Gaia: The Life of an Independent Scientist* (Oxford: Oxford University Press, 2000); see also the guru E. F. Schumacher's *Small Is Beautiful: A Study of Economics as if People Mattered* (London: Sphere Books, 1974).

38. See Elizabeth David, *Mediterranean Food* (1950), *Italian Food* (1954), *French Country Cooking* (1956); Sharon Cadwaller and Judi Ohr, *Whole Earth Cookbook* (1973); Gilly McKay, *The Body Shop: Franchising a Philosophy* (London: Pan, 1986).

39. As in many oral testimonies from the Bradford Heritage Recording Unit, Bradford; I am grateful to Dr Jill Liddington for this reference.

40. On nursing and ancillary services, see Brian Abel-Smith, *A History of the Nursing Profession* (London: Heinemann, 1960); Gerald Larkin, 'The Emergence of the Para-Medical Professions', in Bynum and Porter (eds.), *Companion Encyclopedia of the History of Medicine*, ii; Margaret Stacey, *The Sociology of Health and Healing: A Textbook* (London: Unwin Hyman, 1988), 182–4.

41. Boston Women's Health Book Collective, *Our Bodies Ourselves: A Health Book by and for Women* (Boston: New England Free Press, 1971), ed. Angela Phillips and Jill Rakusen (London: Penguin, 1978); Janet Balaskas and Yehudi Gordon, *Water Birth* (London: Unwin Paperbacks, 1990).

42. Ivan Illich, *Medical Nemesis: The Expropriation of Health* (London: Calder & Boyars, 1975); Gladys T. McGarey, 'The Growth of the American Holistic Medical Association', *British Journal of Holistic Medicine*, 1 (Apr. 1984), 50–1; John Horder, 'Summing Up', ibid. 93–5; Andrew Veitch, 'BMA Look at Alternative Remedies', *The Guardian*, 17 Aug. 1983, 5; British Medical Association, *Alternative Therapy* (London: BMA, 1986).

43. See e.g. S. Levin, A. Katz, and E. Holst, *Self-Care: Lay Initiatives in Health* (London: Croom Helm, 1977), 5; Margaret Stacey, 'Unpaid Workers in the Division of Health Labour', in Stacey, *The Sociology of Health and Healing*; Diane L. Pancoast, Paul Parker, and Charles Froland (eds.), *Rediscovering Self Help: Its Role in Social Care* (Beverly Hills, Calif.: Sage, 1983); David Haber, *Health Care for an Aging Society: Cost Conscious Community Care and Self-Care Approaches* (New York: Hemisphere, 1989); Mildred Baxter, *Health and Lifestyles* (London: Tavistock; New York: Routledge, 1990).

44. NHS Direct, <http://www.nhs.uk>, 1.

45. Diane Hales, *An Invitation to Health* (Pacific Grove, Calif.: Brookes/ Cole, 1999), introd.

46. Biopsychosocial medicine was proposed by George L. Engel, 'The Need for a New Medical Model: A Challenge for Biomedicine', *Science*, 196 (1977), 129–36, repr. as a Classic Paper, *British Journal of Holistic Medicine*, 4 (1989), 37–53; see also Richard Frankel, Timothy Quill, and Susan McDaniel (eds.), *The Biopsychosocial*

Approach: Past, Present, Future (Rochester, NY: Woodbridge, University of Rochester Press, 2003).

47. See e.g. Michio Kushi with Phillip Jannetta, *Macrobiotics and Oriental Medicine: An Introduction to Holistic Health* (Tokyo: Japan Publications, 1991).

48. Waldemar Janusczak, 'Virtual Japan', Channel Four TV, 2 Jan. 2001. Cornaro and Sanctorius would have been astonished.

49. Leon Chaitow, *Body Tonic* (London: Gaia Books, 1995), 1.

50. Lisa Armstrong, 'The Clean Team', *Vogue* (June 1997), 30–3. See also Diane Hales, *An Invitation to Health* (Pacific Grove, Calif.: Brookes/Cole, 1999); [Anita Roddick], *The Body Shop Book of Well-Being: Mind, Body, Soul* (London: Ebury Press, 1998); Amelia Hill and John Arlidge, 'Thin End of a Big Fat Juicy Scam', *The Observer*, 6 Jan. 2002, 11.

51. W. F. F. Kemsley and David Ginsberg, *Expenditure on Hairdressing, Cosmetics and Toilet Necessities*, The Social Survey: Consumer Expenditure Series (London: Central Office of Information, 1949), 6. UK figures from MINTEL, *Teenage Grooming Habits*, in *Teenage Leisure* (London: Mintel International Group, 2002).

52. The economic indices of alternative medicine and the 'well-being' sector require more research than can be given here. On spa travelling, see Alexia Brue, *Cathedrals of the Flesh: My Search for the Perfect Bath* (London: Bloomsbury, 2003); David Meilton and Fabienne Francie, 'Bright-Eyed before Breakfast', *The European*, 29 Apr.–2 May 1993, 19.

53. Global figures, consumer lifestyles, and future trends from Euromonitor, *The World Market for Cosmetics and Toiletries*, Oct. 2005, <http://www.euromonitor.com>.

54. Sander L. Gilman, *Making the Body Beautiful: A Cultural History of Aesthetic Surgery* (Princeton: Princeton University Press, 1999).

55. Obelkevich, 'Men's Toiletries and Men's Bodies in Britain'; Schools Health Educational Unit, *Young People into the Nineties*, book 2: *Health* (Exeter: Schools Health Education Unit, 1993); reviewed in Esther Oxford, 'Young "Take More Care of Hygiene"', *The*

Independent, 25 Jan. 1993, 3; Arrid Extra Dry deodorant survey of 1,000 adults throughout Britain, quoted in John Mullin, 'Summertime and the Living Is Queasy', *The Guardian*, 14 July 1994, 3.

56. Mullin, 'Summertime and the Living Is Queasy'.

57. Euromonitor, 'Consumer Lifestyles in India' and 'Consumer Lifestyles in Turkmenistan', in *Global Markets*, <http://www.euromonitor.com>; Kemsley and Ginsberg, *Expenditure on Hairdressing, Cosmetics and Toilet Necessities*, 1, 5 (table 5), 6.

58. See the classic text by Anthony Giddens, *Modernity and Self-Identity: Self and Society in the Late Modern Age* (Cambridge: Polity Press, 1991). A global survey by the cosmetic surgeon Steven Marquand tested a 'symmetry ratio' of beauty with a 100 per cent identical global response, in *The Human Face*, pt. III, Channel Four TV, 23 Mar. 2001.

59. *The Guardian*, 16 Mar. 2001, The Editor section, 5. Other remedies, notably vaccination and improved animal welfare, are now being sought.

60. *The Hygiene Hypothesis*, a film featuring Dr Erika von Mutius and her East–West Germany study in 1999, from the series *Evolution: The Evolutionary Arms Race* (WGBH Educational Foundation and Clear Blue Sky Productions, 2001); Richard Merritt, *Wild vs. Lab Rodent Comparison Supports Hygiene Hypothesis*, Duke University Medical Center Public Release 919–684–4148 (16 June 2006).

61. UK National Statistics Office (2004): Saving Lives programme of the Health Protection Agency, Communicable Disease Surveillance Centre for the Department of Health, <http://www.dh.gov.uk/PublicationsAndStatistics>. Even before the NHS privatization of hospital cleaners, NHS cleaners were a forgotten workforce; see Duncan Smith, *A Forgotten Sector: The Training of Ancillary Staff in Hospitals* (Oxford: Pergamon Press, 1969), 60–82.

62. See Michael Griffin, 'Mission to Cleanse', in Griffin, *Reaping the Whirlwind: Afghanistan, Al-Qu'ida, and the Holy War* (London: Pluto Press, 2003). Strict fundamentalist ascetic Islamic political regimes (such as the Taliban) reject music, dance, sports, television, and all books except the Qu'r-ān, the baring of any flesh, and the cutting

of any hair, and promote the segregation of men from women, and of all women from public life.

63. Bruno Latour, *We Have Never Been Modern*, trans. Catherine Porter (New York: Harvester/Wheatsheaf, 1993).

64. Lieutenant-Colonel Mervin Willett Gonin, quoted in 'Gagged For It', *Index on Censorship*, vol. 27, pt. 3 (June 1998); repr. in *The Guardian*, The Editor section, 13 June 1998, 12–13.

65. See Richard Wilkinson, *Mind the Gap: Hierarchies, Health and Human Evolution* (London: Weidenfeld & Nicolson, 2000), 3, 11, and *passim*; id., *Unhealthy Societies: The Afflictions of Inequality* (London: Routledge, 1996). Mental health and 'happiness' studies are on the increase. On 'social iatrogenesis', see Illich, *Medical Nemesis*, 25–7. On the iatrogenesis of stress and speed, see id., *Hygienic Nemesis: First Draft* (Cuernavaca: Cidoc Cuaderno, 1974), 8; Carl Honoré, *In Praise of Slow: How a Worldwide Movement Is Challenging the Cult of Speed* (London: Orion, 2004); Paul Glennie and Nigel Thrift, 'Reworking E. P. Thompson's *Time, Work-Discipline and Industrial Capitalism*', *Time and Society*, 5/3 (1996), 275–99. See also Barbara Adam, *Timewatch: The Social Analysis of Time* (Cambridge: Polity Press, 1995); Ronald Frankenberg (ed.), *Time, Health and Medicine* (London: Sage, 1992). An earlier hygiene debate on social or 'free' time took place in during the late 19th century, with legislation that was eroded in the 1970s–1980s by the expanding international economy, and free-trade policies such as the 'relaxation' of Sunday opening hours (now being fiercely contested in France; see Kim Willsher, 'Selling Out Sunday: The Struggle for the Soul of the French Day of Rest', *The Guardian*, Work section, 8 July 2006, 3).

select bibliography

The chapter notes give the full bibliography, and detailed recommendations for further reading. This is a small selection of basic texts, divided into broad themes for easy use: methodology, primary sources, bio-physicality, body-art and cosmetics, purity and asceticism, hot and cold bathing, medical history, and material culture and domestic technology.

Methodology

Adam, Barbara, *Timewatch: The Social Analysis of Time* (Cambridge: Polity Press, 1995).

Braudel, Fernand, *On History (Écrits sur l'histoire)*, trans. Sarah Matthews (London: Weidenfeld & Nicolson, 1980).

Elias, Norbert, *The Civilising Process: Sociogenetic and Psychogenetic Investigations*, trans. Edmund Jephcott (1939; Oxford: Blackwell, 2000).

——*Time: An Essay*, trans. Edmund Jephcott (Oxford: Blackwell, 1993).

Feher, Michel, Ramona Nadeff, NADIA TAZI, and E. ALLIEZ (eds.), *Fragments for a History of the Human Body* (New York: Zone; Cambridge, Mass.: MIT Press, 1989).

Giddens, Anthony, *Modernity and Self-Identity: Self and Society in the Late Modern Age* (Cambridge: Polity Press, 1991).

Shilling, Chris, *The Body and Social Theory* (London: Sage, 1993).

Primary Sources

Buchan, William, *Domestic Medicine: or, A Treatise on the Prevention and Cure of Diseases by Regimen and Simple Medicines* (1769; London, 1803).

Celsus, *De Medicina*, trans. W. G. Spencer, 3 vols. (London: William Heinemann; Cambridge, Mass.: Harvard University Press, 1935).

Ovid, *The Love Poems*, trans. A. D. Melville (Oxford: Oxford University Press, 1990).

Rousseau, Jean-Jacques, *Émile, or, Education*, trans. Barbara Foxley (London: Dent, 1911).

Bio-physicality

Classen, Constance, *Worlds of Sense: Exploring the Senses in History and Across Cultures* (London: Routledge, 1993).

Miller, William Ian, *The Anatomy of Disgust* (Cambridge, Mass.: Harvard University Press, 1997).

Morris, Desmond, *The Naked Ape: A Zoologist's Study of the Human Animal* (London: Jonathan Cape, 1967).

Ridley, Matt, *Nature via Nurture: Genes, Experience and What Makes Us Human* (London: Harper Perennial, 2004).

Body-Art and Cosmetics

Barber, Elizabeth Wayland, *Women's Work: The First 20,000 Years. Women, Cloth, and Society in Early Times* (New York: Norton, 1994).

Chandra, Moti, *Costumes, Textiles, Cosmetics and Coiffure in Ancient and Medieval India* (Delhi: Oriental Publishers, Indian Archaeological Society, 1973).

Ebin, Victoria, *The Body Decorated* (London: Thames & Hudson, 1979).

Sagarin, Edward (ed.), *Cosmetics, Science and Technology* (New York: Interscience, 1957).

Williams, Neville, *Powder and Paint: A History of the Englishwoman's Toilet, Elizabeth I–Elizabeth II* (London: Longmans, Green, 1957).

Purity and Asceticism

Brakke, David, *Athanasius and the Politics of Asceticism* (Oxford: Clarendon Press, 1995).

Brown, Peter, 'Asceticism: Pagan and Christian', in Averil Cameron and Peter Garnsey (eds.), *The Cambridge Ancient History*, xiii: *The Late Empire, AD 337–425* (Cambridge: Cambridge University Press, 1998).

Douglas, Mary, *Purity and Danger: An Analysis of the Concepts of Pollution and Taboo* (1966; London: Routledge & Kegan Paul/Ark, 1984).

Parker, Robert, *Miasma: Pollution and Purification in Early Greek Religion* (Oxford: Clarendon Press, 1983).

Thomas, Keith, 'Cleanliness and Godliness in Early Modern England', in Anthony Fletcher and Peter Roberts (eds.), *Religion, Culture and Society in Early Modern Britain: Essays in Honour of Patrick Collinson* (Cambridge: Cambridge University Press, 1994).

Hot and Cold Bathing

Bonneville, Françoise de, *The Book of the Bath*, trans. Jane Benton (London: Thames & Hudson, 1998).

Corbin, Alain, *The Lure of the Sea: The Discovery of the Seaside in the Western World, 1750–1840*, trans. Jocelyn Phelps (London: Penguin, 1995).

Deakin, Roger, *Waterlog: A Swimmer's Journey through Britain* (London: Vintage, 2000).

Goubert, Jean-Pierre, *The Conquest of Water: The Advent of Health in the Industrial Age* (Cambridge: Polity Press, 1989).

Wright, Lawrence, *Clean and Decent: The History of the Bath and Loo, and of Sundry Habits, Fashions and Accessories of the Toilet Principally in Great Britain, France and America* (London: Routledge and Kegan Paul, 1960).

Yegül, Fikret, *Baths and Bathing in Classical Antiquity* (New York: Architectural History Foundation; Cambridge, Mass.: MIT Press, 1992).

Medical History

Baxter, Mildred, *Health and Lifestyles* (London: Tavistock/Routledge, 1990).

Bynum, W. F., and roy Porter (eds.), *Companion Encyclopedia of the History of Medicine*, 2 vols. (London: Routledge, 1997).

Cooter, Roger (ed.), *Studies in the History of Alternative Science* (London: Macmillan, 1988).

Lloyd, G. E. R., *In the Grip of Disease: Studies in the Greek Imagination* (Oxford: Oxford University Press, 2003).

—— *Polarity and Analogy* (Cambridge: Cambridge University Press, 1966).

Porter, Roy, *The Greatest Benefit to Mankind: A Medical History of Humanity from Antiquity to the Present* (London: HarperCollins, 1997).

—— and DOROTHY PORTER, *In Sickness and in Health: The British Experience 1650–1850* (London: Fourth Estate, 1988).

Tomes, Nancy, *The Gospel of Germs: Men, Women and the Microbe in American Life* (Cambridge, Mass.: Harvard University Press, 1998).

Whorton, James C., *Crusaders for Fitness: The History of American Health Reform* (Princeton: Princeton University Press, 1982).

Material Culture and Domestic Technology

Braudel, Fernand, *Civilisation and Capitalism, 15th–18th Century*, i: *The Structures of Everyday Life*, trans. Sian Reynolds (London: Collins, 1981).

Davidson, Caroline, *A Woman's Work Is Never Done: A History of Housework in the British Isles 1650–1950* (London: Chatto & Windus, 1986).

Horsfield, Margaret, *Biting the Dust. The Joys of Housework*, (London: Fourth Estate, 1997).

Hoy, Suellen, *Chasing Dirt: The American Pursuit of Cleanliness* (New York: Oxford University Press, 1995).

Sarti, Raffaella, *Europe at Home: Family and Material Culture 1500–1800* (New Haven: Yale University Press, 2002).

Vigarello, Georges, *Concepts of Cleanliness: Changing Attitudes in France since the Middle Ages*, trans. Jean Birrell (Cambridge: Cambridge University Press/Éditions de la Maison des Sciences de l'Homme, 1988).

acknowledgements of sources

Chris Saville/Apex News & Pictures: **22**; Archaeological Museum, Florence/The Art Archive/Dagli Orti: **5**; The Art Archive/Dagli Orti: **4**; The Bodleian Library, University of Oxford: John Johnson Collection (Sport 5(7)): **15**; The Bodleian Library, University of Oxford (9419.d.239, p. 81): **18**; British Library (copyright holder not traced): **19**; Kress Collection, Washington, DC, USA/The Bridgeman Art Library: **12**; Kunsthalle, Bremen, Germany/The Bridgeman Art Library: **11**; Musée National du Moyen Âge et des Thermes de Cluny, Paris/ Lauros-Giraudon/The Bridgeman Art Library: **9**; Russell-Cotes Art Gallery and Museum, Bournemouth/The Bridgeman Art Library: **16**; © Kevin Schafer/Corbis: **3**; EfA/C. Tousloukof/ J. Cami: **6**; Jean Paul Gaultier: **23**; Mauro Guerrini: **2**; INDEX/ Pubbli Photo: **8**; Jacques-Henri Lartigue/© Ministère de la Culture-France/AAJHL: **20**; © Bernard Castelein/naturepl.com: **1**; National Archaeological Museum, Athens/photo © Scala 1990: **7**; © Tate, London 2006: **17**; Wellcome Library, London: **10, 13**

In a few instances we have been unable to trace the copyright owner prior to publication. If notified, the publishers will be pleased to amend the Acknowledgements in any future edition.

index

Note: page references in *italic* indicate illustrations. Footnote numbers in brackets are used to indicate the whereabouts on the page of authors/ works who/which are quoted, but not named, in the text.

/

guest honour 62–3
guild system 166
Gully, James Manby 294
gymnasiums 79, 89–93, 100–1, 106, 123–4
gymnastics (callisthenics) 277–8

Hadrian 106, 107
Hahnemann, Samuel 270
hair powder 236
hairstyles 66, 117, 210, 229, 291
Hall, Thomas 196–7 (n. 24)
Haller, Albrecht von 249
Ham Common Concordium 271, 273
Hampton Court Palace 188
Han dynasty 94
Hancocke, John 219
Hans von Waldheim 176
harems 70–1
Harington, Sir John 190
Hassall, Dr Arthur Hill 285–6
Haygarth, Dr John 249
head lice 19–20, 158–9, *160*, 229–30
Health and Cleanliness Council 310
Health and Morals of Apprentices Act 265
Health Education Council 334
health food movement 331–2
Health for All 322
Health of Towns Association 279
Health of Towns Commission 279

health reforms
America 271
in Britain 265, 279–83
magazines and 275–6
Henry VIII, king of England 179, 188
herbalists 52, 268, 269, 270, 414 n. 14
Herbert, George 209
Hercules 77
Here's Health 322
Herod the Great, king of Judea 106–7
Herodicus 91
Herodotus 42–3, 48, 57–8
Hesiod 100
Hetepheres, queen 66
Hill, Christopher 211–12
Himmler, Heinrich 328
Hinduism 32
hip baths 77, 79
Hippias 110–11
Hippocrates 94
Hippocratic Writings 96–7
History of Cold Bathing, The (Floyer) 220
Hitler, Adolf 328
Hoffman, Friedrich 256
holism 3, 332, 335–6
Holmes, Dr Oliver Wendell 278
Holocaust 350–1
homeopathy 270
homeostasis 9–14
Homer 58–9, 63
Hortatus Sanitatis 160